Recent Results in Cancer Research

165

M.W. Büchler · R.J. Heald · B. Ulrich
J. Weitz (Eds.)

Rectal Cancer Treatment

With 56 Figures and 64 Tables

Springer

Prof. Dr. med. Dr. h.c. Markus W. Büchler
PD Dr. med. Jürgen Weitz
Chirurgische Universitätsklinik Heidelberg
Abteilung für Allgemeine, Viszerale, Unfallchirurgie und Poliklinik
Im Neuenheimer Feld 110
69120 Heidelberg, Germany

Prof. Dr. med. Bernward Ulrich
Chirurgie, Krankenhaus Gerresheim
Kliniken der Landeshauptstadt
Gräulinger Straße 120
40625 Düsseldorf, Germany

Professor Richard John Heald OBE
Surgical Director
The Pelican Cancer Foundation
North Hampshire Hospital
Basingstoke, Hampshire
RG24 9NA, UK

Indexed in Current Contents and Index Medicus

ISBN 3-540-23341-5 Springer Berlin Heidelberg New York
ISSN 0080-0015

Library of Congress Control Number: 2005920528

Bibliographic information published by Die Deutsche Bibliothek
Die Deutsche Bibliothek lists this publication in the Deutsche Nationalbibliografie; detailed bibliographic data is available in the Internet at <http: dnd.ddb.de>.

Springer is a part of Springer Science+Business Media
springeronline.com

Editor: Dr. Ute Heilmann, Heidelberg, Germany
Desk editor: Dörthe Mennecke-Bühler, Heidelberg, Germany
Typesetting and Production: LE-TEX Jelonek, Schmidt & Vöckler GbR, Leipzig
Cover design: design&production GmbH, 69121 Heidelberg, Germany

Printed on acid-free paper 21 3150 YL – 5 4 3 2 1 0

Contents

Postoperative Pathophysiology and Choice of Incision

Richard P. Billingham

R.P. Billingham (✉)
Department of Surgery, University of Washington, Seattle WA, USA
e-mail: rbham@u.washington.edu

Abstract

In the few days following major surgical procedures, there are three main physiologic processes which are amenable to surgical management: restoration of fluid and electrolyte homeostasis, management of pain, and attention to gastrointestinal function. New information regarding optimizing the management of these processes is presented, which may accelerate recovery and give improved comfort following abdominal surgery. The type of incision used seems not to be a major factor in such recovery.

During the period immediately following a surgical procedure, numerous physiological processes are at work to achieve restoration of health and function. The three principal processes which require, and are amenable to, surgical management are restoration of fluid and electrolyte homeostasis, management of postoperative pain, and management of gastrointestinal (GI) function. These factors are often interrelated, particularly pain and GI function, because of the fact that narcotic analgesics nearly always required for management of postoperative pain and have a deleterious effect on restoration of GI function. Poor GI motility can, in turn, produce discomfort which may lead to the patient requesting more medication for pain.

The restoration of fluid and electrolyte homeostasis is generally promptly managed after even major elective surgery. The majority of time in the hospital following such procedures is necessary to manage the pain and GI function problems. If pain could be managed without the need for drugs which impair gastrointestinal motility, it is possible that even major abdominal surgery could be done as an outpatient procedure, or with a very brief hospital stay.

Restoration of fluid and electrolyte balance is a multifaceted task, which begins during the preoperative period. Patients often arrive in the operating room somewhat dehydrated, both from the requirement to avoid food and liquids for several hours prior to the time of the operation, as well as the requirement (up to the present time) for a mechanical bowel preparation. This dehydration is sometimes managed by preoperative intravenous hydration, and as well as intraoperatively by vigorous intraoperative provision of fluid. This is done to counteract the perceived preoperative dehydration, as well as to maintain adequate perfusion in the face of peripheral vasodilatation, common after spinal or epidural anesthesia. Parenteral fluid is typically continued during the immediate postoperative period until a urine output of greater than 30 cc per hour is maintained, in order to optimize cardiac and renal function. Once adequate oral intake is established, parenteral fluids can be discontinued.

Several recent studies have challenged these traditional management concepts. Waters and associates, in a randomized blinded trial, reported the use of lactated Ringer's solution versus normal saline intraoperatively at the time of abdominal aortic aneurysm repair [1]. With equal volumes of fluid, they found that the group receiving normal saline developed hyperchloremic acidosis, received more bicarbonate, and required more blood and platelets compared with the lactated Ringer's group, but they found no difference in the duration of hospital stay or duration of requirement for postoperative ventilation. More recently, Lobo et. al., reported the results of a prospective randomized study following elective hemicolectomy with ten subjects in each arm [2]. One group was subjected to "standard management", which consisted of 1 l of normal saline and 2 l of D5 W in the perioperative period, with the test group subjected to some salt and a water restriction, in that they received only 0.5 l of normal saline and 1.5 l of D5 W during the same period. These authors found that the restricted salt and water group had shorter median solid and liquid gastric emptying times, shorter median time to passage of flatus (by 1 day), and shorter median hospital stay (by 3 days!).

Postoperative incisional pain is typically managed through a patient controlled analgesia (PCA) system, whereby the patient presses a button to receive a small dose of intravenous or epidural narcotic [3]. Recently, studies have been done to evaluate the use of continuous local infusion of local anesthesia to the wound edges, but no consensus of efficacy has been reached [4–6].

The cessation of GI function following the combination of surgical stress and narcotic analgesia has been termed "postoperative ileus" or "POI" [7, 8]. This is in distinction to the persistent type of ileus, which impairs intestinal motility and lasts more than a few days. Symptoms of this include lack of appetite, nausea, vomiting, and abdominal cramping, accompanied by physical signs of abdominal and bowel distention. POI is a biphasic response, thought to be "physiologic," involving a short temporary phase, then a brief recovery and a longer phase related to local tissue concentration of inflammatory cells. Postoperatively, this lack of motility typically lasts 0–24 h in the small intestine, 24–48 h in the stomach, and 48–72 h in the large intestine [9].

As mentioned, this has been attributed to the "surgical stress response." Other factors which have been hypothesized as contributory include handling of the bowel at the time of surgery, dehydration of the serosal surfaces, and hypothermia of the intestinal surfaces from evaporation. Pain and the requirement for narcotics have been considered to be contributory factors. Neurologically, POI has been attributed to heightened sympathetic (inhibitory) reflexes. Of these, there are three types: ultra-short reflexes, which are confined to the wall of the gut; short reflexes involving prevertebral ganglia, which provide *efferent* stimuli *to* the *intestines*; and long reflexes, which consist of *afferent* stimuli to *the spinal cord*, which are felt to be most important. It is these long reflexes which may be affected by spinal epidural anesthesia, as well as by abdominal sympathectomy.

Neurotransmitters have also been implicated in the causation of POI. Motilin, substance P, VIP, nitric oxide, corticotropin-releasing factor, and cytokines are all thought to have an inhibitory effect on intestinal transit. Therefore, inhibitors of such substances would potentially improve postoperative function. These neurotransmitters can be stimulated by local (wound) factors, endotoxemia, and "stress," which may be contributed to by surgical manipulation. An intestinal inflammatory response can also stimulate such neurotransmitters. If such factors could be modified, the duration and severity of POI could potentially be ameliorated.

Opioids, both exogenous and endogenous (such as endorphins), inhibit gastric emptying and smooth muscle contraction and cause increases in intraluminal pressure. The gut has opioid receptors, located on presynaptic nerve terminals within the myenteric plexus. When opioids bind to these mu-receptors, decreased propulsive contractions and increased resting tone result. Stimulation of kappa-receptors, also located in the wall of the intestine, may have some role in improving visceral pain relief.

One of the difficulties in studying POI is the problem of defining it and the criteria for its resolution. The presence or absence of bowel sounds does not correlate with resolution of ileus. Passage of flatus has sometimes been used to identify the resolution of the ileus, but is often difficult to reliably identify and record. "Time to resumption of a regular diet" has sometimes been used as an endpoint, but definitions of quantity of food intake, type of food, and what is really meant by "resumption" makes this also problematic to use as a definite end point. Occurrence of the first postoperative bowel movement has also been used to indicate the resolution of ileus, but this usually occurs after the patient has been eating and passing flatus, and sometimes does not occur until after the patient is discharged from the hospital.

Attempts have been made to physiologically identify the time of return of the "migrating myoelectric complex" (MMC), but there seems to be no relationship of such return or with qualitative changes in the MMC, with clinical resolution of POI [9]. Nuclear medicine studies using a gamma camera to measure intestinal transit have also been suggested, but are difficult to put into place as a simple clinical endpoint.

Management of POI includes attempts to minimize the known intraoperative and postoperative causative factors, as well as treatment by symptomatic management and other pharmacologic means. Preventive measures have been aimed at avoidance of the stress response for neurostimulation, and minimization or avoidance of opioids. Treatment of POI, in addition to symptomatic management, has consisted of attempts to block the sympathetic stimulation (or stimulate the parasympathetics), to stop or antagonize neurotransmitters, or to stop or antagonize opioids.

Efforts at prevention of POI have examined the potential effects of different types of anesthesia. General anesthesia is thought to have an insignificant effect, either in causation or prevention, although the use of nitrous oxide has been associated with an increase in the incidence of postoperative nausea and vomiting. A single dose of regional anesthesia (whether spinal or epidural) does not effect the duration of ileus, and intraoperative short-acting opioids, such as fentanyl, are thought to have no effect. Continuous epidural analgesia is thought to blockade afferent and efferent inhibitory reflexes, as well as cause an efferent sympathetic blockade, which may also have an effect on increasing splanchnic blood flow. In addition, this type of analgesia may have a preemptive effect on pain in that it may minimize the requirement for opioids postoperatively. Several studies show that epidural local anesthesia alone seems to have a beneficial effect on the duration of POI, compared to either epidural or narcotics, or the combination of epidural local anesthesia plus narcotics [10, 11]. Low thoracic placement of an epidural, in the T9 to T12 area, is thought to have a better effect on minimizing systemic opioids than lumbar placement, and therefore may have a beneficial role in shortening the duration of POI. Also, use of local anesthetic alone, rather than epidural opioids or a combination of local anesthesia and opioids, has been associated with a shorter duration of POI [10].

However, the use of epidural analgesia has not been universally accepted in most countries for multiple reasons. The first is patient acceptance, in that despite careful explanation, many patients are very concerned about the perception of a needle quite close to their spinal cord. In addition, many anesthesiologists are reluctant to offer this technique, in that it is more time-consuming to provide, compared to the general anesthetic; it requires hospital rounds and maintenance by the anesthesia staff and may be a less common and familiar means of analgesia in some geographic areas. Additionally, for up to 20% of patients, displacement of the epidural catheter, even by a relatively small amount, can interfere with its function during the postoperative period.

Choice of incision has often been felt to associated with greater or lesser amounts of postoperative pain, and if this is true, the less painful incision may reduce the need for narcotic analgesics and therefore have a beneficial effect on the duration of POI. Jeekel and associates reviewed prospective randomized trials in a recent review article, comparing midline, paramedian, transverse, and oblique incisions [12]. They were unable to document any significant difference in postoperative pain, wound infection, or wound dehiscence rates, regardless of incision type. They did find that incisional hernias were slightly more frequent with midline incisions, but only with small incisions; there was no difference between hernia rates between larger incisions, whether transverse, midline, or paramedian. In a study with similar intent, Grantcharov and Rosenberg reviewed 11 randomized controlled trials and seven retrospective studies [13]. They felt that transverse incision resulted in significantly less postoperative pain in three trials using subcostal incisions, but not in the one trial for abdominal aortic surgery. Transverse incisions in other parts of the abdomen were not studied. They did find that the transverse incision was associated with fewer pulmonary complications in seven of nine controlled trials. They also observed the transverse incisions may take 6–15 min longer to make and may be associated with more blood loss. They concluded that the vertical incision is preferable for trauma or when there is increased probability of relaparotomy, such as for a patient with Crohn's disease or undergoing a Hartmann procedure. Lindgren and associates performed a randomized controlled trial for right hemicolectomy for cancer, randomizing 53 patients, of whom 40 completed the study, with 23 vertical and 17 transverse incisions [14]. Those with transverse incisions showed less pain after activity and a lower analgesia requirement, with more rapid improvement in respiratory function. However, there was no indication of a difference of the timing of resolution of POI or the duration of hospital stay.

Many studies have been done regarding the effect of the postoperative use of nasogastric tubes on POI. In a recent analysis of published clinical trials, Cheatham and associates [15] reviewed 26 trials with nearly 4,000 patients, with the finding that only 1 in 20 patients required a nasogastric tube at some point during the postoperative period, and that in those patients managed *without* nasogastric tubes, fever, atelectasis, and pneumonia were significantly less common, and the number of days until first oral intake were significantly fewer. Early feeding has been recommended both for prevention and treatment of ileus in that it is found to stimulate intestinal reflexes, as well as the secretion of intestinal hormones, with the suggestion of a prokinetic effect. This was first reported by Moss in 1981, and since that time, dozens of studies have suggested shortened ileus as a result of early feeding [16–25].

Laparoscopic gastrointestinal surgery has been suggested as a technique which may diminish the duration of ileus, but there appears to be no difference in the resolution of POI between patients after open surgery versus laparoscopic surgery *if* the patients are fed at the same time postoperatively. Hotokezawa and associates evaluated this issue by implanting electrodes in the proximal and distal antrum, proximal to the site of colonic anastomosis and in the distal sigmoid, and measuring the timing of return of electrical impulses [26]. They concluded that there was no difference in the time of return of motility between the laparoscopic and open surgical groups.

Opioid-sparing analgesia, in addition to epidural catheters, has also been associated with diminished duration of POI. Nonsteroidal anti-inflammatory drugs diminish the requirement for opioids by 20–30% and may also have a direct anti-inflammatory effect from inhibition of prostaglandin synthesis [17, 27].

Many attempts have been made to treat POI. Neurotransmitter manipulation has a long history, with guanethidine, a sympathetic inhibitor, and neostigmine, a parasympathomimetic, being used for the treatment of Ogilvie's syndrome, first reported by Hutchison and Griffiths in 1992 [28]. A larger study was reported by Trevisani, Hyman, and Church in 2000, but this does not appear to work on small bowel or for prophylaxis [29]. Many prokinetic agents have been tried, including cisapride, ceruletide, erythromycin, metoclopramide, somatostatin, and bisacodyl [7, 30, 31]. Magnesium salts have been reported efficacious when given orally, but may be difficult for the patient to take in the postoperative period if the patient has any nausea [32].

Selective antagonism of opioid-induced GI side effects is another area which has been explored, attempting to find a pharmaceutical agent which could block the adverse gastrointestinal effects of opioids while preserving pain relief. Three approaches have been explored: First, using centrally acting opioid antagonists with limited oral bioavailability (naloxone); second, using peripherally acting opioid antagonists which have limited penetration of the blood brain barrier (methylnaltrexone); and thirdly, a compound combining both attributes (alvimopan). Alvimopan interferes with the process by which narcotic molecules bind with peripheral mu opioid receptors, and through such antagonism, can prevent the adverse gastrointestinal effects on motility while preserving narcotic analgesic pain relief, since the alvimopan molecule does not cross the blood–brain barrier [33]. In a recent phase III study which was randomized, double-blinded and controlled, the mean time to recovery to GI function was 15–22 h sooner with alvimopan, and the mean time to discharge was 13–20 h sooner compared with placebo [34].

Our current practice to minimize the duration of POI is to use epidural analgesia whenever possible, preferring the thoracic placement of an epidural and the use of local anesthesia alone. We generally use a vertical incision for surgery, and provide intravenous ketorolac until the patient is taking oral intake, and then switch to an oral nonsteroidal anti-inflammatory drug, both efforts to minimize narcotic analgesic use. Nasogastric tubes are avoided entirely, and the patients are offered full liquids on the first postoperative day. As soon as this is tolerated, they are moved to a regular diet on the second or third postoperative day, with discontinuation of the intravenous fluids as soon as possible. Attempts are made to minimize overhydration during the initial postoperative period. We strongly encourage early frequent ambulation. Our patients are discharged a mean of 4.5 postoperative days following major abdominal surgery [24].

In summary, principal physiologic problems in the postoperative period are restoration of fluid and electrolyte homeostasis, pain, and ileus, and they are interrelated. The volume of fluid replacement may be a factor in the duration of POI, as may the choice of incision, although there are no clear data yet to support the latter. Early feeding, opioid-sparing analgesia, and possibly early ambulation are all associated with shortening of the duration of ileus. Sympathetic antagonists, parasympathetic stimulants, or blocking of other neurotransmitters have not been shown to be practical to date. The use of a new antagonist such as alvimopan to block narcotic effects on gastrointestinal motility shows great promise in shortening the duration of ileus.

References

1. Waters JH, Gottlieb A, Schoenwald P, et al. (2001) Normal saline versus lactated Ringer's solution for intraoperative fluid management in patients undergoing abdominal aortic aneurysm repair: an outcome study. Anesth Analg 93:817–822
2. Lobo DN, Dube MG, Neal KR, et al. (2002) Peri-operative fluid and electrolyte management: a survey of consultant surgeons in the UK. Ann R Coll Surg Engl 84:156–160
3. Cataldo P, Senagore A, Kilbride M. Ketorolac and Patient Controlled Analgesia in the Treatment of Postoperative Pain (1993) Surg Gynecol Obst 176:435–438
4. Dowling R, Thielmeier K, Ghaly A, et al. (2003) Improved pain control after cardiac surgery: results of a randomized, double-blind, clinical trial. J Thorac Cardiovasc Surg 126:1271–1278
5. Ilfeld BM, Morey TE, Enneking FK (2003) Portable infusion pumps used for continuous regional analgesia: delivery rate accuracy and consistency. Reg Anesth Pain Med 28:424–432
6. Kulkarni M, Elliot D (2003) Local anaesthetic infusion for postoperative pain. J Hand Surg [Br] 28:300–306

7. Holte K, Kehlet H (2002) Postoperative ileus: progress towards effective management. Drugs 62:2603–2615
8. Kehlet H, Holte K (2001) Review of postoperative ileus. Am J Surg 182(5A Suppl):3S-10S
9. Holte K, Kehlet H (2000) Postoperative ileus: a preventable event. Br J Surg 87:1480–1493
10. Liu SS, Carpenter RL, Mackey DC, et al. (1995) Effects of perioperative analgesic technique on rate of recovery after colon surgery. Anesthesiology 83:757–765
11. Paulson E, Porter M, Helmer S, et al. (2001) Thoracic epidural vs. patient-controlled analgesia in elective bowel resections. Am J Surg 182:570–577
12. Burger JW, van 't Riet M, Jeekel J (2002) Abdominal incisions: techniques and postoperative complications. Scand J Surg 91:315–321
13. Grantcharov TP, Rosenberg J (2001) Vertical compared with transverse incisions in abdominal surgery. Eur J Surg 167:260–267
14. Lindgren PG, Nordgren SR, Oresland T, Hulten L (2001) Midline or transverse abdominal incision for right-sided colon cancer-a randomized trial. Colorectal Dis 3:46–50
15. Cheatham ML, Chapman WC, Key SP, JL S (1995) A meta-analysis of selective versus routine nasogastric decompression after elective laparotomy. Ann Surg 221:469–478
16. Moss G, Regal M, Lichtig L (1986) Reducing postoperative pain, narcotics, and length of hospitalization. Surgery 99:206–209
17. Holte K, Kehlet H (2002) Prevention of postoperative ileus. Minerva Anestesiol 68:152–156
18. Pearl ML, Valea FA, Fischer M, et al. (1998) A randomized controlled trial of early postoperative feeding in gynecologic oncology patients undergoing intra-abdominal surgery. Obstet Gynecol 92:94–97
19. Reissman P, Teoh T, Wexner S, et al. (1995) Is Early oral feeding safe after elective colorectal surgery? Ann Surg 222:73–77
20. Steed HL, Capstick V, Flood C, et al. (2002) A randomized controlled trial of early versus "traditional" postoperative oral intake after major abdominal gynecologic surgery. Am J Obstet Gynecol 186:861–865
21. Binderow S, Cohen S, SD W, Nogueras J (1994) Must early postoperative oral intake be limited to laparoscopy? Dis Colon Rectum 37(6):584–89
22. Bisgaard T, Kehlet H (2002) Early oral feeding after elective abdominal surgery–what are the issues? Nutrition 18:944–948
23. Choi J, O' Connell T (1996) Safe and effective early postoperative feeding and hospital discharge after open colon resection. American Surgeon 62:853–856
24. Melbert R, Kimmins M, JT I, et al. (2002) Use of a critical pathway for colon resections. J Gastrointest Surg 6:745–752
25. Delaney C, Fazio V, Senegore A, et al. (2001) "Fast track" postoperative management protocol for patients with high co-morbidity undergoing complex abdominal and pelvic colorectal surgery. Br J Surg 88:1533–1538
26. Hotokezaka M, Dix J, Mentis EP, et al. (1996) Gastrointestinal recovery following laparoscopic vs. open colon surgery. Surg Endosc 10:485–489
27. Shang AB, Gan TJ (2003) Optimising postoperative pain management in the ambulatory patient. Drugs 63:855–867
28. Hutchinson R, Griffiths C (1992) Acute colonic pseudo-obstruction: a pharmacological approach. Ann R Coll Surg Engl 74:364–367
29. Trevisani GT, Hyman NH, Church JM (2000) Neostigmine: safe and effective treatment for acute colonic pseudo-obstruction. Dis Colon Rectum 43:599–603
30. Bungard TJ, Kale-Pradhan PB (1999) Prokinetic agents for the treatment of postoperative ileus in adults: a review of the literature [In Process Citation]. Pharmacotherapy 19:416–423
31. Miedema BW, Johnson JO (2003) Methods for decreasing postoperative gut dysmotility. Lancet Oncol 4:365–372
32. Kehlet H, Dahl JB (2003) Anaesthesia, surgery, and challenges in postoperative recovery. Lancet 362:1921–1928
33. Taguchi A, Sharma N, Saleem R, et al. (2001) Selective postoperative inhibition of gastrointestinal opioid receptors. NEJM 345:935–940
34. Wolff BG, Michelassi F, Gerkin TM, Group TAS. Alvimopan, a novel, peripherally-acting mu opioid antagonist: results of a double-blind, randomized, placebo-controlled, phase III clinical trial of major abdominal surgery and postoperative ileus (Study 14CL313) (2004) American Surgical Association Annual Scientific Meeting 2004

Fast-Track Colonic Surgery: Status and Perspectives

Henrik Kehlet

H. Kehlet (✉)
Section for Surgical Pathophysiology, Rigshospitalet, Section 4074,
Blegdamsvej 9, 2100 Copenhagen, Denmark
e-mail: henrik.kehlet@rh.dk

Abstract

Multi-modal rehabilitation with an emphasis on preoperative information, reduction of surgical stress responses, optimized dynamic pain relief with continuous epidural analgesia and early mobilization and oral nutrition may reduce hospital stay, morbidity, convalescence, and costs (fast-track surgery). Current results from fast-track colonic surgery suggest that postoperative pulmonary, cardiovascular, and muscle function are improved and body composition preserved as well as a normal oral intake of energy and protein can be achieved. Consequently, hospital stay is reduced to about 2–4 days, with decreased fatigue and need for sleep in the convalescence period. Despite a higher risk for readmissions, overall costs and morbidity seem to be reduced. Existing data from several institutions support the concept of fast-track colonic surgery to improve postoperative organ functions, thereby allowing for early rehabilitation with decreased hospital stay, convalescence, and costs. Further data are needed from multi-national institutions on morbidity, safety, and costs.

Introduction

In the last few decades, several improvements in perioperative care have been developed including newer anesthetic and analgesic techniques to provide early recovery and efficient pain relief [1] and new minimally invasive surgical techniques and pharmacological measures to reduce surgical stress [1, 2]. When these techniques have been combined with an adjustment of the overall perioperative program with regard to use of nasogastric tubes, drains, urinary catheters, and early institution of oral feeding and mobilization, major improvements have been achieved in a variety of surgical procedures [1, 2].

Colonic surgery has usually been associated with a complication rate of 15%–20% and a postoperative hospital stay of 6–10 days, the limiting factors for early recovery and discharge being pain, recovery of gastrointestinal function to allow

Recent Results in Cancer Research, Vol. 165

normal food intake, fatigue, and other organ dysfunctions. In recent years, several efforts have been made to standardize perioperative care protocols after colonic surgery [1–4] in order to achieve earlier restoration of body organ functions, in the hope that need for hospitalization and morbidity subsequently would be reduced. This paper is a short update on the current status of such multimodal rehabilitation programs in elective colonic procedures.

Results

The results are summarized in Table 1.

In all available reports on fast-track colonic surgery, a revised perioperative care program has been instituted with avoidance of nasogastric tubes, early institution of oral feeding and mobilization, optimized multimodal analgesia (most often including continuous epidural analgesia) and a pre-planned program for early discharge.

Table 1. Effects of fast-track colonic surgery on organ functions, hospital stay, convalescence, and costs

		References
Ileus	↓	[3, 7, 8, 9, 10, 12, 14, 16, 17, 18, 19]
Pulmonary function and oxygen saturation	↑	[7]
Exercise capacity	↑	[7, 8]
Muscle strength	↑	[9, 10]
Body composition (lean body mass)	↑	[7, 11]
Oral energy and protein intake	↑	[11]
Cardiopulmonary morbidity	↓	[12]
Hospital stay	↓	[3, 7, 10, 12, 14, 15, 16, 17, 18, 19, 20, 21]
Readmissions	(↑)	[10, 12, 14, 15, 19]
Postoperative fatigue and need for sleep	↓	[10, 13]
Costs	↓	[14]

Ileus

Due to the avoidance of nasogastric tubes with early institution of oral intake facilitated by continuous epidural local anesthetic techniques [5, 6], the duration of ileus has been reduced from usually 4–5 days to about 2 days (Table 1). This is a significant benefit, since discomfort due to abdominal distension is avoided and since early institution of oral nutrition can be instituted, which otherwise has been demonstrated to reduce catabolism and morbidity [1, 2].

Pulmonary Function and Oxygen Saturation

Early institution of mobilization facilitated by optimized pain relief with epidural analgesia has been demonstrated in comparative, nonrandomized studies [7] to improve pulmonary function and oxygen saturation, especially during night time (Table 1).

Exercise Capacity

Fast-track colonic surgery programs have been shown in comparative, nonrandomized studies to improve exercise capacity since the usual approximately 40% deterioration of exercise performance could be avoided [7, 8] (Table 1).

Muscle Strength

In two randomized studies, muscle strength assessed by the force of the quadriceps muscle [9] or handgrip strength [10] was improved by fast-track compared to conventional care colonic surgery (Table 1).

Body Composition

In comparative studies with conventional care, fast-track colonic surgery led to preservation of body composition (lean body mass) as assessed from before to 7–8 days postoperatively [7, 11] (Table 1).

Oral Energy and Protein Intake

An about 40%–50% increase in oral energy and protein intake could be achieved with a fast-track program [11] which may account for the preservation of lean body mass (Table 1).

Cardiopulmonary Morbidity

In a large, comparative, nonrandomized study, a multimodal rehabilitation program decreased cardiopulmonary morbidity compared to conservative treatment [12] (Table 1). These findings may correspond to improved organ functions with less reduced pulmonary function and improved oxygen saturation [7].

Hospital Stay

In all available studies (Table 1), hospital stay was significantly reduced from about 6–10 days to 2–4 days (Table 1). However, in three of these studies, the aim was to restore organ functions, while no aim was made specifically on early discharge [8, 9, 11]. It is important to mention that discharge criteria were unchanged during fast-track programs and the reduced hospital stay is therefore due to earlier achievement of discharge criteria (sufficient pain relief with oral analgesics, normalization of gastrointestinal function allowing normal oral intake, and patient acceptance).

Readmissions

In some, but not all series, an increased rate of admission was observed, but no safety problems were demonstrated, especially in the few patients who had an anastomotic dehiscence diagnosed after discharge (Table 1). Obviously, further data on readmissions and safety aspects are required in large series before final conclusions can be drawn.

Postoperative Fatigue and Convalescence

In the few comparative studies, postoperative fatigue was reduced [10, 13], even in the weeks after discharge, and the need for sleep was also reduced after fast-track care. At the same time, there was no increased need for health care support after discharge with fast-track programs and no increased need for visits to general practitioners (Table 1).

Costs

In the few studies available [14], the early restitution of body organ functions allowing for early discharge and increased convalescence with a potential reduction in morbidity also led to significant cost reductions (Table 1).

Discussion and Conclusions

From the available data on fast-track colonic surgery including a few randomized [9, 10, 11, 15] studies it appears that a revision of the perioperative care program including optimized pain relief with continuous epidural analgesic techniques [6] and enforced early oral nutrition, postoperative mobilization, and comprehensive preoperative information together with a well-defined postoperative nursing care program and discharge plan has led to significant improvements in outcome by reducing organ dysfunctions, cardiopulmonary morbidity, duration of ileus, and subsequently hospital stay. Furthermore, these findings include a potential for improved convalescence with less fatigue and need for sleep, without increased need for health care support and visits to general practitioners.

Additional factors with potential importance for a successful fast-track program include avoidance of perioperative fluid excess [22, 23], which otherwise may increase postoperative morbidity [23]. Although continuous epidural analgesia has been demonstrated to provide benefits after abdominal procedures by improving pain relief [6], reduction of ileus, and postoperative catabolism [5, 6], a few studies with successful fast-track colonic surgery did not use epidural analgesia [15, 19, 20]. Further studies are therefore needed to define the exact role of continuous epidural analgesia. Also, several fast-track programs utilized laparoscopic-assisted colonic resection, but nearly the same results were achieved with a combination of conventional open procedure compared with a fast-track care program [12, 16, 17, 20, 21], although lower costs were claimed with the laparoscopic approach [21, 24]. Further randomized studies are required to compare open versus laparoscopic-assisted colonic surgery in a fast-track program before final conclusions can be made about the potential additional benefits of performing the operation with laparoscopic assisted.

In conclusion, existing data on fast-track colonic surgery are all based on evidence from the single components of perioperative care (preoperative information, short-acting general anesthetics, epidural analgesia, early oral nutrition, enforced mobilization, avoidance of fluid excess, and avoidance of nasogastric tubes and drains) [1, 2] and have subsequently confirmed that conventional discharge criteria can be achieved earlier with subsequently reduced hospital stay. The data also suggest that postoperative medical morbidity can be reduced without an increased risk of surgical (wound and anastomotic) morbidity. These promising data should be extended to other centers in several countries in order to establish safety aspects and cost issues. The results achieved to date with fast-track colonic surgery seem to have major implications for improving care of these often high-risk patients, and the results also serve as a stimulus for development of fast-track programs in other high-risk surgical populations [1, 2].

Acknowledgements. Supported by a grant from Apoteker Fonden af 1991.

References

1. Kehlet H, Dahl JB (2003) Anaesthesia, surgery and challenges for postoperative recovery. Lancet 362:1921–1928
2. Kehlet H, Wilmore DW (2002) Multi-modal strategies to improve surgical outcome. Am J Surg 183:630–641
3. Basse L, Jakobsen DH, Billesbølle P, Werner M, Kehlet H (2000) A clinical pathway to accelerate recovery after colonic resection. Ann Surg 232:51–57
4. Wexner S (1998) Standard perioperative care protocols and reduced length of stay after colon surgery. Am J Coll Surg 186:589–593
5. Holte K, Kehlet H (2002) Epidural anaesthesia and analgesia—effects on surgical stress responses and implications for postoperative nutrition. Clin Nutr 21:199–206
6. Jørgensen H, Wetterslev J, Mønniche S, Dahl JB (2001) Epidural local anaesthetics vs opioid based analgesic regiments on postoperative gastrointestinal paralysis, PONV and pain after abdominal surgery (Cochrane review). Cochrane Library, issue 2, . Oxford: Update Software

7. Basse L, Raskov H, Jakobsen DH, Sonne E, Billesbølle E, Hendel HW, Rosenberg J, Kehlet H (2002) Accelerated postoperative recovery programme after colonic resection improves physical performance, pulmonary function and body composition. Br J Surg :89:446–453
8. Carli F, Mayo N, Clubien K, Schricker T, Trudel J, Bellivau P (2002) Epidural analgesia enhances exercise capacity and health related quality of life after colonic surgery: results of a randomized trial. Anesthesiology 97:540–549
9. Henriksen MG, Jensen MB, Hansen HV, Jespersen TW, Hessov I (2002) Enforced mobilization, early oral feeding, and balanced analgesia improve convalescence after colorectal surgery. Nutrition18:147–152
10. Anderson, ADG, McNaught CE, MacFie J, Tring I, Barker P, Mitchell CJ (2003) Randomized clinical trial of multimodal optimization and standard perioperative surgical care. Br J Surg 90:1497–1504
11. Henriksen MG, Hansen HV, Hessov I (2002) Early oral nutrition after elective colorectal surgery: influence of balanced analgesia and enforced mobilization. Nutrition 18:266–269
12. Basse L, Thorbøl JE, Løssl K, Kehlet H (2004) Convalescence after fast-track versus conventional care of colonic surgery. Dis Colon Rectum 47:271–278
13. Hjort Jakobsen D, Sonne E, Basse L, Bisgaard T, Kehlet H (2004) Convalescence after colonic resection with fast-track vs. conventional care. Scand J Surg (in press)
14. Stephen AE, Berger DL (2003) Shortened length of stay and hospital cost reduction with implementation of an accelerated clinical pathway after elective colonic resection. Surgery 133:277–282
15. Delaney CP, Zutshi M, Senagore AJ, Remzi FH, Hammel J, Fazio VW (2003) Prospective, randomized, controlled trial between a pathway of controlled rehabilitation with early ambulation and diet and traditional postoperative care after laparotomy and intestinal resection. Dis Colon Rectum 46:851–859
16. Senagore AJ, Duepree HJ, Delaney CP, Brady KM, Fazio VW (2003) Results of a standardized technique and postoperative care plan for laparoscopic sigmoid colectomy. A 30-month experience. Dis Colon Rectum 46:503–509
17. Bardram L, Funch-Jensen P, Kehlet H (2000) Rapid rehabilitation in elderly patients after laparoscopic resection. Br J Surg 87:45–45
18. Basse L, Jacobsen DH. Billesbølle P, Kehlet H (2002) Colostomy closure after Hartman's procedure with fast-track rehabilitation. Dis Colon Rectum 45:1661–1664
19. DiFronzo, Yamin N, Patel K, O'Connell TX (2003) Benefits of early feeding and early hospital discharge in elderly patients undergoing open colon resection. J Am Coll Surg 197:747–753
20. Delaney CP, Fazio VW, Senagore AJ, Robinsson B, Halvorson AL, Remzi FH (2001) Fast-track postoperative management protocol for patients with high co-morbidity undergoing complex abdominal and pelvic colorectal surgery. Br J Surg 88:1533–1538
21. Senagore AJ, Duepree HJ, Delaney CP, Dissanaike S, Brady KM, Fazio VW (2002) Cost structure of laparoscopic and open sigmoid colectomy for diverticular disease. Similarities and differences. Dis Colon Rectum 45:485–490
22. Holte K, Sharrock NE, Kehlet H (2002) Pathophysiology and clinical implications of perioperative fluid excess. Br J Anaesth 89:622–632
23. Brandstrup B, Tønnesen H, Beier-Holgersen R, Hjortsø E, Ørding H, Lindorff-Larsen K, Rasmussen MS, Lanng C, Wallin L and the Danish study group on perioperative fluid therapy (2003) Effects of intravenous fluid restriction on postoperative complications: Comparison of two perioperative fluid regimens. Ann Surg 238:641–648
24. Delaney CP, Kiran RP, Senagore AJ, Brady K, Fazio VW (2003) Case-matched comparison of clinical and financial outcome after laparoscopic and/or open colorectal surgery. Ann Surg 238:67–72

Fast-Track Surgery: The Heidelberg Experience

M. Kremer, A. Ulrich, M. W. Büchler, W. Uhl

W. Uhl (✉)
Department of Surgery, St. Josef-Hospital Bochum, Ruhr-University,
Gudrunstr. 56, 44791 Bochum, Germany
e-mail: w.uhl@klinikum-bochum.de

Abstract

Fast-track surgery is an interdisciplinary multimodal concept of minimally invasive surgery or new incision lines and "cutting old plaits" (e.g., the use of drains or tubes). It uses modern intraoperative anesthesia (e.g., fluid restriction) and analgesia, including new drugs and novel ways of administration (e.g., thoracic epidural analgesia) for postoperative pain relief, in combination with the immediate mobilization of the patient and early oral nutrition after the operation. This approach requires a cooperating team of motivated nurses, physiotherapists, anesthesiologists, and surgeons, in addition to continuous improvement of the processes involved. Moreover, extended patient education and information about the procedures and the expected time course are of the highest importance, as the active role of the patient is to be emphasized. This chapter describes the development and implementation of fast-track surgery in colorectal diseases at the Department of Surgery of the University Hospital of Heidelberg, Germany. Preliminary results of fast-track surgery suggest a significant and clear overall benefit for the patient. A shorter hospital stay and reduced systemic morbidity in addition to no increase in postoperative complications on an out-patient basis were found. However, to exclude a "bloody discharge" of the patients, thorough follow-up and quality control are mandatory. Although in the initial phase increased personnel care is necessary, in the new German reimbursement system with G-DRGs (German diagnosis-related groups) fast-track surgery seems to save resources in the long term.

Development of Fast-Track Surgery

Over the past decade, advances in healthcare with an evolution in peri- and postoperative care have led to a new surgical approach, the so-called fast-track surgery. Improved understanding of postoperative physiology in particular has led to reductions in the length of time spent in the hospital after surgery [1, 2], thus saving resources.

In fast-track surgery, a multimodal pathway is applied to patients. In addition to minimally invasive procedures and laparoscopic surgery [3, 4], postoperative stress was reduced to a minimum. Surgeons and anesthesiologists have been using epidural regional anesthetic agents to reduce the stress response associated with elective surgery [5]. An advantage has also been obtained with the use of new pharmacologic agents that control nausea, vomiting, gastric ileus and infection, thereby dramatically reducing the incidence of postoperative complications [6–9].

Such a multimodal approach seems to shorten surgical convalescence following major operative procedures, with dramatically reduced medical morbidity, whereas surgical morbidity is not affected [10, 11].

The Heidelberger Concept

Key factors of fast-track surgery involve thorough patient education, a multidisciplinary team approach to surgical management, epidural anesthetic administration, and early nutrition and ambulation after the procedure.

In accord with the findings and experience of Delaney et al. [11] and Kehlet et al. [12], we developed a modified fast-track surgery concept, which applies to specific clinic-associated routines.

Most important in using fast-track procedures is to gain the cooperation of the patient. Therefore intensive education of the patient preoperatively including written guidelines that describe the future hospital stay, surgical and anesthesiological procedures, milestones of personal recovery, and a set of discharge instructions is given to the patient before the operation. The active role of the patient, guided by a team of specialists, is outlined in Fig. 1.

The trend toward fast-tracking is challenging a number of surgical traditions, including routine use of preoperative bowel preparation and nasogastric tube

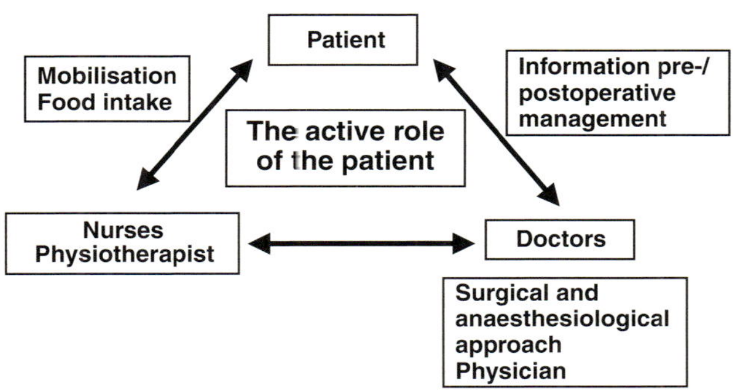

Figure 1. Underlining the importance of active cooperation of the patient with surgeons, anesthesists, nurses, and physiotherapists. Cooperation is achieved by extended preoperative education, minimally invasive surgery and anesthesiology, early mobilization, and early postoperative food intake

decompression. According to the newest findings in evidence-based medicine, preoperative bowel preparation has no advantage. In a review with a total of 1,204 patients, no bowel preparation did not adversely affect mortality, re-operation rate, or wound infection. Furthermore, the rate of anastomotic leakage seemed to be reduced [13].

Similar results were found for the use of nasogastric tubes. The first prospective and randomized study in 1993 showed that nasogastric decompression is not necessary following elective colorectal surgery [14]. However, it was nearly a decade until other studies supporting these findings were published [15, 16], leading now to a reduced use of nasogastric tubes. A meta-analysis of nearly 4,000 patients even demonstrated, surprisingly, that routine use of nasogastric tubes after laparotomy increased the incidence of complications, such as pneumonia and atelectasis, and decreased the time to oral feeding [17].

Therefore the use of nasogastric tubes in our model of fast-track surgery is mostly limited to the day of operation. The tubes are removed within hours after the operation, if there is a reflux of less than 200 ml.

Epidural anesthesia is a key factor, because it blocks the painful stimulus that interferes with postoperative bowel function and contributes to ileus and other potential complications due to immobilization. A review comparing the use of spinal or epidural anesthesia with or without additional general anesthesia and general anesthesia alone demonstrated a significant reduction in postoperative mortality and in the rate of systemic morbidity such as pneumonia, myocardial infarction, bleeding, and transfusion requirements [18].

The combination of therapeutic modalities in fast-track surgery is helpful in overcoming intraoperative factors that tend to delay recuperation. These include blood transfusions which suppress the immune system, and hypothermia, which has been shown to increase the length of hospitalization, particularly for elderly patients [19]. The routine use of drains in several abdominal operations does not improve outcome, as determined by randomized clinical studies [20, 21]. Therefore we perform routine fast-track operations without drains.

Extubation in the OR, early mobilization 6 h after surgery, and drinking of small amounts of noncarbonated liquids 6 h after surgery are implemented in favor of fast recovery.

The first day after the operation, patients receive a protein drink to improve bowel movement; noncarbonated liquids are ad libitum, and soft diet is allowed in the evening. Extended mobilization of at least 50m on the ward is supported by physiotherapists, as are regular respiratory exercizes. The postoperative urinary bladder drainage is removed analogue to the achieved state of mobilization on post-operative day (POD) 1 or 2, according to the findings of controlled trials [22, 23].

As outlined in Table1, on POD 2, the epidural catheter is removed and non-opioid oral analgesia is started. Mobilization and respiratory exercizes are extended, and in the evening the patients get solid food.

On POD 3–5, patients are discharged with instructions to visit their physician the next day and our outpatient clinic one week later. The patients are advised to come to our outpatient clinic immediately if they experience any problems.

Table 1. Scheme of the Heidelberg concept of fast-track surgery (POD, postoperative day)

On the day of operation:
No preoperative bowel preparation
Nasogastric tube only during anesthesia, removed the same day
Thoracic epidural analgesia
Extubation in operating theatre
Start with small amounts of noncarbonated liquids 6 h after surgery
Early mobilization 5 h after surgery

POD 1
Protein drinks/laxative
Early mobilization: walking about 50 m in the ward
Regular respiratory exercise
Liquids ad libitum
Soft diet in the evening

POD 2
Removal of epidural catheter, start with non-opioid oral analgesia
Extended mobilization and regular respiratory exercise
Liquids ad libitum
Solid food

POD 3 till discharge
Oral analgesia
Further extended mobilization
Liquids ad libitum
Solid food

Preliminary Results

To establish the fast-track surgery concept in Heidelberg, the multimodal concept had to be introduced to different disciplines, including nursing and physiotherapist staff. It took nearly one year to implement the modalities of fast-track surgery. From September to November 2003, 26 patients were included in the study.

Based on preliminary results, our concept of fast-track surgery is feasible, ensuring a shorter stay and less systemic morbidity. Patients appeared to have less pain and returned to normal physical activities in a much shorter time than patients managed with traditional techniques.

An important question concerning the early discharge in fast-track surgery is the safety of the patient during the development of abdominal problems in cases of anastomotic leakage. Included in the education of the patient is extensive information about calling our outpatient clinic as well as coming in at any time to our clinic, if any adverse symptoms or signs of complications occur. To date, our patients have suffered no anastomotic leakage, and no adverse effects have been reported when patients were instructed to call the physician if they develop suspicious symptoms at home [24].

Whereas the majority of publications describe the impact of minimally invasive surgery such as laparoscopy-assisted techniques [4, 25] with fast-track surgery, Basse et al. [24] achieved the same results with open colonic resection, suggesting that postoperative recovery may depend more on other factors such as optimal pain relief, early nutrition, and early mobilization and omission of recovery-inhibiting regimens than on the choice of surgical technique itself. These findings concur with our preliminary observations. Therefore minimally invasive surgery must also be questioned if fast-track open surgery can achieve a similar postoperative length of stay.

More studies of the fast-track surgical approach are needed. As it is impossible to randomize and blind patients, nurses, and doctors in a project with multimodal rehabilitation, large multicenter comparative studies must be initiated to evaluate the benefits of the approach of fast-track surgery.

Reimbursement: German DRG (Diagnosis-Related Groups)

Worldwide health care systems are changing significantly, mainly due to limited financial resources. For the reimbursement of hospitalized patients, the diagnosis-related groups that originated in the USA and improved in Australia have been adopted in Germany since 2004. Table 2 gives the data of patients undergoing rectal and colonic/sigmoidal resections with regard to the allowed hospital stay,

Table 2. Reimbursement according to the German diagnosis-related groups (G-DRG). Shown are data of rectal and colonic/sigmoidal resections with regard to the allowed hospital stay, cost weight and earnings with co-morbicity/complications (A) or without (B). Minimal hospital stay varies between 4 and 6 days, whereas the maximum stay is between 28 and 39 days

G-DRG	Hospital stay	Cost weight	Earnings[a]
Rectal resection			
G01A	22.2 (6–39 days)	4.009	12.107 euro
G01B	17.4 (5–30 days)	2.915	8.803 euro
Colonic/sigma resection			
G02A	21.4 (6–39 days)	3.532	10.667 euro
G02B	15.9 (4–28 days)	2.414	7.290 euro

[a] Cost weight × base rate (base rate = 3.020 euro).

cost weight and earnings with co-morbidity and complications (A) and without (B). With regard to hospitalization, the allowed hospital stay ranges from at least 4–6 days and at maximum between 28 and 39 days. If the patient is discharged earlier from the hospital in this financial system, the amount of reimbursement is reduced dramatically for each earlier day. Therefore, this system supports the modern concept of fast-track colorectal surgery only in part. It seems reasonable from the financial aspect not to further reduce hospitalization under 4–6 days in Germany. However, from our clinical point of view, a reduction of hospital stay under 4 days in rectal and colonic fast-track surgery does not show a significant benefit for the patient.

References

1. Pearson SD, Goulart-Fisher D, Lee TH (1995) Critical pathways as a strategy for improving care: problems and potential. Ann Intern Med 123:941–948
2. Archer SB, Burnett RJ, Flesch LV, Hobler SC, Bower RH, Nussbaum MS, Fischer JE (1997) Implementation of a clinical pathway decreases length of stay and hospital charges for patients undergoing total colectomy and ileal pouch/anal anastomosis. Surgery 122:699–703; discussion 703–705
3. Holte K, Kehlet H (2000) Postoperative ileus: a preventable event. Br J Surg 87:1480–1493
4. Chen HH, Wexner SD, Weiss EG, Nogueras JJ, Alabaz O, Iroatulam AJ, Nessim A, Joo JS (1998) Laparoscopic colectomy for benign colorectal disease is associated with a significant reduction in disability as compared with laparotomy. Surg Endosc 12:1397–1400
5. Liu SS, Carpenter RL, Mackey DC, Thirlby RC, Rupp SM, Shine TS, Feinglass NG, Metzger PP, Fulmer JT, Smith SL (1995) Effects of perioperative analgesic technique on rate of recovery after colon surgery. Anesthesiology 83:757–765
6. Tramer MR, Moore RA, Reynolds DJ, McQuay HJ (1997) A quantitative systematic review of ondansetron in treatment of established postoperative nausea and vomiting. Bmj 314:1088–1092
7. Henzi I, Walder B, Tramer MR (2000) Dexamethasone for the prevention of postoperative nausea and vomiting: a quantitative systematic review. Anesth Analg 90:186–194
8. Henzi I, Sonderegger J, Tramer MR (2000) Efficacy, dose-response, and adverse effects of droperidol for prevention of postoperative nausea and vomiting. Can J Anaesth 47:537–551
9. Burke P, Mealy K, Gillen P, Joyce W, Traynor O, Hyland J (1994) Requirement for bowel preparation in colorectal surgery. Br J Surg 81:907–910
10. Bardram L, Funch-Jensen P, Kehlet H (2000) Rapid rehabilitation in elderly patients after laparoscopic colonic resection. Br J Surg 87:1540–1545
11. Delaney CP, Fazio VW, Senagore AJ, Robinson B, Halverson AL, Remzi FH (2001) 'Fast track' postoperative management protocol for patients with high co-morbidity undergoing complex abdominal and pelvic colorectal surgery. Br J Surg 88:1533–1538
12. Kehlet H, Mogensen T (1999) Hospital stay of 2 days after open sigmoidectomy with a multimodal rehabilitation programme. Br J Surg 86:227–230
13. Guenaga KF, Matos D, Castro AA, Atallah AN, Wille-Jorgensen P (2003) Mechanical bowel preparation for elective colorectal surgery. Cochrane Database Syst Rev CD001544
14. Petrelli NJ, Stulc JP, Rodriguez-Bigas M, Blumenson L (1993) Nasogastric decompression following elective colorectal surgery: a prospective randomized study. Am Surg 59:632–635
15. Manning BJ, Winter DC, McGreal G, Kirwan WO, Redmond HP (2001) Nasogastric intubation causes gastroesophageal reflux in patients undergoing elective laparotomy. Surgery 130:788–791
16. Yoo CH, Son BH, Han WK, Pae WK (2002) Nasogastric decompression is not necessary in operations for gastric cancer: prospective randomised trial. Eur J Surg 168:379–383
17. Cheatham ML, Chapman WC, Key SP, Sawyers JL (1995) A meta-analysis of selective versus routine nasogastric decompression after elective laparotomy. Ann Surg 221:469–76; discussion 476–478

18. Rodgers A, Walker N, Schug S, McKee A, Kehlet H, van Zundert A, Sage D, Futter M, Saville G, Clark T, MacMahon S (2000) Reduction of postoperative mortality and morbidity with epidural or spinal anaesthesia: results from overview of randomised trials. BMJ 321:1493
19. Frank SM, Fleisher LA, Breslow MJ, Higgins MS, Olson KF, Kelly S, Beattie C (1997) Perioperative maintenance of normothermia reduces the incidence of morbid cardiac events. A randomized clinical trial. JAMA 277:1127–1134
20. Merad F, Yahchouchi E, Hay JM, Fingerhut A, Laborde Y, Langlois-Zantain O (1998) Prophylactic abdominal drainage after elective colonic resection and suprapromontory anastomosis: a multicenter study controlled by randomization. French Associations for Surgical Research Arch Surg 133:309–314
21. Urbach DR, Kennedy ED, Cohen MM (1999) Colon and rectal anastomoses do not require routine drainage: a systematic review and meta-analysis. Ann Surg 229:174–180
22. Benoist S, Panis Y, Denet C, Mauvais F, Mariani P, Valleur P (1999) Optimal duration of urinary drainage after rectal resection: a randomized controlled trial. Surgery 125:135–141
23. Basse L, Werner M, Kehlet H (2000) Is urinary drainage necessary during continuous epidural analgesia after colonic resection? Reg Anesth Pain Med 25:498–501
24. Basse L, Hjort Jakobsen D, Billesbolle P, Werner M, Kehlet H (2000) A clinical pathway to accelerate recovery after colonic resection. Ann Surg 232:51–57
25. Bokey EL, Moore JW, Chapuis PH, Newland RC (1996) Morbidity and mortality following laparoscopic-assisted right hemicolectomy for cancer. Dis Colon Rectum 39:S24–S28

Rectal Cancer: A Compartmental Disease. The Mesorectum and Mesorectal Lymph Nodes

Susan Galandiuk, Kiran Chaturvedi, Boris Topor

S. Galandiuk (✉)
Section of Colon and Rectal Surgery and Price Institute of Surgical Research,
University of Louisville, and the Digestive Health Center,
University of Louisville Hospital, Louisville KY,40292, USA
e-mail: s0gala01@louisville.edu

Abstract

Even though the technique of total mesorectal excision has been widely used, there have been few detailed descriptions of the distribution of lymph nodes within the rectal mesentery. We describe the results of our anatomic study of lymph node size and distribution within the mesorectum and pelvic side-wall tissue using a fat-clearing solvent in seven male cadavers, and we used a similar technique to examine the mesorectum in a patient who underwent total mesorectal excision after preoperative chemoradiation for a uT3 rectal cancer. In both the cadavers and our patient, the majority of lymph nodes were located within the posterior upper two-thirds of the mesorectum. Few lymph nodes were located in the distal mesorectum or anteriorly. In the cadavers, the majority of lymph nodes were less than 3 mm in diameter. In the patient who had received preoperative chemoradiation, routine tissue processing yielded only four lymph nodes, whereas processing in fat-clearing solvent yielded 25 additional nodes. The majority of these nodes, in contrast to those observed in cadavers, were less than 1 mm in diameter. The majority of mesorectal lymph nodes were located within the upper two-thirds of the posterior mesorectum. Complete removal of nodes in this area may, in part, explain the superior results of total mesorectal excision with respect to local recurrence.

Introduction

The technique of total mesorectal excision, as applied to surgery for rectal cancer, involves the sharp dissection and removal of the entire rectal mesentery and preserves intact the proper rectal fascia that surrounds the mesentery of the rectum posteriorly. This type of surgical approach has resulted in lower rates of local recurrence and increased awareness of pelvic anatomy [1]. It has also heightened our knowledge of the structure of the mesorectum. Surgeons now recognize the role of perirectal lymph nodes in recurrence following surgery for rectal cancer,

Recent Results in Cancer Research, Vol. 165

and the mesorectum as being the first area of tumor drainage for cancer cells. Although details of mesorectal excision were described as early as 1931 by Abel [2], this technique has recently been popularized by Heald [3] and others [4]. Despite the fact that total mesorectum excision has been associated with lower rates of local recurrence than "conventional" blunt dissection techniques [5], little has been published regarding the location, distribution, and size of lymph nodes within the rectal mesentery [6–8].

The Structure of the Mesorectum

Similar to the rectum, the mesorectum is divided into thirds according to the cranio-caudad location: proximal, middle, and distal. In the coronal plane, the mesorectum is divided into quadrants, which are posterior, left lateral, right lateral, and anterior, according to its location with respect to the surrounding pelvic structures. Figure 1 illustrates the upper third of the mesorectum and is shown alongside a computed tomography (CT) scan illustrating the same location. In the upper third of the rectum, total mesorectal excision is least important of all rectal locations, since cancers in this area tend to behave similarly to colon cancers and have a low rate of local recurrence. Figure 2 illustrates the middle third of the rectum in a schematic view with a representative CT scan, showing enlarged lymph nodes with fat stranding in the rectal mesentery. The anterior, posterior, and right and left lateral portions of the rectal mesentery are more pronounced in this location. The lower third of the rectum is shown in Fig. 3.

We wish to report the lymph node distribution, size, and location within the mesentery as based on our cadaver findings [8] as well as our clinical experience in a patient who underwent preoperative chemoradiation.

Methods

Dissections were performed within the Fresh Tissue Dissection Laboratory (Director Robert A. Acland, MD) of the University of Louisville, Department of Surgery. Seven 70- to 90-kg male cadavers were used to perform total mesorectal excision. The rectum, mesorectum, and tissue from the pelvic side walls were dissected free and placed in a fat solvent consisting of 5% glacial acidic acid, 10% buffered formalin, 40% ethyl ether, and 45% ethanol. For the purposes of the cadaver study, the upper anatomic limit of the rectum was considered the point where the taenia coalesced. The pelvic side-wall tissues included the obturator lymph node area and were limited laterally by the external iliac vessels. Our technique was modified from that described by Koren et al. [9] by lengthening the exposure time of specimens in fat-clearing solution from 6 h to 24 h and increasing the volume of ethyl ether from 20% to 40%. Following placement in the fat-clearing solvent, and after incubation for 24 h, specimens were washed, and the rectum opened longitudinally along the anterior surface. The mesorectum was dissected free from the rectum and oriented so that anterior, posterior, and right and left lateral sections could be

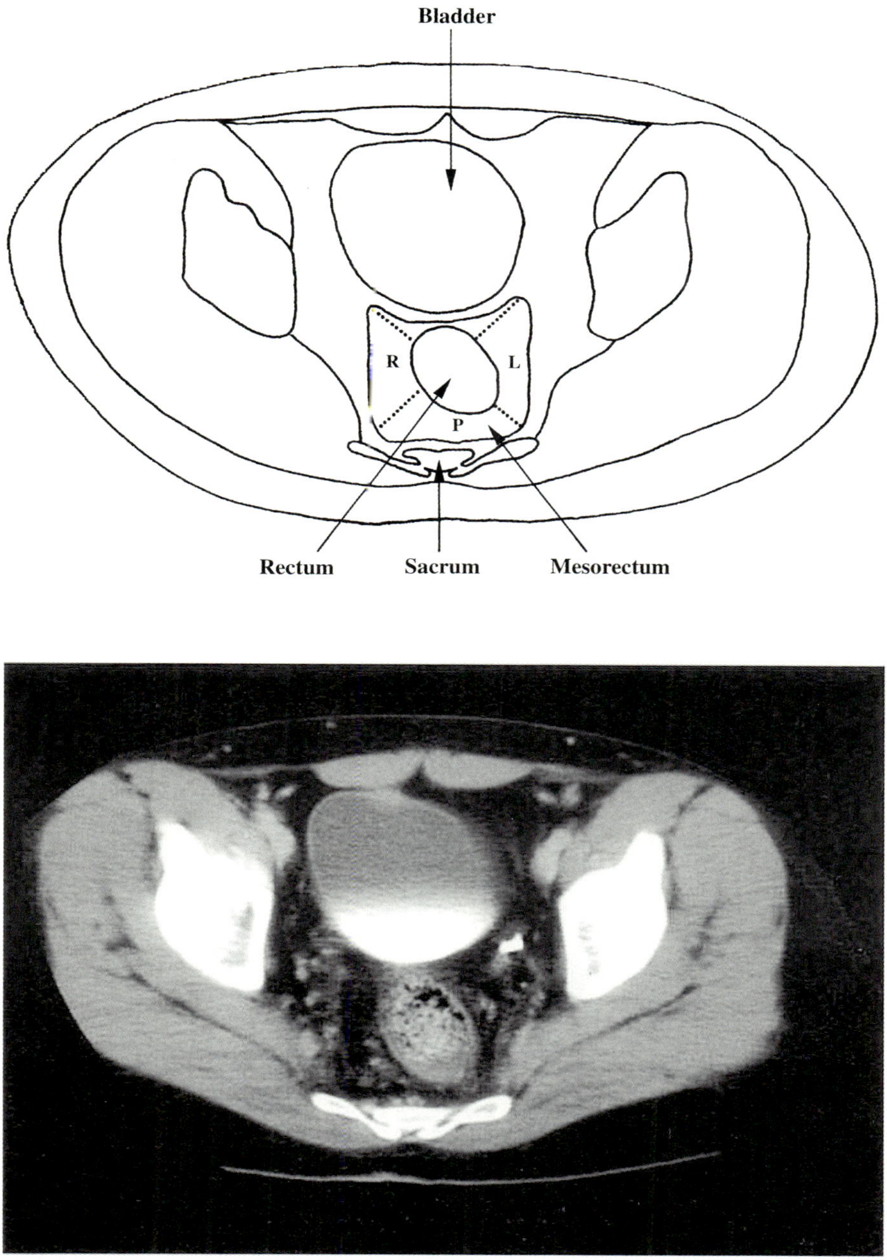

Figure 1. *Top*: Cross-sectional view of the upper third of the rectum. The *dotted lines* separate the posterior (*P*), right lateral (*R*), and left lateral (*L*) portions of the mesorectum. There is no mesorectum anteriorly at this level. (With permission from [8]). *Bottom* Computed tomography (CT) view

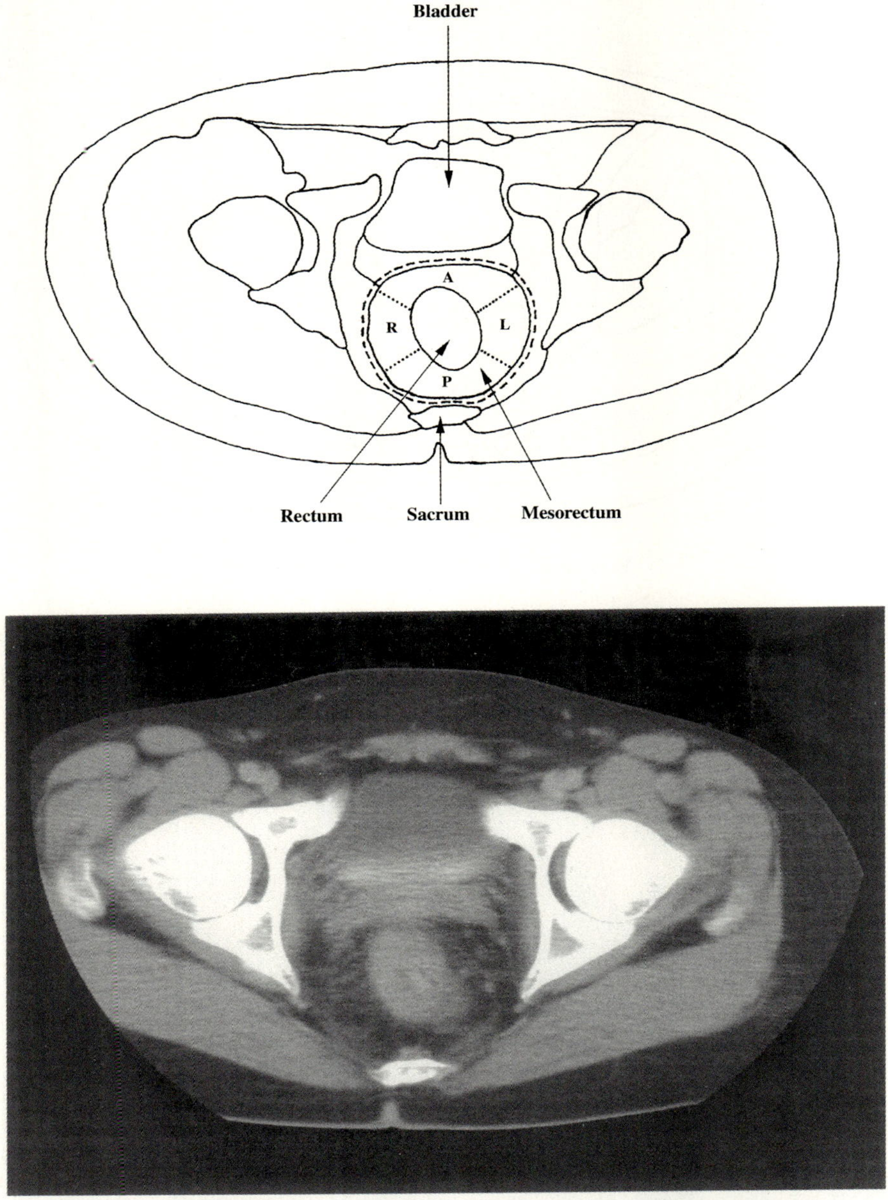

Figure 2. *Top*: Cross-sectional view of the middle third of the rectum. The *dotted lines* separate the posterior (*P*), right lateral (*R*), anterior (*A*), and left lateral (L) portions of the mesorectum. The *dashed line* represents the limits of total mesorectal excision just outside of the proper rectal fascia. Posteriorly, this lies within the presacral space and anteriorly between the sheets of Denonvilliers' fascia. (With permission from [8]). *Bottom*: CT view

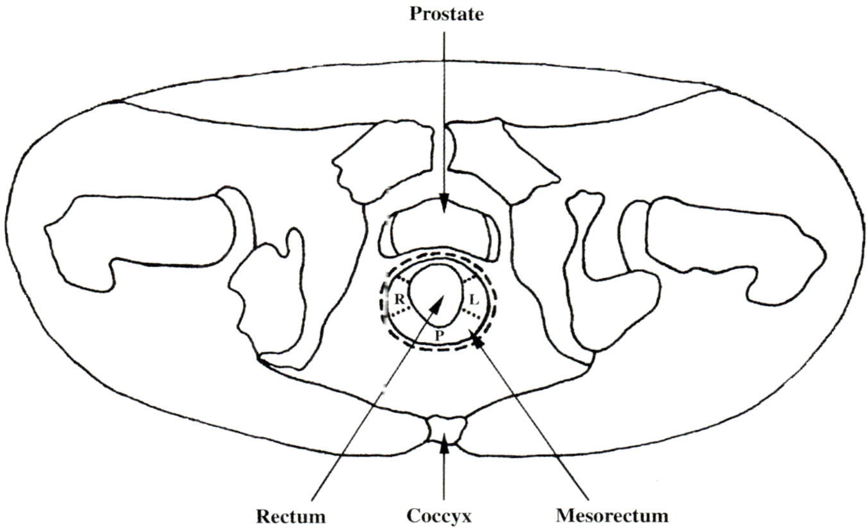

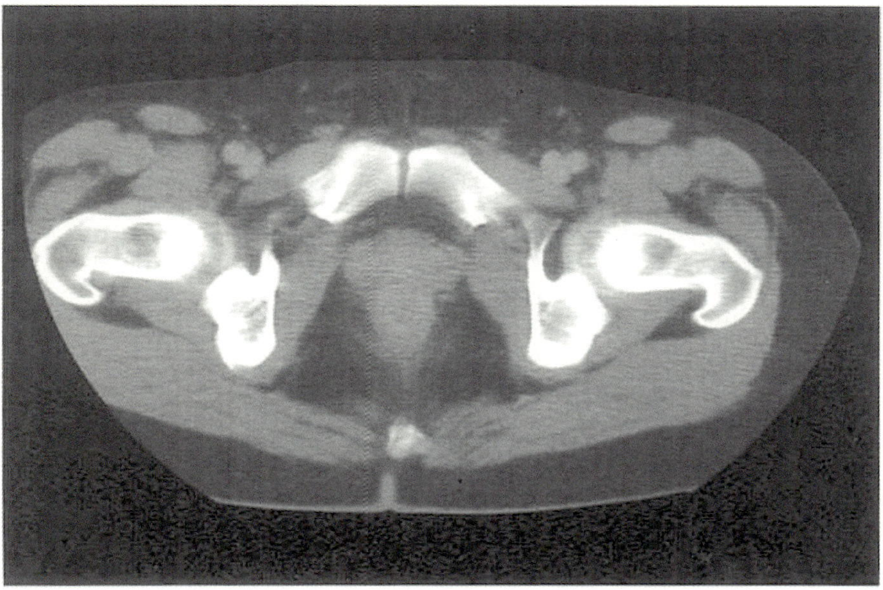

Figure 3. *Top*: Cross-sectional view of the lower third of the rectum. The *dotted lines* separate the posterior (*P*), right lateral (*R*), and left lateral (*L*) portions of the mesorectum. The *dashed line* represents the limits of total mesorectal excision just outside of the proper rectal fascia. Posteriorly, this lies within the presacral space and anteriorly between the sheets of Denonvilliers' fascia. (With permission from [8]). *Bottom*: CT view

identified, labeled, pinned onto a corkboard, and sectioned at 2- to 3-mm intervals. The size and number of lymph nodes in each of the four quadrants of the rectal mesentery were noted. Lymph nodes posterior and anterior to the rectum, right and left laterally, and within the corresponding upper, middle, and lower thirds of the mesorectum were separately noted, as were the size and number of lymph nodes in the pelvic side-wall tissue.

In an additional study, we documented lymph node location, distribution, and size within the mesorectum of a 70-kg man (55 years old) with a uT3 rectal cancer who underwent preoperative chemoradiation using 5-fluorouracil, leucovorin, and 5400 cGy external beam radiation to the pelvis. Total mesorectal excision was performed 5 weeks following the conclusion of his last radiation dose. High ligation of the inferior mesenteric artery and standard total mesorectal excision were performed. Initially, normal processing for lymph node harvest was conducted. Following this, the mesorectum was placed in the same solvent as described for the cadavers. Since it was extremely difficult to identify shrunken lymph nodes against a fatty background, all fibrous tissue was submitted for histological processing and hematoxylin and eosin staining after removing the fat from the specimen.

Results

The fat solvent facilitated the identification of the lymph nodes by showing them as white structures against a yellow background of fat. The majority of lymph nodes within the rectal mesentery were located within the posterior, upper two-thirds of the mesorectum (Table 1). Fifty-six percent of lymph nodes were within the posterior mesorectum, and 50% of lymph nodes were located within the upper two-thirds of the posterior mesorectum. Interestingly, nearly twice as many lymph nodes were located in the pelvic side wall as in the lateral pelvic mesorectum. More than 80% of the lymph nodes in the cadaver mesorectum were less than 3 mm in diameter. The majority of lymph nodes (72%) were 2 mm to 3 mm in size.

In the uT3 rectal cancer patient, normal histological processing yielded four mesorectal lymph nodes. Following processing using the fat-clearing solvent, an additional 25 mesorectal lymph nodes were identified. Twenty-eight lymph nodes were present in the proximal two-thirds of the rectal mesentery, with only one lymph node found in the left portion of the lower third of the rectal mesentery. Similar to the cadaver study, 64% of lymph nodes were located in the posterior two-thirds of the rectal mesentery. The size of the lymph nodes in the radiated tissue was, however, markedly smaller than those in the cadaver study. In the latter, lymph nodes ranged from 2 mm to 3 mm in size, whereas the majority of the lymph nodes in the radiated tissue were 1 mm or less in size. Only one lymph node measured 4 mm in size, and few measured 2 mm or 3 mm in size.

Table 1. Number and location of mesorectal lymph nodes (reprinted with permission from [8])

Mesorectal location	Right lateral		Posterior		Left lateral		Anterior		Total all locations	
	Mean no.	(range)	Mean no.	(range)	Mean no.	(range)	Mean no.	(range)	Mean no.	(range)
Upper third	0.6	(0–3)	3.4	(1–5)	0.6	(0–3)	0	(0)	4.6	(3–9)
Middle third	1.7	(0–3)	3.6	(0–10)	2.1	(1–4)	0.7	(0–3)	8.1	(3–16)
Lower third	0.3	(0–2)	0.6	(0–2)	0.3	(0–1)	0	(0)	1.1	(0–3)
Total no. of mesorectal lymph nodes	2.3	(0–6)	7.6	(1–16)	3.0	(1–6)	0.7	(0–3)	13.6	(6–23)
Lateral side wall	5.9	(3–8)	NA		5.1	(3–13)	NA		11.0	(6–19)
Total mesorectal and side wall	8.1	(5–12)	7.6	(1–16)	8.1	(4–17)	0.7	(0–3)	24.9	(16–41)

Discussion

Most of the nodes detected within the mesorectum were less than 3 mm in diameter. This is important since even small lymph nodes can have deposits of metastatic disease [10]. While the fat-clearing technique is clearly not feasible to use in all patients undergoing preoperative radiation, it clearly provides an additional lymph node yield as compared to routine tissue processing, due to the small size of radiated lymph nodes. Lymph nodes may be difficult to identify, since they are similar in color and consistency to fat. This, combined with preoperative radiation, may make lymph node identification particularly challenging. In the case of the patient presented herein, the increased number of lymph nodes obtained with the fat-clearing technique did not however change the tumor staging. The patient remained lymph-node negative, despite the increase in the number of lymph nodes from four to 29. There are also other factors to consider, such as the toxicity of these fat solvents. Numerous reports have, however, emphasized that at least 13 to 14 lymph nodes are necessary for proper staging in cases of colorectal cancer. Without this, there may be a significant risk of understaging the patient's disease [11, 12]. In select cases, one may wish to consider using such fat-clearing techniques. It is, however, interesting that radiation does *not* change the distribution of lymph nodes within the mesorectum, but only reduces their size. The fact that most lymph nodes within the mesorectum are located within the proximal two-thirds of the mesorectum is supported by data from our cadaver study as well as in the patient treated with preoperative chemoradiation.

Our findings of relatively few lymph nodes in the distal mesorectum may support the fact that sphincter-sparing procedures for rectal cancer are not associated with an increased local recurrence rate. There appear to be very few lymph nodes in this location. Once the entire mesorectum is removed, good oncologic results can be achieved. Although there are numerous lymph nodes in the pelvic side wall, long-term studies have not shown a survival benefit following radical lateral lymphadenectomy, with neither an increase in survival nor a decrease in local recurrence [13, 14].

Our data confirm the small size of normal lymph nodes; more than 80 percent of identified lymph nodes are $\leq$3 mm in diameter. This is particularly important in the context of postoperative pathology reports. Attention to only large lymph nodes may have a significant deleterious impact on staging.

Acknowledgements. This work was supported in part by a J. William Fulbright Scholarship for Boris Topor, M.D., administered by the Bureau of Educational and Cultural Affairs, U.S. Department of State, in cooperation with the Council for International Exchange of Scholars. Modified and expanded from Topor B, Acland R, Kolodko V, Galandiuk S (2003) Mesorectal lymph nodes: their location and distribution within the mesorectum. Dis Colon Rectum 46:779–785.

References

1. Sjödahl R (2001) The role of total mesorectal excision in rectal cancer surgery. Eur J Surg Oncol 27:440–441
2. Abel AL (1931) The modern treatment of cancer of the colon and rectum. Milwaukee Proc 296–300
3. Heald RJ, Husband EM, Ryall RO (1982) The mesorectum in rectal surgery: the clue to pelvic recurrence? Br J Surg 69:613–616
4. Gordon PH (2000) Is total mesorectal excision really important? J Surg Oncol 74:177–180
5. Murty M, Enker WE, Martz J (2000) Current status of total mesorectal excision and autonomic nerve preservation in rectal cancer. Semin Surg Oncol 19:321–328
6. Takahashi T, Ueno M, Azekura K, Ohta H (2000) Lateral node dissection and total mesorectal excision for the rectal cancer. Dis Colon Rectum 43(10 Suppl):S59-S68
7. Bissett IP, Chau KY, Hill GL (2000) Extrafascial excision of the rectum: surgical anatomy of the fascia propria. Dis Colon Rectum 43:903–910
8. Topor B, Acland R, Kolodko V, Galandiuk S (2003) Mesorectal lymph nodes: Their location and distribution within the mesorectum. Dis Colon Rectum 46:779–785
9. Koren R, Siegal A, Klein B, et al (1997) Lymph node-revealing solution: simple new method for detecting minute lymph nodes in colon carcinoma. Dis Colon Rectum 40:407–410
10. Vorburger S, Metzger U (2000) The role of lymph nodes in rectal carcinoma. Zentralbl Chir 125:852–862
11. Tepper JE, O'Connell MJ, Niedzwiecki D, et al (2001) Impact of number of nodes retrieved on outcome in patients with rectal cancer. J Clin Oncol 19:157–163
12. Wong JH, Severino R, Honnebier MB, Tom P, Namiki TS (1999) Number of nodes examined and staging accuracy in colorectal carcinoma. J Clin Oncol 17:2896–2900
13. Moriya Y, Sugihara K, Akasu T, Fujita S (1997) Importance of extended lymphadenectomy with lateral node dissection for advanced lower rectal cancer. World J Surg 21:728–732
14. Yasutomi M, Shindo K, Mori N, Matsuda T (1991) Does the pelvic nodes dissection for the rectal cancer patients make any contribution to the end-results of surgery? [In Japanese] Gan To Kagaku Ryoho 18:541–546

The Pathological Assessment of Total Mesorectal Excision: What Are the Relevant Resection Margins?

Frank Autschbach

F. Autschbach (✉)
Institute of Pathology, Heidelberg University, Im Neuenheimer Feld 220/221, 69120 Heidelberg, Germany
e-mail: Frank_Autschbach@med.uni-heidelberg.de

Abstract

An accurate pathological reporting of rectal cancer specimens has important implications concerning patients' prognosis and further clinical management. Since locoregional recurrence and prognosis in rectal cancer is especially influenced by the extent of extramural tumor spread into the mesorectal lymphovascular fatty tissue, systematic investigation of the status of the circumferential mesorectal resection margin is a point of major importance to determine the completeness of tumor resection. Careful macroscopic assessment of the resection specimen should be performed to monitor the quality of mesorectal excision.

Introduction

Locoregional recurrence and distant metastasis are two major factors which determine a patient's prognosis following curative resection of rectal cancer. While the occurrence of distant metastasis can only indirectly be influenced by surgery and is largely determined by tumor-related factors such as tumor grade and stage, the principal aim of surgical treatment is the prevention of local recurrent disease. Recurrent tumor growth often occurs within the first two years after the operation and mostly presents as a pelvic mass within the excised tumor bed. A number of studies suggest that a major cause of such recurrences is a failure of complete local removal of the tumor. In this context, the quality of the operative procedure performed by the individual surgeon represents one of the most important prognostic factors (Hermanek et al. 1989, 1994, 1995; Hohenberger et al. 1998; Köckerling 1988). The concept of total mesorectal excision (TME), introduced by Heald et al. (Heald et al. 1982; Heald and Ryall 1986), constituted important progress in the surgical treatment of rectal cancer. TME consists of a complete removal of the rectum together with its surrounding mesorectal lymphovascular fatty tissue (mesorectum) by precise sharp dissection along the visceral pelvic fascia ("holy plane") (Heald 1988), to minimize the residual tumor load. It has been shown that careful adherence to this procedure can significantly reduce the rate of locoregional recurrences in rectal cancer.

Types of Resection Margins in Rectal Cancer Specimens

An accurate pathological reporting of rectal cancer resection specimens has important implications for the clinical management and the individual prognosis of the patient. The determination of the completeness of tumor resection is based on the assessment of resection margins by the pathologist. Principal sites which must be considered are the proximal and distal resection margins as well as the deep antiluminal (mesorectal) margin within the plane of dissection, called the lateral, radial, or circumferential resection margin (CRM).

Proximal Resection Margin

Due to the relatively wide proximal safety distance in most rectal cancer specimens (length of resected gut proximal to the tumor usually >15 cm, proximal ligation of the inferior mesenterial artery), involvement of the proximal resection margin by tumor is exceptionally rare. Therefore, this site is generally nonproblematic.

Distal Intramural Resection Margin

The distal resection margin in rectal cancer specimens is more critical, depending on the localization of the tumor (distance from the dentate line). With regard to the question of an adequate distal tumor clearance, two different aspects must be considered: intramural as well as extramural distal tumor spread, including lymphatic spread. Concerning the former type of spread, it has been shown that distal intramural extension is rather uncommon in rectal carcinoma (Shirouzu et al. 1995). In over 95% of cases it is limited to a length of about 1 to 2 cm distal to the endoluminally visible tumor. A distal mural safety margin in this range can thus be considered appropriate for most cases (Maurer et al. 1999; Pollett and Nicholls 1983; Riedl et al. 1995; Shirouzu et al. 1995; Williams et al. 1983). It should be kept in mind that formaldehyde fixation induces a significant shrinkage of the bowel (about twofold), which might result in an underestimation of the length of distal tumor clearance (Goldstein et al. 1999; Hermanek and Gall 1981; Kwok et al. 1996). It is recommended to take measurements on the freshly obtained, native specimen (if possible) and/or to pin the tissue on corkboard before fixation to minimize shrinkage. If the tumor macroscopically approaches the distal mural margin of the specimen, frozen section diagnostics might be considered for pathohistological assessment. Using such precautions, direct involvement of the distal intramural resection margin by tumor is a rare event (Birbeck et al. 2002; Ng et al. 1993). It is noteworthy that even a narrow range of distal mural clearance has no adverse influence on locoregional recurrence rates. However, if distal mural extension is prominent, it is usually associated with a locally advanced tumor stage and poor long-term prognosis, which is largely determined by the occurrence of distant metastasis rather than local recurrence (Pollett and Nicholls 1983; Philips et al. 1984; Shirouzu et al. 1995; Vernava and Moran 1992, Williams et al. 1983).

Circumferential Resection Margin

One important aspect concerning the growth pattern of rectal carcinoma is its tendency for extramural radial spread into the mesorectal lymphovascular fatty tissue. Radial tumor spread may be continuous and expansive, displaying a "pushing" type of the invasive margin (Fig. 1), but not rarely (>20%) also includes irregular, infiltrative, and discontinuous modes of spread with tumor deposits extending to the CRM and/or the serosa (Fig. 2). It has been shown that an infiltrative pattern of growth is correlated with poor prognosis in colorectal cancer (Jass et al. 1986) and constitutes an adverse prognostic factor which is independent of tumor stage (Compton et al. 2000). By histology, various often co-existing modes of extramural tumor spread occur, including continuous and discontinuous infiltrates within the perirectal fatty tissue, extramural venous invasion, lymphangiosis carcinomatosa and lymph node metastasis (Fig. 3). Although most mesorectal tumor deposits are located at the level of or proximal to the cancer, discontinuous extra-

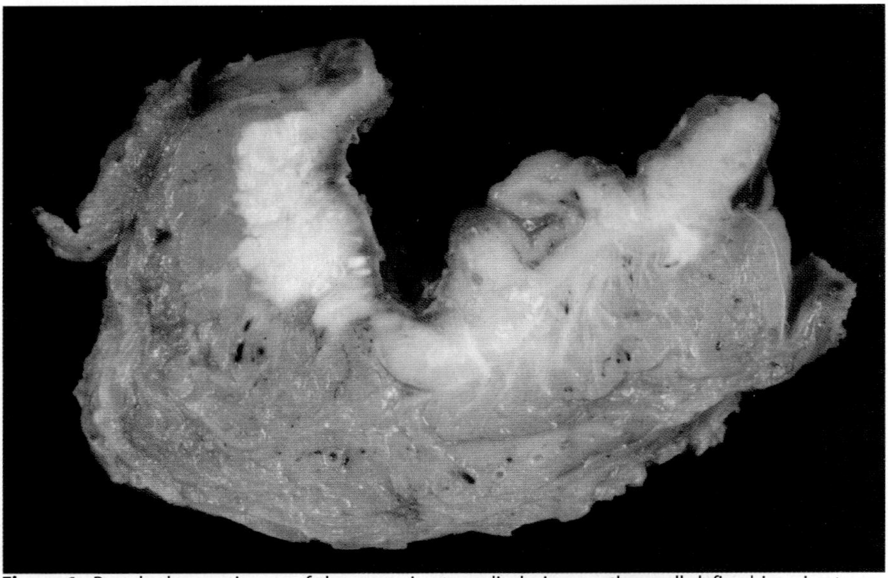

Figure 1. Rectal adenocarcinoma of the expansive type displaying a rather well defined invasive tumor margin. Tumor formations (*gray-white color*) infiltrate the mesorectal fatty tissue (pT3), but do not approach the circumferential (mesorectal) resection margin

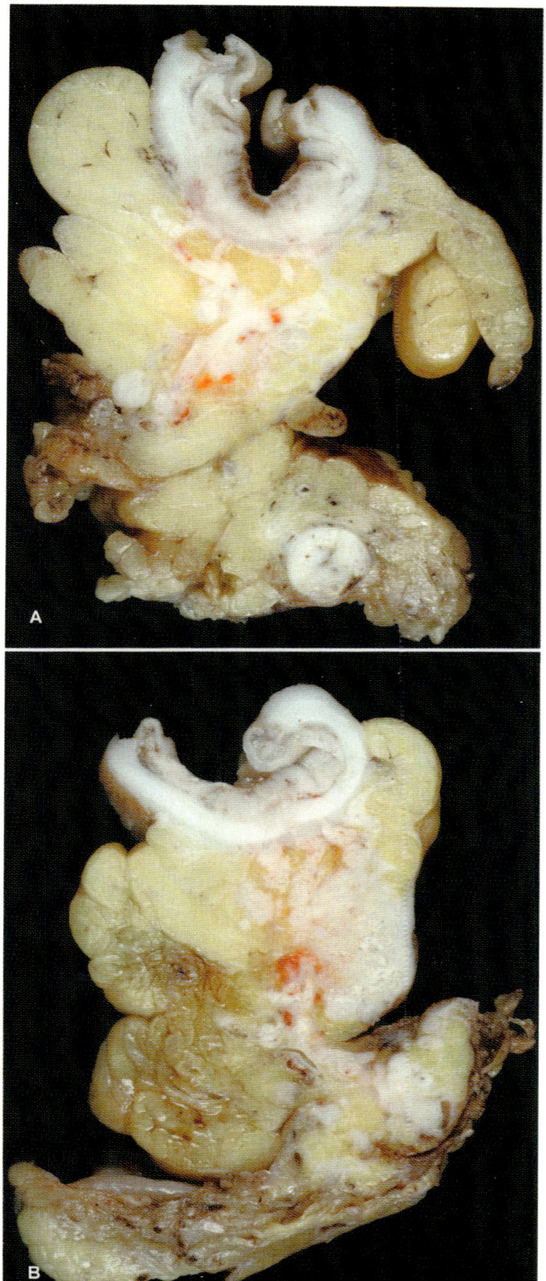

Figure 2A, B. Adenocarcinoma of the infiltrative type displaying an irregular and discontinuous mode of spread with extramural tumor deposits extending to the circumferential resection margin (*bottom*) and to the lateral serosal aspects (*left* and *right*) of this specimen (rectosigmoid)

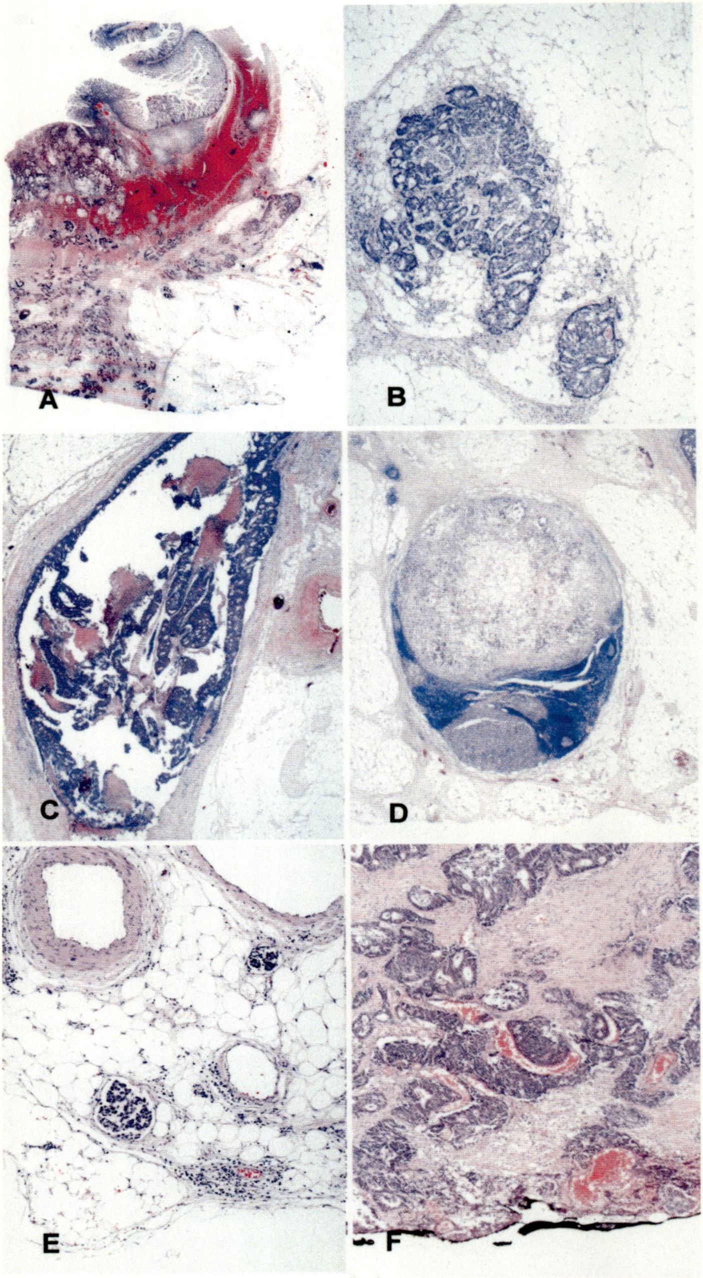

Figure 3A–F. Histopathological modes of mesorectal tumor spread in rectal adenocarcinoma. **A** Continuous spread. **B** Discontinuous mesorectal deposits. **C** Extramural venous invasion. **D** Lymph node metastasis. **E** Lymphangiosis carcinomatosa in the immediate vicinity of the circumferential resection margin (*bottom*). **F** Direct involvement of the circumferential resection margin. H&E stains

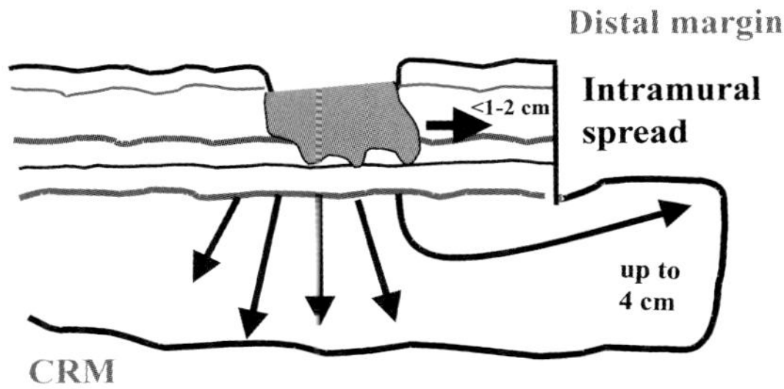

Figure 4. Intra- and extramural spread in recta cancer

mural tumor spread has been shown to involve also regions distal (up to 4 cm) to the main tumor mass (>10%) (Heald and Ryall 1986; Scott et al. 1995) (Fig. 4).

The demonstration of significantly reduced local recurrence rates and increased patient survival after total mesorectal excision for rectal cancer (Heald et al. 1982, 1998; Heald and Ryall 1986; Heald et al. 1998; Hohenberger et al. 1998; Kapiteijn et al. 2001; Köckerling et al. 1998; MacFarlane et al. 1993; Wibe et al. 2002) strongly indicate that recurrence is mainly caused by an inadequate resection of extramural tumor deposits within the mesorectal lymphovascular fatty tissue using standard surgical procedures.

One of the basic reports demonstrating the importance of lateral tumor spread and the prognostic significance of CRM involvement in rectal cancer was published in 1986 by Quirke and colleagues. They investigated a series of 52 rectal carcinomas (operated by standard procedures) where they embedded the whole tumor area after serial transverse slicing of the specimens. The extent of mesorectal spread was determined, including morphometric measurements. The outer limit of the tumor was defined as the most lateral penetration of the mesorectum, either by continuous or discontinuous tumor extension. An involvement of the CRM was considered when tumor directly infiltrated the CRM or reached this margin within a distance of less than 1 mm (Quirke et al. 1986; Quirke and Dixon 1988) . The CRM was involved in 27% of the cases investigated in that study. Most importantly, those authors found that CRM involvement was associated with a local recurrence rate of 85%, in contrast to a recurrence rate of only 3% in the group of CRM-negative cases (median follow-up: 23 months). Involvement of the CRM was associated with increasing Dukes' stage, decreasing tumor differentiation, and an infiltrative tumor margin.

In a further study on 141 cases, these results were confirmed (Adam et al. 1994). Tumor involvement of the CRM was seen in 25% of cases with potentially curative resection, and the frequency of local recurrence was again significantly higher in CRM-positive cases compared to CRM-negative cases (78% vs. 10%, respectively; median follow-up, 5 years). The authors performed a multivariate analysis of several pathological variables and demonstrated that an involvement of the CRM is one of the most important factors independently influencing both local recurrence and survival.

The important prognostic significance of the circumferential margin status in rectal cancer has been confirmed independently by other groups (Cawthorn et al. 1990; DeHaas-Kock 1996; Ng et al. 1993). In a recent follow-up study from Leeds, UK (Birbeck et al. 2002), the investigators could formally validate that a tumor distance of 1 mm or less to the CRM is associated with a significantly increased risk of local recurrence. All major modes of tumor spread contributed to this increased risk, except for a CRM involvement by tumor deposits within a lymph node, a result which has also been confirmed by others (Nagtegaal et al. 2002).

Since total mesorectal excision was not systematically performed in the series mentioned above, the relevance of CRM involvement in patient subgroups treated exclusively by TME has been debated. A recent study by the Norwegian Rectal Cancer Group addressed this point in a series of 686 patients who underwent TME (Wibe et al. 2002). Although the overall recurrence rate and the percentage of CRM involvement were comparably reduced (7% and 9.5%, respectively), this study proved that involvement of the CRM by a distance of 1 mm or less is associated with significantly higher rates of locoregional recurrence, distant metastasis, and tumor-related death, even after TME (22% recurrence in CRM-positive vs. 5% in CRM-negative cases; exponential increase with decreasing CRM). A further recent study from the Netherlands independently confirmed that CRM involvement in TME-treated patients is of prognostic significance with regard to local recurrence (especially TNM stage III patients), distant metastasis, and survival (Nagtegaal et al 2002). Those authors found that a tumor distance of less than 2 mm from the circumferential margin is already associated with a significantly increased recurrence risk and should be considered a CRM involvement.

Macroscopic Assessment of Mesorectal Excision

Since the introduction of TME surgery, it has become clear that considerable regional differences exist between surgical departments with regard to the oncological quality of resection as well as local recurrence rates. In this context, it has been proposed that a macroscopic assessment of the mesorectal excision should be included in pathology reports to monitor the surgical practice (Hermanek et al. 2003). Due to the problem of distal mesorectal spread, carcinomas of the middle and lower thirds of the rectum require a total excision of the mesorectum down to the pelvic floor. A partial TME can be considered for the treatment of carcinomas of the upper third, provided that the mesorectum is transected at least 3 cm distal to the aboral margin of the tumor (measured on the fresh non-stretched specimen, corresponding to an in situ distance of about 5 cm) and has a right-angled configuration of the transection line (avoidance of so-called "coning" of the mesorectum). Concerning the circumferential aspect, an optimal/complete mesorectal excision is characterized by a good bulk of mesorectum with a smooth, lipoma-like surface with no or only minor defects/incisions (not deeper than 5 mm). Suboptimal/nearly complete excisions have a moderate bulk of mesorectum with a slightly irregular surface, circumscript defects, and probably some minor degree of coning. Incomplete mesorectal excisions of poor quality are characterized by a little bulk of mesorectum with a highly irregular surface, larger defects (>1 cm^2), or deep incisions down onto the muscularis propria and/or prominent coning (Hermanek et al. 2003; Nagtegaal and Van Krieken 2002; Nagtegaal et al. 2002; Quirke 1998). The evaluation of surface defects is facilitated by serial transverse slicing of the tumor area (photodocumentation is recommended) and might be supplemented by recently published stain marking techniques (Sterk et al. 2000). Concerning the relevance of such type of assessment, a recent study on 180 cases by the Dutch Colorectal Cancer Group (Nagtegaal et al. 2002) could demonstrate that incomplete mesorectal excision is related to advanced T-stages and is associated with a high incidence of CRM involvement (>40%). However, even in cases without demonstrated CRM involvement, significant differences in outcome between cases with a complete/nearly complete versus incomplete mesorectum were observed. These results indicate a prognostic relevance of this macroscopic parameter, which should be investigated in more detail in future studies.

Conclusions

The pathological reporting of rectal cancer resection specimens should adhere to standardized protocols. The quality of mesorectal excision and the status of the circumferential resection margin should receive special attention (Fig. 5). Such information has important implications concerning a patient's prognosis and further clinical management.

Pathology items for the reporting of rectal carcinoma

Tumor
- **localization and size**
- **gross configuration**
- **gross invasion**
- **gross distance from resection margins**

- **histological type**
- **grade of differentiation**
- **vascular/lymphatic invasion**

- **number of examined and confirmed positive lymph nodes**

Gross assessment of the quality of the mesorectal excision	**Gross and histological assessment of invasion depth and distance to the distal and circumferential margins**
Complete, nearly complete, incomplete Partial TME: Distance between distal margin of tumor and distal transection line (>3cm) Angle of transection Coning	Serial transverse slicing of tumor area Systematic tissue sampling Morphometric measurements (distance of tumor to CRM in mm)

TNM-classification, R-classification

Figure 5. Pathological reporting of rectal carcinoma

References

Adam IJ, Mohamdee MO, Martin IG, Scott N, Finan PJ, Johnston D, Dixon MF, Quirke P (1994) Role of circumferential margin involvement in the local recurrence of rectal cancer. Lancet 344:707–711

Birbeck KF, Macklin CP, Tiffin MJ, Parsons W, Dixon MF, Finan PJ, Johnston D, Quirke P (2002) Rates of circumferential margin involvement vary between surgeons and predict outcomes in rectal cancer surgery. Ann Surg 235:449–457

Cawthorn SJ, Parums DV, Gibbs NM, A'Hern RP, Caffarey SM, Broughton CIM, Marks CG (1990) Extent of mesorectal spread and involvement of lateral resection margin as prognostic factors after surgery for rectal cancer. Lancet 335:1055–1059

Compton C, Fenoglio-Preiser CM, Pettigrew N, Fielding LP (2000) American Joint committee on cancer prognostic factors consensus conference—colorectal working group. Cancer 88:1739–1757

DeHaas-Kock DFM, Baeten CGMI, Jager JJ, Langendijk JA, Schouten LJ, Volovics A, Arends JW (1996) Prognostic significance of radial margins of clearance in rectal cancer. Br J Surg 83:781–785

Hall NR, Finan PJ, Al-Jaberi T, Tsang CS, Brown SR, Dixon MF, Quirke P (1998) Circumferential margin involvement after mesorectal excision of rectal cancer with curative intent. Predictor of survival but not local recurrence? Dis Colon Rectum 41:979–983

Goldstein N, Soman A, Sacksner J (1999) Disparate surgical margin lengths of colorectal resection specimens between in vivo and in vitro measurements. Anat Pathol 111:349–351

Heald RJ (1988) The holy plane of rectal surgery. J Royal Soc Med 81:503–508

Heald RJ, Ryall RDH (1986) Recurrence and survival after total mesorectal excision for rectal cancer. Lancet 1:1479–1482

Heald RJ, Husband EM, Ryall RDH (1982) The mesorectum in rectal cancer surgery—the clue to pelvic recurrence? Br J Surg 69:613–616

Heald RJ, Moran BJ, Ryall RDH, Sexton R, MacFarlane JK (1998) Rectal cancer. The Basingstoke experience of total mesorectal excision, 1978–1997. Arch Surg 133:894–899.

Hermanek P, Gall FP (1981) Der aborale Sicherheitsabstand bei der sphinctererhaltenden Rektumresektion. Chirurg 52:25–29

Hermanek P, Guggenmoos-Holzmann, Gall FP (1989) Prognostic factors in rectal carcinoma. A contribution to the further development of tumor classification. Dis Colon Rectum 32:593–599

Hermanek P, Wiebelt H, Riedl S, Staimmer D, Hermanek P, und die Studiengruppe Kolorektales Karzinom (SGKRK) (1994) Langzeitergebnisse der chirurgischen Therapie des Coloncarcinoms. Ergebnisse der Studiengruppe Kolorektales Karzinom (SGKRK). Chirurg 65:287–297

Hermanek P, Wiebelt H, Staimmer D, Riedl S, and the German Study Group Colo-Rectal Carcinoma (SGCRC) (1995) Prognostic factors of rectum carcinoma—experience of the German multicentre study SGCRC. Tumori 81 Supplement:60–64

Hermanek P, Hermanek P Hohenberger W, Klimpfinger M, Köckerling F, Papadopoulos T (2003) The pathological assessment of mesorectal excision: implications for further treatment and quality management. Int J Colorectal Dis 18:335–341

Hohenberger W, Schick CH, Göhl J (1998) Mesorectal lymph node dissection: is it beneficial? Langenbeck's Arch Surg 383:402–408

Jass JR, Atkin WS, Cuzick J, Bussey HJ, Morson BC, Northover JM, Todd IP (1986) The grading of rectal cancer: historical perspectives and a multivariate analysis of 447 cases. Histopathology 10:437–459

Kapiteijn E, Marijnen CAM, Nagtegaal ID, Putter H, Steup WH, Wiggers T, Rutten HJT, Pahlmann L, Glimelius B, Van Krieken HJM, Leer JWH, Van de Velde CJH, for the Dutch Colorectal Cancer Group (2001) Preoperative radiotherapy combined with total mesorectal excision for resectable rectal cancer. N Engl J Med 345:638–646

Köckerling F, Reymond MA, Alterdorf-Hofmann A, Dworak O, Hohenberger W (1988) Influence of Surgery on metachronous distant metastases and survival in rectal cancer. J Clin Oncol 16:324–329

Kwok SPY, Lau WY, Leung KL, Liew CT, Li AKC (1996) Prospective analysis of the distal margin of clearance in anterior resection for rectal carcinoma. Br J Surg 83:969–972

Maurer CA, Renzulli P, Meyer JD, Büchler MW (1999) Rektumkarzinom. Optimierung durch partielle oder totale Mesorektumentfernung. Zentralbl Chir 124:428–435

MacFarlane JK, Ryall RDH, Heals RJ (1993) Mesorectal excision for rectal cancer. Lancet 341:457–460.
Nagtegaal ID, Van Krieken JHJM (2002) The role of the pathologist in the quality control of diagnosis and treatment of rectal cancer—an overview. Eur J Cancer 38:964–972
Nagtegaal ID, Marijnen CAM, Kranenbarg EK, Van de Velde CJH, Van Krieken JHJM, for the Pathology Review Committee and the Cooperative Clinical Investigators (2002) Circumferential margin involvement is still an important predictor of local recurrence in rectal carcinoma. Not one millimeter but two millimeters is the limit. Am J Pathol 26:350–357
Nagtegaal ID, Van de Velde CJH, Van der Worp E, Kapiteijn E, Quirke P, Van Krieken JHJM, and the Pathology Review Committee for the Cooperative Clinical Investigators of the Dutch Colorectal Cancer Group (2002) Macroscopic evaluation of rectal cancer resection specimen: clinical significance of the pathologist in quality control. J Clin Oncol 20:1729–1734
Ng IOL, Luk ISC, Yuen ST, Lau PWK, Pritchett CJ, Ng M, Poon GP, Ho J (1993) Surgical lateral clearance in resected rectal carcinomas. A multivariate analysis of clinicopathologic features. Cancer 71:1972–1976
Phillips RKS, Hittinger R, Blesovsky L, Fry JS, Fielding LP (1984) Local recurrence following curative surgery for large bowel cancer: II. The rectum and rectosigmoid. Br J Surg 71:17–20
Pollett WG, Nicholls RJ (1983) The relationship between the extent of distal clearance and survival and local recurrence rates after curative anterior resection for carcinoma of the rectum. Ann Surg 198:159–163
Quirke P (1998) The pathologist, the surgeon and colorectal cancer-get it right because it matters. Progress Pathol 4:201–213
Quirke P, Dixon MF (1988) How I do it. The prediction of local recurrence in rectal adenocarcinoma by histopathological examination. Int J Colorect Dis 3:127–131
Quirke P, Durdey P, Dixon MF, Williams NS (1986) Local recurrence of rectal adenocarcinoma due to inadequate surgical resection. Histopathological study of lateral tumour spread and surgical excision. Lancet 2:996–999
Riedl S, Wiebelt H, Bergmann U, Hermanek P (1995) Postoperative Komplikationen und Letalität in der chirurgischen Therapie des Coloncarcinoms. Ergebnisse der deutschen Multizenterstudie der Studiengruppe Kolorektales Karzinom (SGKRK). Chirurg 66:597–606
Scott N, Jackson P, Al-Jaberi T, Dixon MF, Quirke P, Finan PF (1995) Total mesorectal excision and local recurrence: a study of tumour spread in the mesorectum distal to rectal cancer. Br J Surg 82:1031–1033
Shirouzu K, Isomoto H, Kakegawa T (1995) Distal spread of rectal cancer and optimal distal margin of resection for sphincter-preserving surgery. Cancer 76:388–92
Vernava AM, Moran M (1992) A prospective evaluation of distal margins in carcinoma of the rectum. Surg Gynecol Obstet 163:101–103
Wibe A, Eriksen MT, Syse A, Myrvold HE, Soreide O. on behalf of the Norwegian Rectal Cancer Group (2002) Total mesorectal excision for rectal cancer—what can be achieved by a national audit? Colorectal Disease 5:471–477
Wibe A, Rendedal PR, Svensson E, Norstein J, Eide TJ, Myrvold HE, Soreide O, on behalf of the Norwegian Rectal Cancer Group (2002) Prognostic significance of the circumferential resection margin following total mesorectal excision for rectal cancer. Br J Surg 89:327–334
Williams NS, Dixon MF, Johnston D (1983) Reappraisal of the 5 centimetre rule of distal excision for carcinoma of the rectum: a study of distal intramural spread and of patients' survival. Br J Surg 70:150–154

Is the Lateral Lymph Node Compartment Relevant?

Moritz Koch, Peter Kienle, Dalibor Antolovic, Markus W. Büchler, Jürgen Weitz

M. Koch (✉)
Department of Surgery, University of Heidelberg, 69120 Heidelberg, Germany
e-mail: moritz_koch@med.uni-heidelberg.de

Abstract

Lateral pelvic lymphadenectomy is routinely performed in advanced lower rectal cancers by Japanese surgeons, whereas in the western world it has not progressed to a frequently performed technique. Claimed benefit for this extensive surgery is an improved locoregional control; on the other hand, low positive lateral lymph node yields, questionable prognostic significance, and high morbidity (urinary and sexual dysfunction) are main reasons against this procedure. Clinical results published on lateral lymphadenectomy in the literature are conflicting. Due to major improvements in local control and survival of rectal cancer patients mainly based on preoperative radiotherapy and total mesorectal excision (TME), only a few patients may profit from lateral lymph node dissection. This article gives an overview of the current status and the clinical relevance of the lateral lymph node compartment in rectal cancer surgery.

Introduction

The clinical and prognostic significance of the lateral pelvic lymph node compartment remains a controversial issue in rectal cancer surgery. Lateral pelvic lymphadenectomy is usually performed in urologic and gynecologic operations [1, 2]. This procedure was first described in rectal cancer surgery in the early fifties, but until now it has not progressed to a frequently performed operative technique in western countries. On the other hand, lateral lymph node dissection is used as a standard procedure for lower rectal cancers in Japan.

A postulated benefit of lateral pelvic lymphadenectomy is an improved locoregional control by excision of both the mesenteric and extramesenteric lymphatic drainage, resulting in an increased overall survival of rectal cancer patients. Opponents of the method name low positive lateral lymph node yields, questionable prognostic significance, and high morbidity (urinary and sexual dysfunction) as main reasons for not performing this procedure. Clinical results published on

Recent Results in Cancer Research, Vol. 165

lateral lymphadenectomy in the literature are conflicting. Furthermore there is significant disagreement on aspects of surgical anatomy and definitions.

This article gives an overview of the current status and of the clinical relevance of the lateral lymph node compartment in rectal cancer surgery.

Anatomy and Definition of the Lateral Lymph Node Compartment

Takahashi et al. distinguish between three planes located around the rectum [3]. The inner space is surrounded by the visceral pelvic fascia on the posterior side and Denonvilliers fascia on the anterior side; the autonomic pelvic nerve plexuses are located below these fascias laterally on both sides. The intermediate space is bordered by the parietal pelvic fascia on the posterior side and the internal iliac arteries and their branches on the anterior and lateral sides. The outer space finally is located outside the internal iliac arteries and their branches. These anatomic structures act as a barrier to lymphatic drainage, whereas the lateral ligaments on both sides of the mesorectum are an exception to this rule. Although the lateral ligament is not a clear anatomic entity, it is clinically an important pathway for lymphatic and blood vessels and for parasympathetic and sympathetic nerve fibers forming visceral branches from the pelvic plexuses.

Two main pathways are important for lymphatic drainage of the middle and lower rectum: the superior lymphatic drainage along the inferior mesenteric artery and the lateral lymphatic drainage along the internal iliac artery [3–5]. Lymphatic flow from the rectum mainly goes upwards within the inner space along the inferior mesenteric artery. As total mesorectal excision usually incorporates complete removal of the inner space, all lymphatic spread of rectal cancer within this compartment is removed. Some lymphatic vessels, mostly from the lower rectum, penetrate into the intermediate and outer space via the lateral ligaments and ascend along the internal iliac arteries. This region is called the lateral lymph node compartment.

According to the Japanese Classification of Colorectal Carcinoma, Ueno et al. classified the lateral pelvic lymph node compartment into five regions: the middle rectal root region (along the middle rectal artery), the internal iliac region (along the internal iliac artery), the obturator region (along the obturator nerve and vessels), the common iliac region (along the common iliac artery), and the external iliac region (along the external iliac region) [5]. Canessa et al., on the other hand, subdivided the lateral pelvic lymph nodes into three surgical groups (presacral, obturator, and hypogastric) [6]. In that study using cadaveric dissection of the lateral pelvic lymph node compartment, they found the highest number of lymph nodes in the obturator group [6]. A major problem of the published studies is that several different classifications and definitions of the lateral pelvic lymph node compartment were used, which makes comparisons of the results difficult.

Incidence and Prognostic Significance of Lateral Lymphatic Spread in Rectal Cancer

The incidence of lateral lymph node metastasis in rectal cancer reported in the literature ranges from 4% to 30%, depending mainly on tumor height and tumor stage [3, 5, 7–12]. The highest rate of metastatic lateral lymph nodes is detected in patients with lower rectal cancer (below peritoneal reflection) and with advanced tumor stage [7, 8, 11]. Comparison and interpretation of the data of the published studies is difficult because of variation in patient selection, definitions, and statistical analysis. Lateral nodal involvement in rectal cancer is often associated with a positive lymph node status in the routinely dissected lymph nodes (e.g., perirectal lymph nodes). This makes the analysis of the prognostic significance of lateral lymphatic spread itself somewhat more difficult.

In a large retrospective series of 448 rectal cancer patients, Moriya et al. found that patients with Dukes' C tumor at or below the peritoneal reflection showed perirectal spread alone in 69% and perirectal spread plus lateral spread in 23%; lateral spread alone was found in 4% [13]. Although lateral node metastasis is considered an important prognostic factor among Japanese surgeons, there was no significant difference in disease-free survival of patients with only upward lymph node metastasis compared to those with lateral node metastasis and upward lymph node metastasis reported by Moriya et al. [13]. These observations were confirmed by Takahashi et al. who, in a retrospective series of 764 rectal cancer patients, could demonstrate that lateral lymph node metastasis alone (without perirectal or upward lymph node involvement) occurred in only 16 patients (2%). As all of those patients underwent lateral lymph node dissection, resulting in a five-year survival rate of 75%, the authors concluded that patients with lateral lymph node metastasis could be cured by this procedure.

Several retrospective clinical studies revealed a prognostic significance of lateral lymphatic spread in rectal cancer and an improved survival of rectal cancer patients after resection with extended lateral lymph node dissection compared to conventional resection without lateral lymph node dissection [5, 9, 11, 14]. In order to prevent urinary and sexual dysfunction after extended lateral lymph node dissection, Mori et al. combined autonomic nerve-preserving (ANP) resection with lateral lymph node dissection in patients with lower rectal cancer, stage UICC III [8]. They also observed a significantly improved 5-year survival rate in the ANP resection group compared to the patient group with extended lateral lymph node dissection [8].

Ueno et al. examined lateral (iliac) lymph nodes from 70 consecutive patients with low rectal cancer for occult microscopic metastasis using serial sectioning [5]. They detected occult microscopic foci in 5 patients (7%), whereas the overall incidence of lateral spread was 24% (17/70 patients), and the highest incidence of positive lymph nodes was found in the middle rectal root region along the middle rectal artery [5]. With the use of immunohistochemistry Shimoyama et al. examined lateral lymph nodes of 57 patients with low rectal cancer classified histopathologically as tumor-free, and detected lateral lymph node micrometastases in 11 (19.3%) patients [15]. These 11 patients with lateral lymph node micrometastases showed a significantly higher recurrence rate and had a worse overall survival compared to the 46 patients without lateral lymph node metastases [15].

Since there are no data from prospective randomized controlled trials available in the literature, the prognostic and clinical significance of lateral lymph node metastasis remains unclear.

Therapeutic and Clinical Consequences

The above cited studies were mainly performed by surgeons in Japan, where lateral lymph node dissection is widely used for advanced lower rectal cancer with the aim to decrease the local recurrence rate [3]. Hojo et al. compared conventional excision with extended excision (plus lateral lymph node dissection) of middle and lower rectal cancers and showed a significantly lower local recurrence rate for the lateral dissection group in Dukes' C patients (23.6% vs. 32.8%). However, a major drawback of this study is that the overall local recurrence rate was rather high compared to results of recent studies without lateral lymphadenectomy [14]. The extended resection performed in Japan resulted in a high rate of genitourinary dysfunction, as the pelvic autonomic nervous system (hypogastric nerves and pelvic plexus) was often sacrificed during lateral lymph node dissection [16]. As a consequence of this, nerve-sparing surgery with wide pelvic lymphadenectomy was introduced from 1984 onwards [7]. Several reports from Japanese surgeons have demonstrated various types of pelvic autonomic nerve preservation procedures (depending on the extent of the local tumor) which resulted in improved urinary and sexual function compared to previous results [7, 10, 16]. Uyama et al. demonstrated that lateral lymph node dissection with autonomic nerve preservation for lower rectal cancer can also be performed laparoscopically [17]. However, it is still unclear which patients benefit from extended lateral lymph node dissection and which patients do not need such extensive surgery [7]. Therefore Ueno et al. examined prognostic variables in rectal cancer patients with lateral lymph node metastasis and showed that the most important factors for poor prognosis and outcome are: distant metastases, the total number of involved lymph nodes, circumferential resection margin, and age [12]. The search for prognostic parameters defining patient subgroups who truly profit from this aggressive surgical approach remains ongoing.

In contrast, surgeons in western countries advocate total mesorectal excision (TME), proposed by Heald in 1982, as the standard surgical method to achieve good local control and to preserve autonomic nerve function in rectal cancer [18, 19]. Another argument against performing lateral lymph node dissection is that lateral lymph node metastases primarily reflect systemic spread rather than regional disease [20]. Combined treatment modalities, e.g., TME together with preoperative radiotherapy, have led to a very effective therapeutic concept in rectal cancer in recent years, resulting in a low local recurrence rate and improved survival [21, 22]. Accordingly Watanabe et al. suggested that preoperative radiotherapy may be an alternative to extended lateral lymphadenectomy [23]. In his retrospective study, 115 patients with low rectal cancer were divided into different therapy groups, and there was no difference between the group with radiotherapy (without lateral lymph node dissection) and the group with lateral lymph node dissection (without radiotherapy) in terms of overall survival, disease-free survival, and recurrence rate [23]. These results were later confirmed in a study by Koda et al. [24]. However, until now, no prospective randomized controlled trial had been conducted comparing lateral lymphadenectomy with TME and radiotherapy. One randomized controlled trial compared lateral node dissection versus nerve-preserving resection (without lateral node dissection) in patients with rectal cancer after preoperative radiotherapy [25]. In that study, no difference in survival and local recurrence rate was observed between the two treatment groups, and the authors concluded that lateral node dissection is not necessary in terms of curability for patients with advanced lower rectal cancer who undergo preoperative radiotherapy [25]. However, lateral node dissection still remains the standard treatment for advanced lower rectal cancer in Japan, as the results are similar to TME with prior radiotherapy. Havenga et al. demonstrated that standardized surgery is probably the most important prognostic factor in rectal cancer treatment [26]. They analyzed 691 patients with rectal cancer from three international centers in the United States, Europe, and Japan and could demonstrate similar survival and local recurrence rates in all three centers [26].

New intraoperative staging procedures such as sentinel lymph node mapping in rectal cancer are currently under examination in order to evaluate their prognostic and therapeutic significance [27].

In conclusion, due to major improvements in local control and survival of rectal cancer patients on the basis of preoperative radiotherapy and total mesorectal excision, only a certain subgroup of rectal cancer patients may profit from more aggressive surgical approaches such as lateral lymph node dissection. In the future, sentinel lymph node mapping may facilitate a further individualization of therapy allowing the selection of patients who would gain prognostic and therapeutic benefit from lateral lymph node dissection.

References

1. DiSaia PJ, Creasman WT (1999) Clinical gynecologic oncology. Chicago: Mosby-Year Book
2. Heidenreich A, Varga Z, von Knobloch R (2002) Extended pelvic lymphadenectomy in patients undergoing radical prostatectomy: high incidence of lymph node metastasis. J Urol 167:1681–1686
3. Takahashi T, Ueno M, Azekura K, Ohta H (2000) Lateral node dissection and total mesorectal excision for rectal cancer. Dis Colon Rectum 43(Suppl):S59–S68
4. Morikawa E, Yasutomi M, Shindou K, Matsuda T, Mori N, Hida J, et al (1994) Distribution of metastatic lymph nodes in colorectal cancer by the modified clearing method. Dis Colon Rectum 37:219–223
5. Ueno H, Yamauchi, Hase K, Ichikura T, Mochizuki H (1999) Clinicopathological study of intrapelvic cancer spread to the iliac area in lower rectal adenocarcinoma by serial sectioning. Br J Surg 86:1532–1537
6. Canessa CE, Miegge LM, Bado J, Silveri C, Labandera D (2004) Anatomic study of lateral pelvic lymph nodes: implications in the treatment of rectal cancer. Dis Colon Rectum 47:297–303

7. Morita T, Murata A, Koyama M, Totsuka E, Sasaki M (2003) Current status of autonomic nerve-preserving surgery for mid and lower rectal cancers. Dis Colon Rectum 46(Suppl):S78–S88
8. Mori T, Takahashi K, Yasuno M (1998) Radical resection with autonomic nerve presentation and lymph node dissection techniques in lower rectal cancer surgery and its results: the impact of lateral lymph node dissection. Langenbeck's Arch Surg 383:409–415
9. Dong XS, Xu HT, Yu ZW, Liu M, Cui BB, Zhao P, et al (2003) Effect of extended radical resection for rectal cancer. World J Gastroenterol 9:970–973
10. Hida J, Yasutomi M, Tokoro T, Kubo R (1999) Examination of nodal metastases by a clearing method supports pelvic plexus preservation in rectal cancer surgery. Dis Colon Rectum 42:510–514
11. Fujita S, Yamamoto S, Akasu T, Moriya Y (2003) Lateral pelvic lymph node dissection for advanced lower rectal cancer. Br J Surg 90:1580–1585
12. Ueno H, Mochizuki H, Hashiguchi Y, Hase K (2001) Prognostic determinants of patients with lateral nodal involvement by rectal cancer. Ann Surg 234:190–197
13. Moriya Y, Sugihara K, Akasu T, Fujita S (1997) Importance of extended lymphadenectomy with lateral node dissection for advanced lower rectal cancer. World J Surg 21:728–732
14. Hojo K, Sawada T, Moriya Y (1989) An analysis of survival and voiding, sexual function after wide iliopelvic lymphadenectomy in patients with carcinoma of the rectum, compared with conventional lymphadenectomy. Dis Colon Rectum 32:128–133
15. Shimoyama M, Yamazaki T, Suda T, Hatakeyama K (2003) Prognostic significance of lateral lymph node micrometastases in lower rectal cancer. Dis Colon Rectum 46:333–339
16. Saito N, Koda K, Takiguchi N, Oda K, Soda H, Nunomura M et al (1999) Nerve-sparing surgery for advanced rectal cancer patients: special reference to Dukes C patients. World J Surg 23:1062–1068.
17. Uyama I, Sugioka A, Matsui H, Fujita J, Komori Y, Hanai T et al (2001) Laparoscopic lateral node dissection with autonomic nerve preservation for advanced lower rectal cancer. J Am Coll Surg 193:579–584
18. Heald RJ, Husband EM, Ryall RD (1982) The mesorectum in rectal cancer surgery: the clue to pelvic recurrence? Br J Surg 69:613–616
19. Heald RJ, Ryall RD (1986) Recurrence and survival after total mesorectal excision for rectal cancer. Lancet 28:1479–1482
20. Enker WE, Thaler HT, Cranor ML, Polyak T (1995) Total mesorectal excision in the operative treatment of carcinoma of the rectum. J Am Coll Surg 181:335–346
21. Swedish Rectal Cancer Trial (1997) Improved survival with preoperative radiotherapy in resectable rectal cancer. . N Engl J Med 336:980–987
22. Kapiteijn E, Marijnen CA, Nagtegaal ID, Putter H, Steup WH, Wiggers T, et al (2001) Preoperative radiotherapy combined with total mesorectal excision for resectable rectal cancer. N Engl J Med 345:638–646
23. Watanabe T, Tsurita G, Muto T, Sawada T, Sunouchi K, Higuchi Y, et al (2002) Extended lymphadenectomy and preoperative radiotherapy for lower rectal cancers. Surgery 132:27–33
24. Koda K, Saito N, Oda K, Takiguchi N, Sarashina H, Miyazaki M (2004) Evaluation of lateral lymph node dissection with preoperative chemo-radiotherapy for the treatment of advanced middle to lower rectal cancers. Int J Colorectal Dis 19:188–94
25. Nagawa H, Muto T, Sunouchi K, Higuchi Y, Tsurita G, Watanabe T, et al (2001) Randomized, controlled trial of lateral node dissection vs. nerve-preserving resection in patients with rectal cancer after preoperative radiotherapy. Dis Colon Rectum 44:1274–1280
26. Havenga K, Enker WE, Norstein J, Moriya Y, Heald RJ, van Houwelingen HC, et al (1999) Improved survival and local control after total mesorectal excision or D3 lymphadenectomy in the treatment of primary rectal cancer: an international analysis of 1411 patients. Eur J Surg Oncol 25:368–374
27. Mulsow J, Winter DC, O'Keane JC, O'Connell PR (2003) Sentinel lymph node mapping in colorectal cancer. Br J Surg 2003; 90:659–667

Diagnostics of Rectal Cancer: Endorectal Ultrasound

Hanns-Peter Knaebel, Moritz Koch, Tobias Feise, Axel Benner, Peter Kienle

P. Kienle (✉)
Department of Surgery, University of Heidelberg, INF 110, 69120 Heidelberg, Germany
e-mail: Peter_Kienle@med.uni-heidelberg.de

Abstract

In rectal cancer, accurate preoperative staging is essential to adequately select patients for different therapeutic regimes. Endosonography has been proven to be an accurate staging modality in multiple prospective studies. A recent large retrospective study, however, has cast doubt on the actual accuracy of endorectal ultrasound for staging rectal cancer in everyday clinical routines. The results of endosonographic staging of rectal tumours over a period of 10 years at the Department of Surgery of the University of Heidelberg are presented. In a first time period, 424 patients with rectal cancer were staged by endosonography and the data recorded prospectively. The examinations were exclusively done by four surgeons with high experience and scientific interest in endosonography. The second time period comprises 332 patients with rectal tumours (including adenomas) having undergone endosonography by six different examiners after introduction of this staging method into the clinical routine. The data here were analysed retrospectively. Accuracy, sensitivity, specificity, and positive and negative predictive values were calculated for the T and N classifications for both series. In the second series, eight factors which have been postulated to influence staging accuracy in the literature were included in a regression analysis in order to identify relevant factors for staging inaccuracies. Accuracy for staging of the T classification was 81% in the first series versus 71.7% in the second series. In the regression analysis of the second series, status post-chemoradiation proved to be the most significant factor for staging inaccuracy ($p<0.0002$). When excluding all patients having undergone chemoradiation, the accuracy for staging of the T classification rose to 76%. A major problem of endosonography in this second series was overstaging; the T category was overestimated in 76 cases (22.9% of patients). The main error here was overstaging of adenomas as cancerous lesions (45.5% of all adenomas) and T2-cancers as more advanced cancers (42.2% of all T2-cancers). When excluding the adenomas from this analysis, the accuracy increased to 73.5%. Accuracy for staging of the N classification was 76% in the first series versus 71% in the second series. Status post-chemoradiation again was a relevant factor ($p<0.0003$);

Recent Results in Cancer Research, Vol. 165

when excluding these patients the accuracy increased to 73%. The accuracy of endosonography for rectal tumours decreases after introduction of the method into the everyday clinical routine. Nonetheless, apart from magnetic resonance imaging with an endorectal coil, rectal endosonography is still the most accurate staging modality for rectal tumours and allows adequate selection of patients for different therapeutic regimes. As the major problem of rectal endosonography is overstaging, more patients are likely to undergo overtreatment rather than undertreatment. Endosonography is inaccurate in staging patients having undergone chemoradiation.

Introduction

Accurate preoperative staging is essential for planning adequate oncologic treatment in patients with rectal cancer, as different stages of the disease require different therapeutic strategies [1–4]. Early cancer stages in selected patients may be treated solely by local excision without lymphadenectomy [5–8]. Patients with advanced rectal cancer (T3 or T4 and all lymph node-positive cases), on the other hand, are now recommended to undergo neoadjuvant treatment followed by rectal resection with total mesorectal excision. The Swedish and the Dutch Rectal Cancer Trials have both shown that neoadjuvant chemoradiation improves local tumour control in patients with rectal cancer [9, 10].

Endorectal ultrasound has established itself as a reliable staging modality for rectal cancer in the last ten years [1, 2, 11]. However, there is now debate on the actual accuracy of this method in daily practice. Most of the earlier, smaller prospective studies demonstrated impressive results for endosonographic staging in rectal cancer [12–15], but a recent large analysis of 545 patients revealed an accuracy of only 69% for assessing the level of wall infiltration (T classification) in the routine setting [16].

In this chapter we present our own results of endosonographic staging in rectal cancer over a period of over 10 years, focussing on pitfalls of the method. Moreover, we review the literature in order to put this staging modality in perspective to other standard staging modalities.

Patients and Methods

From January 1988 until June 1996, 424 patients undergoing endosonography for rectal cancer at the Surgical Department of the University of Heidelberg were examined in a prospective study and documented accordingly. Only patients undergoing surgery with subsequent pathohistological work-up were included, as pathohistological staging served as the gold standard to evaluate endosonographic staging accuracy. Only four surgeons with high experience and scientific interest in endosonography performed the examinations. The results of this study have in part been published [17] and will therefore only be referred to briefly in this chapter.

After the introduction of rectal endosonographic staging into our daily routine, the overall accuracy of endosonographic staging seemed to decrease. A retrospective analysis was therefore initiated to evaluate the results and to identify possible risk factors for poorer staging results of rectal tumours. Again only patients undergoing surgery with subsequent pathohistological work-up were included, as pathohistological staging served as the gold standard. From August 1996 to December 2001, 332 patients fulfilled the inclusion criteria [109 (32.8%) female and 223 (67.2%) male patients]. The average age of these patients was 61 years.

Endosonography was done with a rigid endosonographic probe with a rotating 7 MHz or 10 MHz scanner (Bruel und Kjaer, Type 1846, Bruel u. Kjaer Instruments Inc. Marlborough, MA) which generates a 360° image of the rectal wall. The examination was performed in the lithotomy position after cleansing the rectum with an enema. The endosonography device was generally blindly advanced beyond the tumour and then slowly withdrawn while scanning. In cases of higher-grade stenosis, a rigid rectoscope was inserted and used to visualise the lumen, thus facilitating the advancement of the endosonography device through the rectoscope. Acoustic coupling was achieved with the help of a water-filled balloon placed over the transducer.

Endosonographic T-staging was done according to the criteria of Hildebrandt and Feifel [14] (Table 1). In contrast to that classification, differentiation of T1-cancers from adenomas was done on the basis of their echogenicity: hyperechoic, homogenous lesions were considered benign, whereas hypoechoic, inhomogeneous lesions were classified malignant [18] (Fig. 1). Staging accuracy was deter-

Table 1. Corresponding histopathologic and endosonographic T category according to Hildebrandt and Feifel

pT category (TNM classification)	uT category
pT0 No evidence for malignant lesion	uT0 Normal 5-layer structure of rectal wall
pT1 Tumour infiltrates mucosa or submucosa	uT1 Inner hypoechoic layer protrudes or is interrupted (mucosa), middle hyperechoic layer is intact
pT2 Tumour infiltrates muscularis propria	uT2 Middle hyperechoic layer is perforated (border mucosa/ submucosa), the outer hypoechoic layer (muscularis propria) is infiltrated but not perforated
pT3 Tumour perforates muscularis propria and infiltrates perirectal fatty tissue	uT3 Infiltration of outer hyperechoic layer (borders perirectal fatty tissue)
pT4 Tumour perforates visceral peritoneum or infiltrates other organs	uT4 Tumour infiltrates other organs

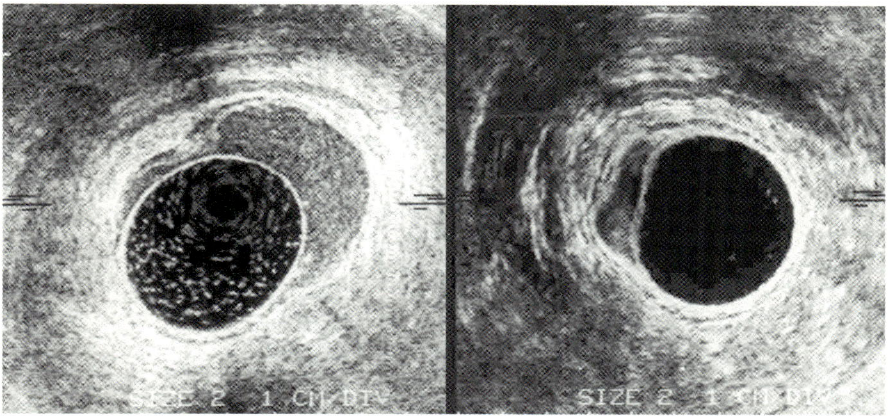

Figure 1. Endosonographic differentiation of an adenoma (*left*), which is homogenous and hyperechoic from a T1 cancer (*right*), which is inhomogeneous and hypoechoic

mined for the T and N category. Sensitivity, specificity, and positive and negative predictive values were calculated for nodal involvement and for different stages of the T classification. Tumours infiltrating other organs were analysed in relation to all earlier tumour stages, as patients with such advanced tumours generally undergo neoadjuvant chemoradiation (uT4 vs. uT1–3). Tumours confined to the rectal wall were compared to tumours having infiltrated beyond the bowel wall because this is relevant for indicating neoadjuvant radiotherapy (short protocol 5×5 Gray, uT1,2 vs. uT3,4). Furthermore the ability to differentiate tumours confined to the mucosa from further progressed tumours (uT1 vs. uT2–4) and the differ-

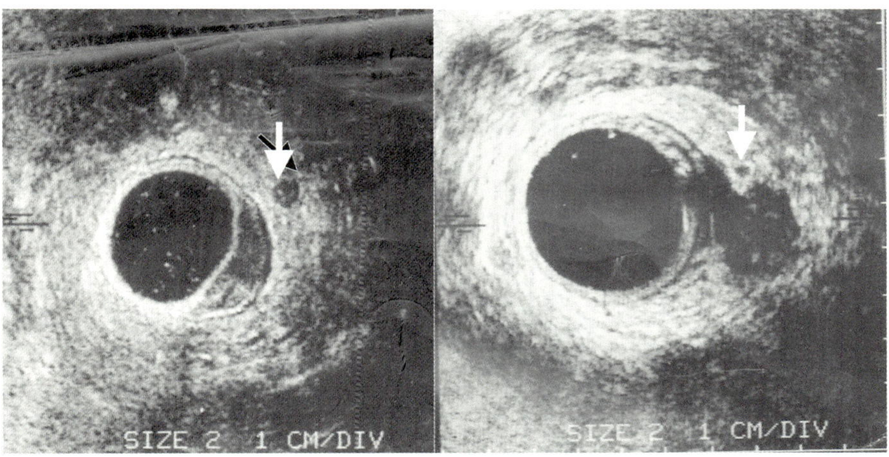

Figure 2. Endosonographic image of infiltrated lymph node (*left image arrow*) and possible staging errors (*right image arrow* indicating vessels and artefacts) in patients with rectal cancer

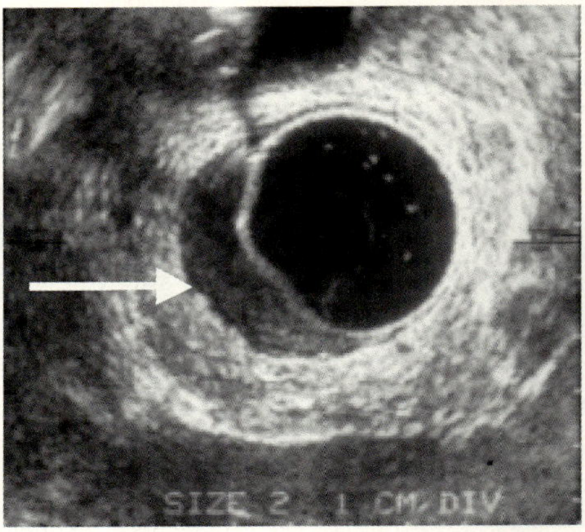

Figure 3. Endosonographic image of a beginning uT3 rectal cancer (*arrow* depicts the beginning infiltration of the outer hyperechoic layer which corresponds to the perirectal fatty tissue)

entiation of adenomas from cancerous lesions (uT0 vs. uT1–4) were analysed, as these may be relevant for indicating local excision versus oncological resection.

Lymph nodes were classified as malignant if they were hypoechoic or had the same echogenicity as the tumour and if they had round or oval borders; size was not used as a criterion for infiltrated lymph nodes [19] (Figs. 2, 3).

To identify possible risk factors for poor staging, all factors complicating or impairing the examination were evaluated [20]. The more common factors were then further analysed in a regression analysis to see whether these had statistical influence on the staging results [21]. The parameters tested in the logistic regression analysis are given in Table 2. As status post-chemoradiation is known to significantly influence all staging modalities [22], an additional stratified analysis was done including only patients without pre-staging chemoradiation.

Table 2. Parameters tested for influence on staging accuracy of endosonography in rectal cancer

Parameter I	*Beginning* uT3-stage[a] (Fig. 3)
Parameter II	Cancer arising within an adenoma
Parameter III	Tumour not completely traversable, only limited assessment possible
Parameter IV	Inflammation/desmoplastic reaction
Parameter V	Ulceration
Parameter VI	Mucinous differentiation
Parameter VII	Status post-probe excision within last 2 weeks
Parameter VIII	Status post-chemoradiation

[a] In this case the examiner could not specifically decide whether this was still a uT2 or indeed already a uT3 cancer. In order to exclude understaging which may result in patients not undergoing neoadjuvant therapy, these cases are generally classified as uT3 in our department.
In order to document the difficulty in distinguishing these cases from simple uT2 cancers, the term "beginning" is always added.

Results

First Series [17]

Overall accuracy for staging of the T category in these 424 patients was 81% (Table 3); for staging of the N category it was 76% (Table 4). In this series only histologically confirmed rectal cancers but no adenomas were included

Second Series

Overall accuracy in this series including rectal adenomas was 71.7% (Table 5). In 18 patients endosonography underestimated the T category, resulting in an understaging in 5.4% of cases. The most relevant error here was understaging of T4 cancers, which occurred in 20%. The major problem of endosonography, however, was overstaging; the T category was overestimated in 76 cases (22.9% of

Table 3. Comparison of preoperative endosonographic (u) versus postoperative histological (p) staging of the T classification in patients with rectal cancer (first series). Sensitivity, specificity, positive predictive value (PPV), and negative predictive value (NPV) are given for assessment of bowel wall penetration

	n	pT1	pT2	pT3	pT4
uT1	51	**44**	6	1	0
uT2	114	14	**83**	17	0
uT3	222	2	33	**182**	5
uT4	37	0	0	3	**34**
•	424	60	122	203	39
Sensitivity	92.5%				
Specificity	80.7%				
PPV	86.4%				
NPV	89.1%				

Table 4. Comparison of preoperative endosonographic (u) versus postoperative histological (p) staging of the N classification in patients with rectal cancer (first series). Sensitivity, specificity, positive predictive value (PPV), and negative predictive value (NPV) are given for assessment of nodal involvement

	n	pN-	pN+
uN-	238	**186**	52
uN+	171	46	**125**
•	409	232	177
Sensitivity	70.6%		
Specificity	80.1%		
PPV	73.1%		
NPV	78.1%		

Table 5. Comparison of preoperative endosonographic (u) versus postoperative histological (p) staging of the T classification in patients with rectal tumours (second series). Sensitivity, specificity, positive predictive value (PPV), and negative predictive value (NPV) are given for assessment of bowel wall penetration (excluding adenoma cases)

	n	pT0	pT1	pT2	pT3	pT4
uT0	20	**18**	1	0	1	0
uT1	31	6	**22**	1	0	2
uT2	65	3	4	**47**	11	0
uT3	176	5	1	33	**135**	2
uT4	40	1	3	2	18	**16**
•	332	33	31	83	165	20
Sensitivity	92.9%					
Specificity	65.4%					
PPV	81.4%					
NPV	85%					

Table 6. Comparison of preoperative endosonographic (u) versus postoperative histological (p) staging of the T classification in patients with rectal tumours excluding patients having undergone chemoradiation. Sensitivity, specificity, positive predictive value (PPV), and negative predictive value (NPV) are given for assessment of bowel wall penetration (excluding adenoma cases)

	n	pT0	pT1	pT2	pT3	pT4
uT0	19	**17**	1	0	1	0
uT1	31	6	**22**	1	0	2
uT2	61	0	4	**46**	11	0
uT3	132	2	1	21	**106**	2
uT4	19	0	0	0	11	**8**
•	262	25	28	68	129	12
Sensitivity	90.7%					
Specificity	76.8%					
PPV	85.2%					
NPV	84.8%					

patients). The main error here was overstaging of adenomas as cancerous lesions (45.5% of all adenomas) and T2 cancers as more advanced cancers (42.2% of all T2 cancers). When excluding the adenomas from this analysis, the accuracy increased to 73.5%.

When excluding the patients having undergone chemoradiation, the results improved significantly. The accuracy for staging the T classification increased to 76%, and the rate of overstaging decreased considerably (Table 6). On the other hand, when looking at the group of 70 patients who had undergone neoadjuvant chemoradiation, this accuracy was merely 55.7%. Of 21 cases endosonographically staged as uT4, only eight were later confirmed pathohistologically (38.1%).

Table 7. Comparison of preoperative endosonographic (u) versus postoperative histological (p) staging of the N classification in patients with rectal tumours (second series). Sensitivity, specificity, positive predictive value (PPV), and negative predictive value (NPV) are given for assessment of nodal involvement

	n	pN-	pN+	pNx
uN-	201	**150**	43	8
uN+	120	47	**70**	3
uNx	11	7	4	0
•	332	204	117	11
Sensitivity			62.0%	
Specificity			76.0%	
PPV			59.8%	
NPV			77.7%	

When looking at the capability of distinguishing adenomas and T1 cancers from further advanced tumours, none of the tested parameters including status post-chemoradiation revealed any significant influence on endosonographic staging accuracy. However, when analysing the ability to assess wall penetration (T1,2 cancers combined v T3,4 cancers combined), the following parameters had a significant influence on staging accuracy: parameter II (cancer arising within an adenoma, p=0.03), parameter VII (status post-probe excision within last 2 weeks, p=0.01), and parameter VIII (status post-chemoradiation, p<0.0001). When looking at the capability of distinguishing between T4 cancers from all less-progressed stages, only parameter VIII again showed a highly significant influence on staging accuracy (p<0.0002).

Lymph node staging was correct in 71% of cases (Table 7). Understaging was more common than overstaging (38% vs. 23.8%). Only pre-staging chemoradiation was significantly associated with poorer lymph node staging (p=0.0003). When excluding the patient group having undergone pre-staging chemoradiation, lymph node staging accuracy increased to 73%.

Discussion

The two presented series suggest that endosonographic staging may not be as accurate in clinical routine as previously thought. The accuracy for assessing the T classification in our first prospectively followed series exceeded the accuracy in the second retrospectively analysed series by nearly 10%. This can only partially be explained by taking into account that there were considerably more patients having undergone chemoradiation in this second series following the more widespread introduction of neoadjuvant therapy in advanced tumour stages in recent years. Even when excluding all patients having undergone pre-staging chemoradiation in the second series, the accuracy for assessing the T classification is still 5% less than in the first series.

A further explanation for the discrepant findings in our two series is the different clinical settings in which these results were generated. The first series was accumulated in a prospective study, and the examinations were exclusively done by four surgeons with high experience and scientific interest in rectal endosonography [17]. The second series is the retrospective analysis of the results after having introduced this method into clinical routine. Six different surgeons performed the examinations over this period of time, but there were no further scientific goals associated with it. The data were not prospectively followed, resulting in a lack of feedback on the accuracy of the method. There are numerous other examples in the literature demonstrating that impressive results of a diagnostic modality in previous prospective studies cannot be always reproduced in everyday clinical routines [23, 24].

Our findings are in part supported by the largest study on endosonography published to date. In this recent retrospective analysis, Garcia-Aguilar et al. found an accuracy of only 69% for staging of the T category, and concluded that endosonographic staging is probably not as accurate in staging of rectal cancer as previously thought [16]. However, in that study all patients having undergone pre-staging radiotherapy were excluded, which should have actually improved the results in comparison to other studies. When excluding those cases in our analysis, the accuracy for staging of the T category increased to 76%, which is considerably better than in the above-mentioned study but still considerably worse than in most other previously published prospective studies, including our own. In conclusion, the accuracy for endosonography in everyday clinical practice is obviously not as good as previously suggested in smaller prospective studies.

However, when looking at alternative diagnostic procedures, rectal endosonography is still the most accurate staging modality for rectal cancer apart from magnetic resonance imaging (MRI) with an endorectal coil [25–28]. The systematic review by Kwok et al. including 4,897 patients clearly demonstrates that endosonography is superior in staging the T classification in comparison to computed tomography (CT) and standard MRI [29]. In regard to the assessment of the N classification, MRI is comparable to endosonography but CT again is less accurate. Most of the analysed studies actually included less than 100 patients, and most of these were prospectively conducted. This may explain why the results in most of these studies for all staging modalities were better than in the two largest series in the literature, those by Garcia-Aguilar and us, but the reasons for this have already been discussed.

Endosonography is obviously not capable of adequately assessing patients who have undergone neoadjuvant therapy [22, 30, 31]. This is of minor importance, as the decision for indicating neoadjuvant therapy is made beforehand, and staging afterwards has only very limited if any consequences. Endosonography is accurate enough to select patients for different therapeutic strategies even in everyday practice. Less than 5% of patients with T2 cancers and less than 10% of patients with T3 cancers were understaged in our series, meaning that only a minority of patients could have potentially had too little treatment (only local excision or lack of neoadjuvant treatment). On the other hand, the considerable amount of overstaging results in a relevant number of patients receiving more treatment than they actually require. This was especially relevant in adenomas and T2 cancers, where over 40% were overstaged, meaning that a considerable number of patients had an oncologic resection instead of limited resection (in case of an adenoma) or superfluous chemoradiation (in case of a T2 cancer) . However, over one-third of the patients with overstaged T2 cancers showed lymph node infiltration on postoperative histology, which on its own is an indication for oncologic surgical resection and adjuvant therapy, thereby reducing the number of patients being subjected to overtreatment in this group.

Lymph node staging remains a problem, as there are still no stringent criteria to identify malignant infiltration. The size criterion has been proven inaccurate, as enlarged lymph nodes are often only inflammatory, and vice versa, small lymph nodes can still harbour metastases [32, 33]. This problem applies to all staging modalities, and there is no real solution in sight. The only definite solution here would be guided fine-needle biopsy of all identified nodes, but this is hardly practicable [34]. Endosonography has one specific problem in regard to lymph node staging; scanning depth is limited and therefore more distant lymph nodes may be overlooked. Nonetheless, this is obviously not clinically relevant, as lymph node staging accuracy is still as good with endosonography as with all other staging modalities apart from endo-MRI.

In times of increased rationing of health care services, endosonography has one major advantage over all other staging modalities—it is by far the cheapest method to stage rectal cancer [35, 36]. However, about 10% of rectal cancers cannot be adequately assessed by endosonography due to higher-grade stenosis. 3D-endosonography may prove valuable in this setting, as it allows staging of nontraversable tumours [37–39]. Moreover, preliminary studies have shown an increased accuracy for this method compared to standard endosonography. Nonetheless, MRI and CT still have their place in the staging of rectal cancer, especially for detection of distant metastases and for local staging of advanced tumour stages. Furthermore there is now new data suggesting that high-resolution MRI may be advantageous in identifying a subgroup of patients within the T3 classification with a higher risk of recurrence, by defining lateral spread [40].

References

1. Chawla AK, Kachnic LA, Clark JW, Willett CG (2003) Combined modality therapy for rectal and colon cancer. Semin Oncol 30 Suppl 9:101–112
2. Gibbs P, Chao MW, Tjandra JJ (2003) Optimizing the outcome for patients with rectal cancer. Dis Colon Rectum 46:389–402
3. Påhlman L (2000) Neoadjuvant and adjuvant radio- and radio-chemotherapy of rectal carcinomas Int J Colorectal Dis 15:1–8
4. Midgley R, Kerr D (1999) Colorectal cancer Lancet 353:391–399
5. Biggers OR, Beart RW Jr, Ilsrup DM (1986) Local excision of rectal cancer. Dis Colon Rectum 29:374–377
6. Buess G, Kipfmuller K, Naruhn M, Braunstein S, Junginger T (1987) Endoscopic microsurgery of rectal tumors. Endoscopy 19 Suppl 1:38–42
7. Mentges B, Buess G, Effinger G, Manncke K, Becker HD (1997) Indications and results of local treatment of rectal cancer. Br J Surg 84:348–351

8. Cohen AM (1994) Transrectal ultrasonography and operative selection for early carcinoma of the rectum. J Am Coll Surg 179:513–517
9. Swedish Rectal Cancer Trial (1997) Improved survival with preoperative radiotherapy in resectable rectal cancer. N Engl J Med 336:980–987
10. Kapiteijn E, Marijnen CA, Nagtegaal ID, Putter H, Steup WH, Wiggers T, Rutten HJ, Pahlman L, Glimelius B, van Krieken JH, Leer JW, van de Velde CJ; Dutch Colorectal Cancer Group (2001) Preoperative radiotherapy combined with total mesorectal excision for resectable rectal cancer. N Engl J Med 345:638–646
11. Adams DR, Blatchford GJ, Lin KM, Ternent CA, Thorson AG, Schristensen MA (1999) Use of preoperative ultrasound staging for treatment of rectal cancer. Dis Colon Rectum 42:159–166
12. Glaser F, Schlag P, Herfarth C (1990) Endorectal ultrasonography for the assessment of invasion of rectal tumours and lymph node involvement. Br J Surg 77:883–887
13. Herzog U, von Flue M, Tondelli P, Schuppisser JP (1993) How accurate is endorectal ulrasound in preoperative staging of rectal cancer? Dis Colon Rectum 36:127–134
14. Hildebrandt U, Feifel G (1985) Preoperative staging of rectal cancer by intrarectal ultrasound. Dis Colon Rectum 28:42–46
15. Beynon J, Mortensen NJ, Rigby HS (1988) Rectal endosonography, a new technique for the preoperative staging of rectal carcinoma. Eur J Surg Oncol 14:297–309
16. Garcia-Aguilar J, Pollack J, Lee SH, Hernandez de Anda E, Mellgren A, Wong WD, Finne CO, Rothenberger DA, Madoff RD (2002) Accuracy of endorectal ultrasonography in preoperative staging of rectal tumors. Dis Colon Rectum 45:10–15
17. Kienle P, Glaser F, Kuntz C, Düx M, Herfarth C (1997) Endosonography, CT and MRI in the diagnostic concept of rectal carcinoma. Langenbecks Arch Chir Suppl. 114:477–479
18. Kuntz Ch, Glaser F, Buhr HJ, Herfarth C (1993) Endorectal ultrasound in diagnosis and therapy planning of broad-base rectal adenomas Chirurg 64:290–294
19. Glaser F, Layer G, Zuna I, von Gaik G, Schlag P, Herfarth C (1990) Preoperative assessment of perirectal lymph nodes by ultrasound. Chirurg 61:587–591
20. Akasu T, Sugihara K, Moriya Y, Fujita S (1997) Limitations and pitfalls of transrectal ultrasonography for staging of rectal cancer. Dis Colon Rectum 40 (suppl): S10–S15
21. Coughlin SS, Trock BJ, Criqui MH (1992) The logistic modeling of sensitivity, specificity, and predictive value of a diagnostic test. J Clin Epidemiol 45:1–7
22. Vanagunas A, Lin DE, Stryker SJ (2004) Accuracy of endoscopic ultrasound for restaging rectal cancer following neoadjuvant chemoradiation therapy. Am J Gastroenterol. 99:109–112
23. Bosing N, Schumacher B, Frieling T, Ohmann C, Jungblut R, Lubke H, Bohner H, Verreet P, Roher HD (2003) Endoscopic ultrasound in routine clinical practice for staging adenocarcinomas of the stomach and distal esophagus. Chirurg 74:214–221
24. Butch RJ, Stark DD, Wittenberg J, Trepper JE, Saini S, Simeone JF, Mueller PR, Ferrucci JT Jr. (1986) Staging rectal cancer by MR and CT. Am J Radiol 146:1155–1160
25. Gualdi GF, Casciani E, Guadalaxara A, d'Orta C, Polettini E, Pappalardo G (2000) Local staging of rectal cancer with transrectal ultrasound and endorectal magnetic resonance imaging. Comparison with histologic findings. Dis Colon Rectum 43:338–345
26. Kim NK, Kim MJ, Yun SH, Min SJ (1999) Comparative study of transrectal ultrasonography, pelvic computerized tomography and magnetic resonance in preoperative staging of rectal cancer. Dis Colon Rectum 42:750–775
27. Kramann B, Hildebrandt U (1986) Computed tomography versus endosonography in the staging of rectal carcinoma: a comparative study. Int J Colorect Dis 1:216–218
28. Romano G (1985) Intrarectal ultrasound and computed tomography in the pre-and postoperative assessment of patients with rectal cancer. Br J Surg 72 Suppl: S117–S119
29. Kwok H, Bissett IP, Hill GL (2000) Preoperative staging of rectal cancer. Int J Colorectal Dis 15:9–20
30. Rau B, Hünerbein M, Barth C, Wust P, Haensch W, Riess H, Felix R, Schlag PM (1999) Accuracy of endorectal ultrasound after preoperative radiochemotherapy in locally advanced rectal cancer. Surg Endosc 13:980–984
31. Williamson PR, Hellinger MD, Larach SW, Ferrara A (1996) Endorectal ultrasound of T3 and T4 rectal cancers after preoperative chemoradiation. Dis Colon Rectum 39:45–49
32. Hermanek P, Marzoli GP (1994) Local therapy of rectal carcinoma. eds: Hermanek P, Marzoli GP, Springer Verlag Berlin
33. Boscaini M, Masoni L, Montori A (1986) Transrectal ultrasonography: three years' experience. Int J Colorectal Dis 1:131–139

34. Milsom JW, Czyrko C, Hull TL, Strong SA, Fazio VW (1994) Preoperative biopsy of pararectal lymph nodes in rectal cancer using endoluminal ultrasonography. Dis Colon Rectum 37:364–368
35. Harewood GC, Wiersema MJ (2002) Cost-effectiveness of endoscopic ultrasonography in the evaluation of proximal rectal cancer. Am J Gastroenterol 97:874–882
36. Vining DJ (1998) Rectal imaging and cancer. Semin Surg Oncol. 15:72–77
37. Ivanow KD, Diacov CD (1997) Three dimensional endoluminal ultrasound: new staging technique in patients with rectal cancer. Dis Colon Rectum 40:47–50
38. Hunerbein M, Pegios W, Rau B, Vogl TJ, Felix R, Schlag PM (2000) Prospective comparison of endorectal ultrasound, three-dimensional endorectal ultrasound, and endorectal MRI in the preoperative evaluation of rectal tumors. Preliminary results. Surg Endosc 14:1005–1009
39. Kim JC, Cho YK, Kim SY, Park SK, Lee MG (2002) Comparative study of three-dimensional and conventional endorectal ultrasonography used in rectal cancer staging. Surg Endosc 16:1280–1285
40. Brown G, Kirkham A, Williams GT, Bourne M, Radcliffe AG, Sayman J, Newell R, Sinnatamby C, Heald RJ (2004) High-resolution MRI of the anatomy important in total mesorectal excision of the rectum AJR Am J Roentgenol 182:431–439

Preoperative Staging of Rectal Cancer: The MERCURY Research Project

G. Brown, I. R. Daniels

G. Brown (✉)
Department of Radiology, The Royal Marsden Hospital, Downs Road,
Sutton SM2 5PT, UK
e-mail: gina.brown@rmh.nthames.nhs.uk

Abstract

The development of a surgical technique that removes the tumour and all local draining nodes in an intact package, namely total mesorectal excision (TME) surgery, has provided the impetus for a more selective approach to the administration of preoperative therapy. One of the most important factors that governs the success of TME surgery is the relationship of tumour to the circumferential resection margin (CRM). Tumour involves the CRM in up to 20% of patients undergoing TME surgery, and results in both poor survival and local recurrence. It is therefore clear that the importance of the decision regarding the use of pre-operative therapy lies with the relationship of the tumour to the mesorectal fascia. In addition, a high-spatial-resolution MRI technique will identify tumours exhibiting other poor prognostic features, namely, extramural spread >5 mm, extramural venous invasion by tumour, nodal involvement, and peritoneal infiltration. The potential benefits of a selective approach using MRI-based selection criteria are evident. That is, over 50% of patients can be treated successfully with primary surgery alone without significant risk of local recurrence or systemic failure. Of the remainder, potentially dramatic improvements may be achieved through the use of intensive and targeted preoperative therapy aimed not only at reducing the size of the primary tumour and rendering potentially irresectable tumour resectable with tumour-free circumferential margins, but also at enabling patients at high risk of systemic failure to benefit from intensive combined modality therapy aimed at eliminating micrometastatic disease.

Introduction

The increasingly wide array of imaging technologies now available to stage primary rectal cancer renders it necessary to determine the most clinically and cost-effective means of staging rectal cancer. This review will examine the evidence basis for

Recent Results in Cancer Research, Vol. 165

staging rectal cancer and the potential role of imaging in demonstrating important known prognostic variables prior to surgery.

Endoluminal Ultrasound

Endoluminal ultrasound (EUS) has long been regarded as the staging method of choice in local assessment of primary rectal cancer. Its advantages include convenient accessibility, as in many instances it is part of the initial assessment performed by the colorectal surgeon in conjunction with the digital rectal examination (DRE). EUS has been advocated as a method of identifying early-stage tumours that may be safely treated by surgery alone and in identifying T3 tumours requiring preoperative therapy. It is of undoubtedly great importance in assessing early tumours, and has been shown to be of high accuracy in selecting early-stage T1 tumours suitable for local excision (Mackay et al. 2003). However, there are significant limitations in the assessment of tumours that are T2 or greater. Problems with maintaining an orthogonal plane of the probe with respect to the tumour may in many instances result in substantial overstaging with overestimation of tumour depth (Akasu et al. 1997). The inability of this modality to interrogate the whole of the mesorectum and most critically to assess the interface between tumour and the mesorectal margin limits its value in detecting patients at risk of R1 or R2 resection (Bartram and Brown 2002). The poor performance of EUS in staging nodes has been demonstrated in a study using node-wise correlation (Spinelli et al. 1999), confirming the inability of EUS to detect positive nodes <5 mm in diameter. Most EUS probes will not identify lymph nodes that measure <5 mm in diameter beyond the immediate vicinity of the rectal wall, and the inherent small field of view limits EUS assessment of mesorectal tumour deposits that can occur high above the level of the tumour. Important surgical landmarks, namely the point of attachment of the peritoneal reflection, mesorectal fascia, Denonvilliers fascia, and pelvic sidewall nodes and lymph nodes are similarly not shown by this modality.

In a prospective study, the accuracy of high-resolution MRI, DRE, and EUS in identifying favourable, unfavourable, and locally advanced rectal carcinomas was compared prospectively against the gold standard of pathological findings in resection specimens. The potential impact of each staging modality on the preoperative treatment pathway was then compared, for clinical benefit and cost-effectiveness. MRI performed better than EUS and DRE in the assessment of depth of extramural invasion, nodal involvement, and in prediction of CRM status (Brown et al. 2004). By contrast, DRE (which depends on the subjective appreciation of tumour mobility or fixity) performed poorly, understaging 47% of cases (Brown et al. 2004). In our experience, EUS tended to overestimate tumour depth, and these limitations have been noted by others (Hulsmans et al. 1992; Akasu et al. 1997). These difficulties result from the obliquity of the probe in relation to the lesion and the difficulty in separating peritumoural inflammation or fibrosis from true tumour (Maier et al. 1997). Few previous EUS studies have assessed its accuracy in TME specimens, and its inherent small field of view has limited its usefulness in assessing the whole mesorectum.

Computed Tomography

Published studies to date have shown computed tomography (CT) to be inferior to EUS in local staging (Harewood et al. 2002). Recent years have seen the development of multidetector CT with sub-millimetre voxel size achievable on modern machines. The high spatial resolution achieved is not accompanied by a similarly high contrast resolution, and it thus remains doubtful whether the high spatial resolution in itself will improve accuracy, since the inherent contrast resolution is poor (Fig. 1). This results in difficulty delineating the true local extent of tumour

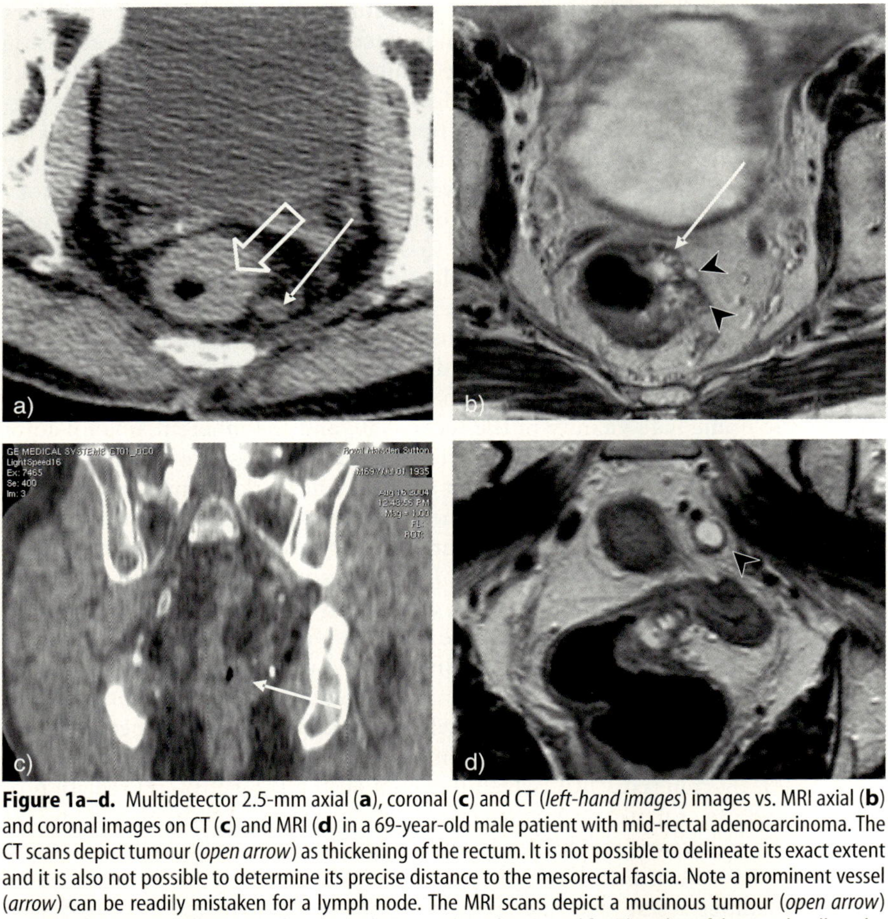

Figure 1a–d. Multidetector 2.5-mm axial (**a**), coronal (**c**) and CT (*left-hand images*) images vs. MRI axial (**b**) and coronal images on CT (**c**) and MRI (**d**) in a 69-year-old male patient with mid-rectal adenocarcinoma. The CT scans depict tumour (*open arrow*) as thickening of the rectum. It is not possible to delineate its exact extent and it is also not possible to determine its precise distance to the mesorectal fascia. Note a prominent vessel (*arrow*) can be readily mistaken for a lymph node. The MRI scans depict a mucinous tumour (*open arrow*) which is of higher signal intensity than muscularis propria and perirectal fat. The edge of the rectal wall can be seen (*arrow*) and thus the precise depth of extramural spread of tumour can be measured (*arrowhead*). The coronal CT shows tumour (*arrow*) but it is not possible to relate the extent of spread to the mesorectal fascia. The coronal MR image (**d**) depicts an encapsulated lymph node containing high signal intensity mucinous tumour >1 mm from the mesorectal fascia (*arrowhead*)

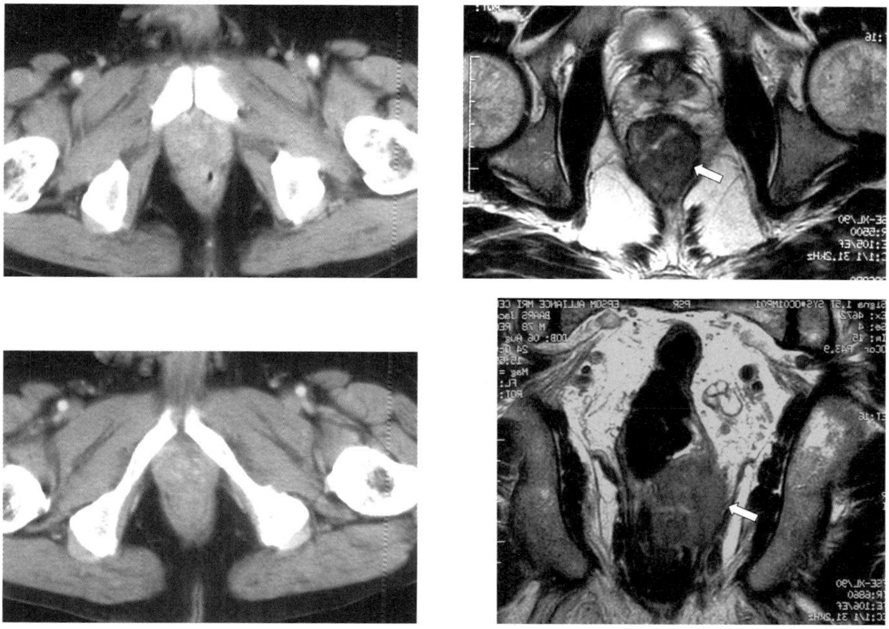

Figure 2. Low tumour on CT compared with MRI

and indeed in distinguishing tumour from normal anatomic structures. Tumour assessment using CT relies on the assessment of indirect features of tumour such as apparent thickening or "loss of tissue planes", irregularity of the border of the rectal wall, and strands of soft tissue extending into perirectal fat (Thoeni 1989; Thoeni et al. 1981). These findings are nonspecific and may be due to fibrosis, inflammation, and desmoplasia. With intravenous contrast enhancement, tumour enhances but inflammatory tissue, desmoplastic reaction, and normal peritumoral hypervascularity all enhance, leading to substantial problems with overstaging. Invasion into adjacent structures may be difficult to assess, as loss of fat planes may occur due to congestion of vessels and lymphatics, inflammation, and absence of intrapelvic fat in cachectic patients (Thoeni 1989). Thus sensitivity for local invasion is poor and ranges from 48% to 55% (Mehta et al. 1994).

Lack of contrast between the planes is a particular problem for low rectal tumours, which are of similar attenuation to the levators and sphincter complex and thus impossible to delineate (Fig. 2). Furthermore, the inability to consistently depict the mesorectal fascia on CT makes this an ineffective technique when assessing the potential mesorectal resection margins, except in extensive disease in which the mesorectal fascia has been has invaded and thickened (Grabbe et al. 1983).

18FDG-PET Imaging

18-FDG positron emission tomography (PET) imaging is an important new tool that will undoubtedly play an important role in staging and follow-up of colorectal cancer. Its role in local staging of the primary tumour is limited since the high metabolic activity of the primary tumour masks the spatial and anatomical information required for local T-, N-staging as well as assessment of the mesorectal margin status.

However, its role in the preoperative work-up of patients by the demonstration of unsuspected extra-pelvic metastatic disease is increasingly recognised, and this will influence the early instigation of systemic therapy as well as potential resection of isolated extrapelvic metastatic disease. However, it is in the follow-up of patients with colorectal cancer that PET is of major importance, and a number of studies have demonstrated that PET is a cost-effective technique in evaluating recurrent colorectal cancer (Lonneux et al. 2002; Rohren et al. 2002; Rollins 2002; Ruers et al. 2002; Simo et al. 2002; Valk et al. 1999). The technique can detect subtle lesions that are not always appreciated on CT. A meta-analysis of the use of PET in the evaluation of recurrent disease concluded that a change of management results in 29% of patients (Huebner et al. 2000).

However, in the pelvis both MRI and 18-FDG PET are needed and provide complimentary information. Caution must be applied in using 18-FDG PET alone to detect local recurrence without detailed anatomic corroboration of a positive PET scan, particularly since inflammatory changes, and changes relating to radiotherapy as well as bowel and bladder activity, may give both false positive and false negative results if 18-FDG PET is used alone (Haberkorn et al. 1991) (Fig. 3).

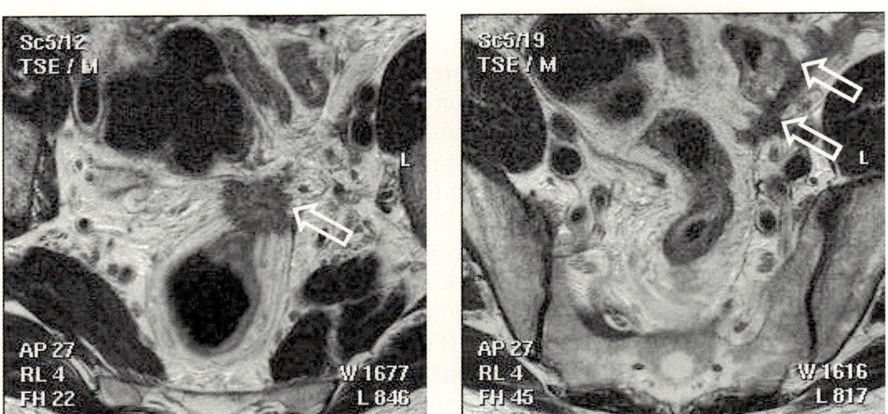

Figure 3. Example of PET negative recurrence shown on MRI

Primary Rectal Tumour Staging Using MRI

In the 1980s and early 1990s, MRI results in staging rectal cancer were disappointing (de Lange 1994; Hadfield et al. 1997; McNicholas et al. 1994; Okizuka et al. 1996; Thaler et al. 1994; Wallengren et al. 1996). Poor spatial and contrast resolution contributed to results that could not be shown to be superior to CT or EUS. Furthermore, patient numbers in each of the MRI studies were too small to determine a statistically significant level of agreement with histopathological staging. A large multi-centre study performed in the US (Zerhouni et al. 1996) evaluated the staging accuracy of MRI using a body coil in 79 patients with rectal cancer; the staging accuracy in this study was only 58%. Chan et al. (1991), Imai (1999), and Schnall et al. (1994) evaluated the endorectal coil in staging rectal cancers. Although patient numbers were small and the studies contained disproportionately high numbers of early rectal cancers, these studies did demonstrate the potential of MRI in depicting the layers of the bowel wall. The studies also noted that the T2-weighted images provided better contrast between the tumour and the rectal wall than could be obtained with T1-weighted images. However there are major problems with using endorectal coil techniques in assessing rectal tumours. Firstly, appropriate positioning of the coil is difficult, particularly for mid- and upper-third rectal tumours. Secondly, bulky or stricturing tumours are not assessable, and thirdly images obtained are suboptimal due to only a limited assessment of the mesorectum and distortion of the rectum caused by the probe itself.

Fortunately, in recent years, the parallel developments of the phased array multi-element surface coils (Fig. 4) and fast T2-weighted spin echo sequences as well as advances in magnetic field gradients have enabled high-spatial-resolution and high-contrast-resolution scanning with acceptable scan duration.

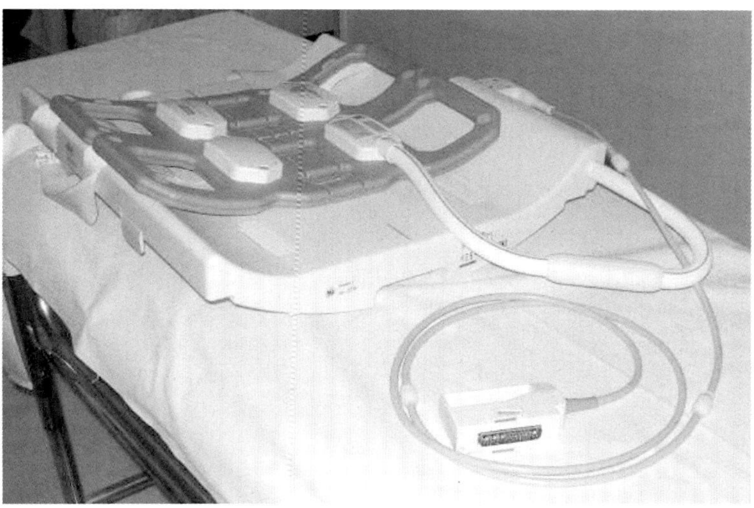

Figure 4. Pelvic phased array surface coil

Table 1. Parameters for high-spatial-resolution images

Field of view	160 mm
Number of slices	24
Interleaved/contiguous	Interleaved
Echo train length/TSE factor	16
Time to repetition	> 3,000 and <6,000 (shortest)
Phase-encoding direction	R to L
Scan time	7:48 s
Rectangular field of view %	100%
Slice thickness/gap	3 mm/no gap
Number of rest slabs/drive	None
Time to echo	100
Matrix 256/256	256 × 256

By limiting the field of view to between 160 and 180 mm and slice thickness to 3 mm, and by planning scans orthogonal to the rectal wall and tumour, high spatial- and contrast-resolution scans can be obtained that depict the tumour and its relation to the muscle coat, mesorectal fascia that shows direct agreement with that of corresponding histopathology measurements (Brown et al. 1999). Using the scanning technique summarised in Table 1 and a surface pelvic coil rather than an endorectal coil, an in-plane resolution can be achieved similar to that obtained with an endorectal coil (0.6×0.6 mm in plane). The images obtained depict the layers of the rectal wall, and no patient preparation is necessary for MRI scanning of the rectum (Fig. 5). An advantage of using this technique has been the ability to image

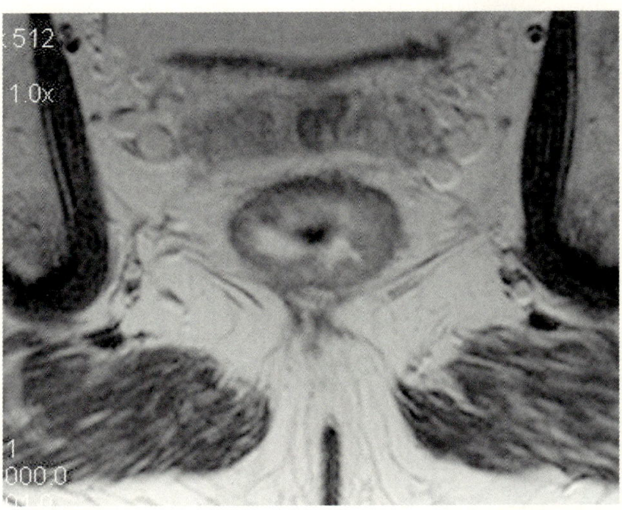

Figure 5. Bowel wall layers shown on MRI

a relatively large area of the perirectal tissue, and thus the whole of the mesorectum can be assessed. On the FSE T2-weighted images, perirectal fat is of higher signal than tumour, allowing clear visualisation of tumour extension into fat. Having penetrated the bowel wall, these tumours can spread over a large distance in the perirectal fat, a feature not appreciated by direct visualisation sigmoidoscopy or EUS. This MRI technique can therefore assess all patients rather than a subgroup, and also provides more information that is relevant to preoperative treatment planning than other staging methods. Adenocarcinoma is shown very distinctly as intermediate signal intensity material, and the morphological spectrum shown on MRI reflects the range of morphology observed by histopathologists.

Preoperative Assessment of Prognostic Factors

With such clear depiction of tumour and normal anatomy, we have focused on the ability of MRI to identify pathological prognostic factors.

Relationship of Tumour to the Mesorectal Margin

In 1982, the importance of the lateral circumferential margin involvement by tumour and its relation to local recurrence was prospectively investigated (Quirke et al. 1986). The risk of local recurrence in CRM-positive patients was significantly higher than in CRM-negative patients and, compared with CRM-negative patients, the risk of death was three times higher. Moreover, CRM-positive patients had only a 15% 5-year survival. The CRM status has emerged as one of the most important prognostic determinants in the practice of successful rectal cancer surgery and as the basis for the success of the TME. An involved CRM, defined as tumour observed <1 mm from the resection margin, predicts for local recurrence, distant metastasis, and poor survival even after TME (Hall et al. 1998). In the Leeds single institution series of 586 patients, those with an involved CRM had a significantly higher risk of local recurrence and lower overall survival than those who had a clear CRM (Birbeck et al. 2002). Similar figures were seen in the Norwegian series of 686 patients where CRM involvement increased the risk of developing local recurrence by a factor of 12, distant metastasis by a factor of 4.7, and mortality by a factor of 3.7 (Wibe et al. 2002). Thus CRM involvement is an important prognostic factor whose value does not diminish with TME. The CRM status may also be used as an immediate measure of the quality of both the preoperative strategy and the surgery.

When high-spatial-resolution techniques are employed, the mesorectal fascia is clearly depicted and the relationship of tumour to this fascia shows good agreement with that of histopathology. If a potential circumferential margin is defined as involved if tumour lies within 1 mm of the mesorectal fascia, this predicts for subsequent margin involvement by tumour, and agreement with histopathologic CRM status is 92% (Kappa = 0.81; 95% confidence interval for Kappa is 0.62 to 0.91) (Brown et al. 2003a).

Extramural Depth and T Stage

Dukes' 1958 paper (Dukes and Bussey 1958) highlighted the importance of extent of extramural spread in the prediction of local recurrence as well as survival. Survival figures for Dukes' B cases were 89.7% for slight spread, 80% for moderate spread, and 57% for extensive spread. The measurement is taken from the outer edge of the longitudinal muscle layer.

Another important feature is that once spread beyond the bowel wall occurs, the incidence of lymph node invasion increases, rising from 14.2% in tumours confined to the bowel wall to 43.2% in those tumours extending beyond the bowel wall (Dukes and Bussey 1958). Regardless of lymph node status, it has been shown by the St Marks group that survival was 97% in those tumours with no spread beyond the bowel wall (Jass et al. 1986).

In 1993, an optional modification of the TNM system was proposed to take into account the importance of extramural spread as a means of distinguishing between otherwise heterogeneous groups of T3 tumours (Hermanek et al. 1993). This also included a separate classification of T4 tumours to distinguish between peritoneal perforation (pT4b) and invasion of adjacent pelvic structures (pT4a) (Hermanek et al. 1993). The advantage of such subcategorisation was to allow the collection of additional important prognostic data without altering the definitions of the existing TNM categories. Hermanek also noted the importance of incorporating independent prognostic factors whilst retaining an intact TNM system, and postulated that a future sophisticated prognostic index incorporating such data may be used to assign patients to various prognostic groups. In doing so, this could enable the better design of future trials by appropriate stratification based on all relevant prognostic factors. This approach has highlighted the need to separate T3 tumours according to extent of extramural spread. In 2001, a study evaluating the prognostically inhomogeneous pT3 rectal carcinomas data on over 1400 patients was analysed following radical surgery alone (Merkel et al. 2001). The category pT3 was subdivided according to the histological measurement of the maximal tumour invasion beyond the outer border of the muscularis propria: pT3a (up to 5 mm) and pT3b (more than 5 mm). The cancer-related 5-year survival rates were 85.4% for tumours with less than 5 mm spread compared to 54.1% for tumours with >5 mm spread ($p<0.0001$). Lymph node-negative tumours with <5 mm spread and pT2 patients showed very similar high 5-year survival rates (91.2% vs. 93.6%, respectively) as did lymph nodepositive tumours with <5 mm spread and pT2 patients (77.8% vs. 82.8%, respectively). The subdivision of pT3 thus enables the identification of a subgroup of patients in whom 5-yr survival is >85% and for whom routine preoperative therapy is unlikely to provide a significant benefit (Merkel et al. 2001).

Using a high-resolution technique, it has been shown that thin-slice MRI can be used to measure the depth of extramural spread accurately and shows good correlation with corresponding pathology measurements in resection specimens (Brown et al. 1999). By careful correlation of preoperative images with histopathology sections, criteria for T staging have been derived. When these criteria were tested prospectively, direct agreement between preoperative MR measurements and histopathology measurements was reaffirmed. Furthermore, 87% of patients with tumour spread >5 mm beyond the bowel wall were correctly identified by preoperative MRI. Discrepancies in measurement of extramural depth between histology and MRI differing by >3 mm were seen in a few patients after long-course radiotherapy. In addition, depth of extramural spread may be difficult to accurately correlate in tumours that produced erosion or destruction of the muscularis propria (Brown et al. 2003a).

Lymph Node Status

The influence of the number of lymph nodes involved by tumour on prognosis has been well shown (Jass et al. 1986; Wolmark et al. 1986), and a major challenge for any imaging modality lies in the ability to predict lymph node status prior to surgery. However, a significant limitation of any imaging technique is the ability to demonstrate nodes that contain microscopic tumour foci (<3 mm diameter tumour clusters within nodes). By both morphologic and functional criteria, these nodes are difficult to detect with certainty. Notwithstanding these limitations, the rejection of the traditionally favoured size criteria for determining nodal status in favour of morphological criteria has resulted in improvements in the accuracy of nodal staging. Using definitions based on the border or heterogeneity of signal within nodes, it is possible to predict final nodal status with greater accuracy than

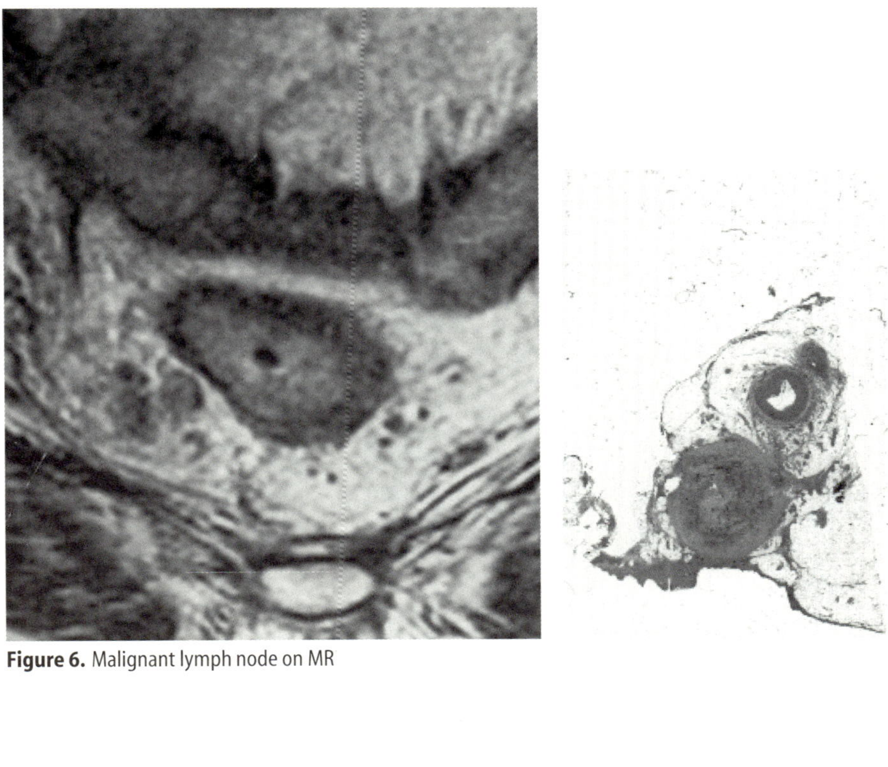

Figure 6. Malignant lymph node on MR

using size criteria. These criteria were developed by careful matching of nodes seen in vivo with nodes harvested from the surgical specimen (Brown et al. 2003b). When nodes are defined as malignant, if either an irregular border is demonstrated or mixed signal intensity is present within the node (Fig. 6), superior accuracy is obtained, resulting in sensitivity of 85% and a specificity of 97%. When these criteria were applied in a prospective study, agreement with histological N stage was 85% (kappa=0.68).

Extramural Venous Invasion

Spread in to large extramural veins carries a very poor prognosis. In one series, the corrected 5-year survival for Dukes' stage C patients with invasion of large extramural veins was only 8%, and invasion of extramural veins was associated with a low 5-year survival rate of 33% (Talbot et al. 1981). Others have reaffirmed this observation (Bokey et al. 1999; Horn et al. 1990, 1991). Moreover in models using step-wise selection of prognostic indicators, extramural venous invasion has been shown to retain independent prognostic significance (Bokey et al. 1999; Harrison et al. 1994).

The formation of discrete tubular projections of tumour extending into perirectal fat which appears to be following the course of a perirectal vessel corresponds to extramural venous invasion (Fig. 7), and when detected is highly predictive of venous invasion on subsequent histopathological assessment (Brown et al. 2003a). Often, the sagittal image shows dramatic demonstration of direct extramural invasion by tumour with characteristic serpiginous growth of tumour by direct spread extramurally along the course of the superior rectal vein (Fig. 8). Paradoxically,

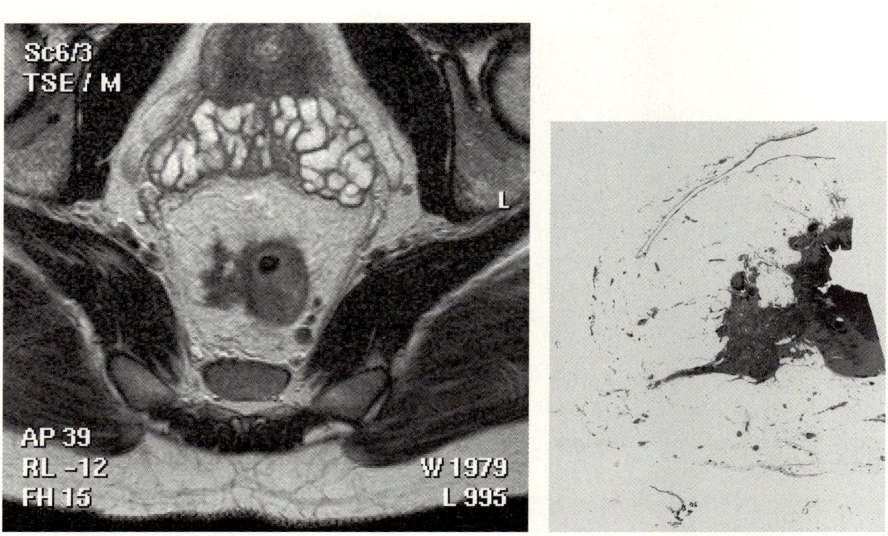

Figure 7. Extramural venous invasion

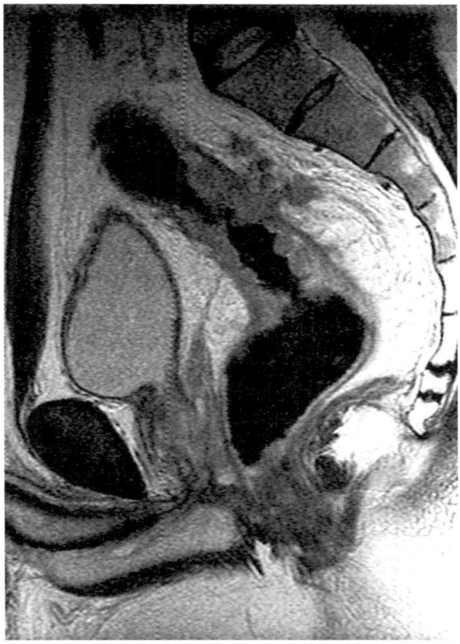

Figure 8. Superior rectal vein invasion

such clear observations of extramural venous invasion shown on MRI may be difficult to corroborate on histology, since obliteration of normal venous architecture may make it difficult to appreciate that tumour lies along the course of a vein, particularly on transverse sectioning of the specimen, which may simply show apparent tumour nodules (Fig. 8).

Peritoneal Perforation

This is defined as perforation of the peritoneal membrane by tumour, and the consequent spillage of tumour cells is presumed to result in both local recurrence and transcoelomic dissemination. Local peritoneal involvement was detected in 25.8% (54/209) of cases (Shepherd et al. 1997). This is an independent prognostic factor and predicts for local recurrence after surgery for upper and middle rectal cancer (Shepherd et al. 1997).

The typical appearance on MRI is that of anterior nodular extension of intermediate signal intensity through the fine low-signal-intensity peritoneal reflection at or above the level of its attachment to the anterior surface of the rectum (Fig. 9). Review of histological sections of cases missed by MR shows instances when tumour cells on the surface of the peritoneum or within a cleft of peritoneum invaginating the mesorectum cannot be delineated on MR. On the other hand, MR images may indicate nodular infiltration through the peritoneum, but histological examina-

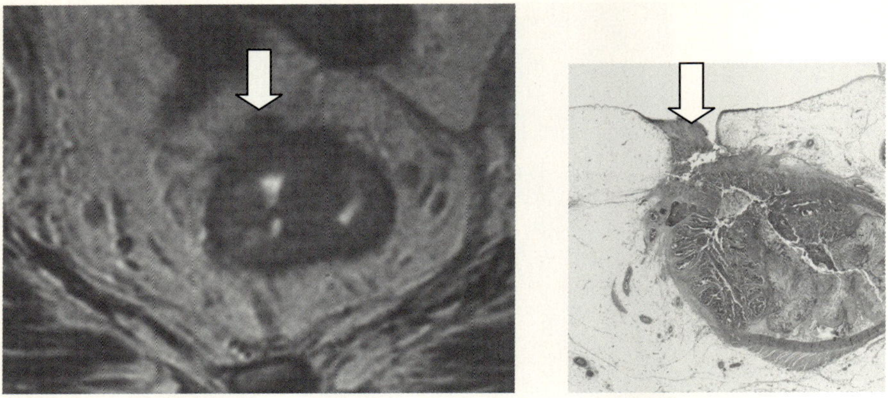

Figure 9. Peritoneal invasion

tion in some cases will show tumour close to the peritoneal surface with an intact peritoneum stretched over the tumour. Thus, although MRI may very accurately show tumour in relation to the level of peritoneal reflection, the determination of actual peritoneal perforation by tumour may not be as reliable as the detection of other prognostic factors.

Developing Imaging-Based Preoperative Strategies

The majority of histopathologic prognostic features are consistently seen using high-spatial-resolution MRI, and although the technique is limited by inability to identify microscopic (<2 mm) lymph node involvement and microscopic extramural venous invasion, it is believed that the prognostic implications for missing such disease may not be as great compared with the ability to identify tumours that are at risk of R1 and R2 resection or tumours at risk of systemic failure by virtue of increasing extramural depth, N2 disease, peritoneal perforation, or large vein invasion by tumour. As a consequence, a targeted preoperative strategy has been developed to tailor treatment according to risk of local or distant failure or both. The most optimal treatment approach will need to be determined by future phase III randomised trials, but an MRI-based selective approach has recently been tested in a phase II trial (Chau et al. 2003). The preoperative strategy employed in this trial is summarised in Fig. 10). In a recent audit of our experience employing an MRI-based preoperative strategy, we observed that MRI was able to reliably distinguish between patients at risk of systemic or local failure (any of the following: potential R1 or R2 resection, T3 disease >5 mm, extramural venous invasion, N2 disease) compared with those at minimal or no risk of local or systemic failure (all of the N0 or N1 disease). Furthermore, the preoperative use of MRI to select patients for primary surgery without neoadjuvant therapy resulted in no instances of R1 or R2 resections. The use of intensive preoperative therapy increased the number of resections performed with curative intent to 87% (95% CI = 83%–90%)

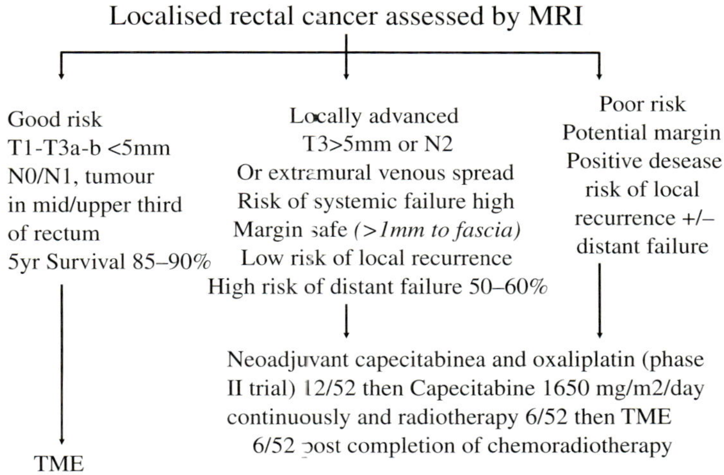

Figure 10. Preoperative strategy

with an overall R1/R2 rate for the entire group of 298 patients undergoing surgery of 8% (95% CI = 5%–11%).

The benefits of a selective approach using MRI-based selection criteria are thus self-evident. That is, over 50% of patients can be treated successfully with primary surgery without significant risk of local recurrence or systemic failure. Of the remainder, potentially dramatic improvements may be achieved through the use of intensive and targeted preoperative therapy aimed not only at reducing the size of the primary tumour and rendering potentially irresectable tumour resectable with tumour-free circumferential margins, but also to enable patients at high risk of systemic failure to benefit from intensive combined modality therapy aimed at eliminating micrometastatic disease.

The MERCURY Research Project

The MERCURY Study (*M*agnetic R*e*sonance Imaging and *R*ectal *C*ancer E*u*ropean Equivalence Stud*y*) was launched in January 2002 to demonstrate the feasibility and reproducibility of high-resolution MRI in multiple centres and its equivalence to the corresponding whole-mount histopathological section. The study completed accrual for its primary endpoint of equivalence of MRI with histopathology in November 2003 and will report in 2005. The technique, if shown to be successful, could be a crucial predictor of the CRM status and lead to the identification of patients who are likely to benefit from neo-adjuvant therapy in the multicentre setting. Similarly with the identification of those independent pathological factors that are associated with disease recurrence, the validation of an MRI pre-operative staging system, based upon the ability of MRI staging to predict not only the status of the mesorectal margin but also to identify known adverse features verified on pathology, would allow future stratification of patients into prognostic groups. Such information would be advantageous in the development of future adjunctive and neo-adjunctive trials in rectal cancer.

The study encompasses a European network of multi-disciplinary teams, in collaborating centres that are capable of submitting quality-controlled data and images. This study completed its targeted accrual of patients from the 11 participating centres by October 2003, and for the first time this study is demonstrating that surgeons, radiologists, and pathologists can recruit consecutive patients with rectal cancer in a prospective study. The underlying principles of this study were those of quality control and an elimination of selection bias by registering nearly all rectal cancer patients treated at the 11 participating centres during the 2-year duration of the study. We believe that the combination of high-quality radiological assessment, targeted pre-operative therapy, optimum TME surgery assessed by pathological quality control, and the comparison of the radiological and pathological findings will form a robust database for future research and teaching.

References

Akasu T, Sugihara K, Moriya Y, Fujita S (1997) Limitations and pitfalls of transrectal ultrasonography for staging of rectal cancer. Dis Col Rec 40:S10–15

Bartram C, Brown G (2002) Endorectal ultrasound and magnetic resonance imaging in rectal cancer staging. Gastroenterol Clin North Am 31:827–839

Birbeck KF, Macklin CP, Tiffin NJ, Parsons W, Dixon MF, Mapstone NP, Abbott CR, Scott N, Finan PJ, Johnston D, Quirke P (2002) Rates of circumferential resection margin involvement vary between surgeons and predict outcomes in rectal cancer. surgery Ann Surg, 235:449–457

Bokey EL, Ojerskog B, Chapuis P, Dent O, Newland RC, Sinclair G (1999) Local recurrence after curative excision of the rectum for cancer without adjuvant therapy: role of total anatomical dissection. Br J Surg 86:

Brown G, Davies S, Williams GT, Bourne MW, Newcombe RG, Radcliffe AG, Blethyn J, Dallimore NS, Rees BI, Phillips CJ, Maughan TS (2004) Effectiveness of preoperative staging in rectal cancer: digital rectal examination, endoluminal ultrasound, or magnetic resonance imaging? Br J Cancer 91:23–29

Brown G, Radcliffe AG, Newcombe RG, Dallimore NS, Bourne MW and Williams GT (2003a) Preoperative assessment of prognostic factors in rectal cancer using high-resolution magnetic resonance imaging. Br J Surg 90:355–364

Brown G, Richards CJ, Bourne MW, Newcombe RG, Radcliffe AG, Dallimore NS, Williams GT (2003b) Morphologic predictors of lymph node status in rectal cancer with use of high-spatial-resolution MR imaging with histopathologic comparison. Radiology 227:371–377

Brown G, Richards CJ, Newcombe RG, Dallimore NS, Radcliffe AG, Carey DP, Bourne MW, Williams GT (1999) Rectal carcinoma: thin-section MR imaging for staging in 28 patients. Radiology 211:215–222

Chan TW, Kressel HY, Milestone B, Tomachefski J, Schnall M, Rosato E, Daly J (1991) Rectal carcinoma: staging at MR imaging with endorectal surface coil: Work in progress. Radiology 181:461–467

Chau I, Cunningham D, Tait AD, Brown G, Tebbutt N, Hill M, Wotherspoon A, Norman A, Massey A, Oates J (2003) Twelve weeks of neoadjuvant capecitabine (cap) and oxaliplatin (ox) followed by synchronous chemoradiation (CRT) and total mesorectal excision (TME) in MRI defined poor risk locally advanced rectal cancer resulted in promising tumour regression and rapid symptomatic relief. Proc Am Soc Clin Oncol 22:71

de Lange EE (1994) Staging rectal carcinoma with endorectal imaging: how much detail do we really need? [editorial; comment] Radiology 190:633–635

Dukes CE, Bussey HJ (1958) The spread of cancer and its effect on prognosis. Cancer 12:309–320

Grabbe E, Lierse W, Winkler R (1983) The perirectal fascia: morphology and use in staging of rectal carcinoma. Radiology 149:241–246
Haberkorn U, Strauss LG, Dimitrakopoulou A, Engenhart R, Oberdorfer F, Ostertag H, Romahn J, van Kaick G (1991) PET studies of fluorodeoxyglucose metabolism in patients with recurrent colorectal tumors receiving radiotherapy. J Nucl Med 32:1485–1490
Hadfield MB, Nicholson AA, MacDonald AW, Farouk R, Lee PW, Duthie GS, Monson JR (1997) Preoperative staging of rectal carcinoma by magnetic resonance imaging with a pelvic phased-array coil. Br J Surg 84:529–531
Hall NR, Finan PJ, al-Jaberi T, Tsang CS, Brown SR, Dixon MF, Quirke P (1998) Circumferential margin involvement after mesorectal excision of rectal cancer with curative intent Predictor of survival but not local recurrence? Dis Col Rect 41:979–983
Harewood GC, Wiersema MJ, Nelson H, Maccarty RL, Olson JE, Clain JE, Ahlquist DA, Jondal ML (2002) A prospective, blinded assessment of the impact of preoperative staging on the management of rectal cancer. Gastro 123:24–32
Harrison JC, Dean PJ, el-Zeky F, Vander Zwaag R (1994) From Dukes through Jass: pathological prognostic indicators in rectal cancer. [See comments]. Hum Path 25:498–505
Hermanek P, Henson DE, Hutter RV, Sobin LH (1993) UICC TNM supplement 1993. A commentary on uniform use. Springer, Berlin, Heidelberg, New York
Horn A, Dahl O, Morild I (1990) The role of venous and neural invasion on survival in rectal adenocarcinoma. Dis Col Rect 33:598–601
Horn A, Dahl O, Morild I (1991) Venous and neural invasion as predictors of recurrence in rectal adenocarcinoma. Dis Col Rect 34:798–804
Huebner RH, Park KC, Shepherd JE, Schwimmer J, Czernin J, Phelps ME, Gambhir SS (2000) A meta-analysis of the literature for whole-body FDG PET detection of recurrent colorectal cancer. J Nucl Med 41:1177–89
Hulsmans FH, Bosma A, Mulder PJ, Reeders JW, Tytgat GN (1992) Perirectal lymph nodes in rectal cancer: in vitro correlation of sonographic parameters and histopathologic findings. Radiol 184:553–60
Imai Y (1999) MR imaging of rectal cancer using endorectal surface coil: histopathological correlation. Nippon Igaku Hoshasen Gakkai Zasshi—Nippon Acta Radiologica, 59:458–66
Jass JR, Atkin WS, Cuzick J, Bussey HJ, Morson BC, Northover JM, Todd IP (1986) The grading of rectal cancer: historical perspectives and a multivariate analysis of 447 cases. Histopathol 10:437–59
Lonneux M, Reffad AM, Detry R, Kartheuser A, Gigot JF, Pauwels S (2002) FDG-PET improves the staging and selection of patients with recurrent colorectal cancer. Eur J Nucl Med Mol Imaging 29:915–21
Mackay SG, Pager CK, Joseph D, Stewart PJ, Solomon MJ (2003) Assessment of the accuracy of transrectal ultrasonography in anorectal neoplasia. Br J Surg 90:346–350
Maier AG, Barton PP, Neuhold NR, Herbst F, Teleky BK, Lechner GL (1997) Peritumoral tissue reaction at transrectal US as a possible cause of overstaging in rectal cancer: histopathologic correlation. Radiol 203:785–789
McNicholas MM, Joyce WP, Dolan J, Gibney RG, MacErlaine DP, Hyland J (1994) Magnetic resonance imaging of rectal carcinoma: a prospective study. Br J Surg 81:911–914
Mehta S, Johnson RJ, Schofield PF (1994) Staging of colorectal cancer. Clin Radiol 49:515–523
Merkel S, Mansmann U, Siassi M, Papadopoulos T, Hohenberger W, Hermanek P (2001) The prognostic inhomogeneity in pT3 rectal carcinomas. Int J Colorectal Dis 16:298–304
Okizuka H, Sugimura K, Yoshizako T, Kaji Y, Wada A (1996) Rectal carcinoma: prospective comparison of conventional and gadopentetate dimeglumine enhanced fat-suppressed MR imaging. J Mag Res Imag 6:465–471
Quirke P, Durdey P, Dixon MF, Williams NS (1986) Local recurrence of rectal adenocarcinoma due to inadequate surgical resection: Histopathological study of lateral tumour spread and surgical excision. Lancet 2:996–999
Rohren EM, Paulson EK, Hagge R, Wong TZ, Killius J, Clavien PA, Nelson RC (2002) The role of F-18 FDG positron emission tomography in preoperative assessment of the liver in patients being considered for curative resection of hepatic metastases from colorectal cancer. Clin Nucl Med 27:550–555
Rollins G (2002) PET scans improve management decisions, reduce unnecessary surgery in recurrent colorectal cancer. Rep Med Guidel Outcomes Res 13:7–9

Ruers TJ, Langenhoff BS, Neeleman N, Jager GJ, Strijk S, Wobbes T, Corstens FH, Oyen WJ (2002) Value of positron emission tomography with [F-18]fluorodeoxyglucose in patients with colorectal liver metastases: a prospective study. J Clin Oncol 20:388–395

Schnall MD, Furth EE, Rosato EF, Kressel HY (1994) Rectal tumor stage: correlation of endorectal MR imaging and pathologic findings. [See comments]. Radiology 190:709–714

Shepherd NA, Baxter KJ, Love SB (1997) The prognostic importance of peritoneal involvement in colonic cancer: a prospective evaluation. Gastroenterol 112:1096–1102

Simo M, Lomena F, Setoain J, Perez G, Castellucci P, Costansa JM, Setoain-Quinquer J, Domenech-Torne F, Carrio I (2002) FDG-PET improves the management of patients with suspected recurrence of colorectal cancer Nucl Med Commun 23:975–982

Spinelli P, Schiavo M, Meroni E, Di Felice G, Andreola S, Gallino G, Belli F, Leo E (1999) Results of EUS in detecting perirectal lymph node metastases of rectal cancer: the pathologist makes the difference. Gastrointest Endo 49:754–758

Talbot IC, Ritchie S, Leighton MH, Hughes AO, Bussey HJ, Morson BC (1981) Spread of rectal cancer within veins Histologic features and clinical significance. Am J Surg 141:15–17

Thaler W, Watzka S, Martin F, La Guardia G, Psenner K, Bonatti G, Fichtel G, Egarter-Vigl E, Marzoli GP (1994) Preoperative staging of rectal cancer by endoluminal ultrasound vs. magnetic resonance imaging. Preliminary results of a prospective, comparative study. Dis Col Rect, 37:1189–1193

Thoeni RF (1989) CT evaluation of carcinomas of the colon and rectum. Radiol Clin of No Am 27:731–741

Thoeni RF, Moss AA, Schnyder P, Margulis AR (1981) Detection and staging of primary rectal and rectosigmoid cancer by computed tomography. Radiology 141:135–138

Valk PE, Abella-Columna E, Haseman MK, Pounds TR, Tesar RD, Myers RW, Greiss HB, Hofer GA (1999) Whole-body PET imaging with [18F]fluorodeoxyglucose in management of recurrent colorectal cancer. Arch Surg 134:503–511; discussion 511–513

Wallengren NO, Holtas S, Andren-Sandberg A (1996) Preoperative staging of rectal carcinoma using double-contrast MR imaging. Technical aspects and early clinical experiences. Acta Radiologica 37:791–8

Wibe A, Rendedal PR, Svensson E, Norstein J, Eide TJ, Myrvold HE, Soreide O (2002) Prognostic significance of the circumferential resection margin following total mesorectal excision for rectal cancer. Br J Surg 89:327–34

Wolmark N, Fisher B, Wieand HS (1986) The prognostic value of the modifications of the Dukes' C class of colorectal cancer. An analysis of the NSABP clinical trials. Ann Surg 203:115–122

Zerhouni EA, Rutter C, Hamilton SR, Balfe DM, Megibow AJ, Francis IR, Moss AA, Heiken JP, Tempany CM, Aisen AM, Weinreb JC, Gatsonis C, McNeil BJ (1996) CT and MR imaging in the staging of colorectal carcinoma: report of the Radiology Diagnostic Oncology Group II. Radiology 200:443–451

Rectal Cancer Management: Europe Is Ahead

R. J. Heald, I. Daniels

R.J. Heald · I.R. Daniels (✉)
Pelican Cancer Foundation, North Hampshire Hospital, Basingstoke, UK
e-mail: Jennifer@pelicancancer.org

For most of the twentieth century it was simply accepted that the 'Miles operation' or abdominoperineal resection (APR) was so mutilating that it had to be as 'curative' or 'radical' as was possible. In reality, the 'devil was in the detail'.

Until the total mesorectal excision (TME) controversy, almost nothing was published about dissection *around* a rectal cancer. The arbitrary 5-cm distal margin along the muscle tube, formerly considered necessary for sphincter preservation, has long been abandoned, although the relevance or irrelevance of the internal iliac nodes still provokes some controversy which lingers on, in both Japan and Italy. Ten years ago local recurrence rates between 25% and 50% were standard, and recurrence within the pelvis was by far the most common presentation of recurrence and by far the cruellest mode of death.

It is a special reason for pride in European clinical research that it is a German study which has answered finally the most important question in rectal cancer this decade—should chemoradiotherapy (CRT) be given before or after surgery? TME surgery largely emanated from England, whilst the value of adjuvant radiotherapy was originally championed and proven in Sweden. Now the German study has succeeded where it proved impossible on the other side of the Atlantic. This German study, currently awaiting publication, demonstrates dramatically how very much superior preoperative neo-adjuvant therapy is to the postoperative. The dictates of the U.S. NIH on one side of the Atlantic and the German Cancer Society on the other now need to be fundamentally modified, and many workers now seriously question the value of routine postoperative radiotherapy. At the same time the seminal work of Hermanek is being fully recognised as having pointed clearly toward the primacy of surgical technique and audit in the drive to achieve better results.

TME is becoming widely accepted as the standard operation for rectal cancer, and the discussion is moving toward an exciting new chapter in the development of surgical education. The principal practical weapon has become the video camera, and the measurement of progress is the meta-analysis of results from whole populations. Many years ago the distinguished American professor Bill Silen made the following prescient observation in *The Lancet*:

Recent Results in Cancer Research, Vol. 165

> 'The likelihood that a proper prospective randomised controlled trial (PRCT) will ever be carried out to see whether TME provides an advantage over conventional surgery for rectal cancer is essentially nil. Possibly meta-analysis will help...In my view it is unconscionable to dismiss comparisons with retrospective controls when the procedure is SO superior in terms of both Local Recurrence and Survival.'

The impossibility of applying prospective randomised trial techniques to the detail of technical surgery has been a major impediment to its establishment as the new 'gold standard'. No PRCT has ever been successfully mounted to underpin a complex advance in surgical technique. Furthermore, significant confusion stems from the development of alternative technologies such as laparoscopic surgery. These are to some extent amenable to PRCT methods, and trials are continuing, but it is likely that the inherent difficulties of applying PRCT methods to surgical techniques will make every trial suspect in one way or another. It is impossible for example even to compare optimal open with optimal laparoscopic cancer surgery, because so few surgeons are optimal at both, whilst different surgeons on the two sides of a trial invalidate that trial completely since one group may simply be technically better than the other. It is important to understand that TME is an oncological principle that is theoretically achievable by either open or laparoscopic methods; these trials will add nothing to the most crucial controversy—the detail of the excision of the tumour and the paramount importance of attention to detail.

A few years after Professor Silen's statement, Professor Hans Troidl described the invitation to a Canadian Professor of Surgery (John MacFarlane) to review and audit independently the Basingstoke data as a 'milestone in surgical objectivity'. Professor John MacFarlane, from the University of British Columbia, published in August 1988 the second set of data from his independent audit of the results in Basingstoke, where TME has been a surgical priority for over twenty years. These data comprised a personal series of 519 consecutive surgical cases with adenocarcinoma treated for cure or palliation (Heald et al. 1998). The largest group was 465 anterior resections (ARs) with low stapled anastomosis (407 TME and 58 mesorectal transactions). The remainder comprises 37 abdominoperineal (AP) resections, 10 Hartmann resections, four local excisions, and three laparotomy only. Preoperative radiotherapy had been used in only 49 cases (7 AP, 38 AR, three Hartmann, one laparotomy). Cancer-specific survival (CSS) rate of all surgically treated cases is 68% at 5 years and 66% at 10 years. There was a 6% local recurrence (LR) at 5 years (2%–10% at 95% confidence interval [95% CI]), and 8% at 10 years (2%–14% at 95%CI). In 405 'curative' resections the LR rate is 3% and 4% and the CSS rate 80% and 78% at 5 years and 10 years, respectively. All patients were followed regularly until death. The principal risk factors for recurrence include the necessity to perform an AP as opposed to AR (for LR), Dukes' stage (for CSS), and extramural vascular invasion (EVI0; for LR and CSS).

Substantial improvements on all previously published, comprehensive, unselected consecutive series appeared were beyond all doubt by this data. In addition, it became clear that low LR rates from better surgery had a substantial effect on overall survival. Many LRs after conventional surgery are the result of regrowth of local mesorectal residues; when these were the only residual disease present at the time of surgery, their optimal removal would have led to actual cure. Thus local control equates with cure in such cases, and better local control leads to more cures. This is exactly what Hermanek had pointed out. Directly comparable results are now published from German workers, which further confirm what can be achieved by better surgery (Merkel et al. 2000).

TME is a system of cancer management that defines the block of tissue to be excised and describes the surgical detail of how this is to be achieved. It is now more readily comprehended by non-surgeons because of the development by specialist MRI radiologists of images that are far superior to anything previously achievable. These demonstrate, for the first time, the contours of the mesorectum and the distribution of the cancer within it. Such imaging will in the future provide a rational basis for selecting those cases for pre-operative therapy when the mesorectal margin is in danger of being breached during surgery or when there are pelvic deposits outside the mesorectal fascia.

The TME concept can be extended now to embrace a multidisciplinary four-stage process:

1. Accurate local staging using body-coil fine-slice MRI
2. Targeted pre-operative therapy in selected cases
3. Precision surgery
4. Macroscopic assessment of the quality of surgical excision and histopathological audit of the process

For the colorectal surgeon, TME comprises five basic principles:

1. Perimesorectal 'Holy Plane' sharp dissection with diathermy and scissors under direct vision
2. Specimen-oriented surgery and histopathology, of which the object is an intact mesorectum with no tearing of the surface and no circumferential margin involvement (CMI)—naked eye or microscopic
3. Quirke-style pathology audit for CMI as the principal outcome measure. Combined with objective assessment of the whole specimen, this confirms the success or failure of the surgery
4. Recognition during surgery and preservation of the autonomic nerve plexus, on which sexual and bladder function depend
5. A major increase in anal preservation and reduction in the number of permanent colostomies
6. Stapled low pelvic reconstruction, usually using Moran triple stapling technique plus short colon pouch anastomosis to low rectum or anal canal (Moran et al. 1994)

Total mesorectal excision and precise perimesorectal plane dissection are being introduced in all the major countries of Europe. Increasingly the specimen is being audited by the detailed histopathology of Quirke and Dixon (1998). The most significant new evidence comes from joint publication from the Stockholm Colorectal Cancer Group and the Basingstoke Bowel Cancer Research Project. In

The Lancet in July 2000, the first report was published ever to show a major impact of a teaching and surgical video-workshop programme on cancer outcomes in a whole population. Both the permanent colostomy rate and the local recurrence rate had been more than halved for the entire population of Stockholm County (Lehander et al. 2000). The 5-year follow up on the series will be published shortly, and analysis of subsequent developments is interesting. The most assiduous attendees at the 11 Stockholm workshops are now performing one-half of all the rectal cancer surgery in Stockholm—all with local recurrence rates below 5% in 'curative' cases. A major publication has also been presented from Norway (Wibe et al 2003) where a somewhat similar teaching programme was introduced, and a Danish study is also completed. Individual surgeon's series such as those already published in the USA by Enker and in New Zealand by Hill show strikingly similar results to those in Basingstoke. Hill called what is essentially an identical technique 'extra fascial excision', and he also published similar results on all outcome parameters. Certainly the initial widespread dismissal of the early Basingstoke results with single-figure local recurrence rates as 'inconceivable' are now set aside by others achieving exactly the same. In all the individual surgeon series, there is a significant improvement on the multi-surgeon series, as would be anticipated for a technique that is technically demanding and challenging.

It is now generally accepted in Europe and in many parts of the world that more precise surgery directed toward total mesorectal excision is the principal determinant of outcome and the principal hope for improvement. The author has undertaken over 300 television workshop demonstration operations in more than 25 countries. TME has become the national standard in Norway, Sweden, Denmark, and the Netherlands. In the larger countries—Germany, France, and the UK—official guidelines support the TME concept. In Germany major studies are ongoing to introduce it and even embrace the specialisation and audit routines necessary to eliminate the surgeon variability that Hermanek et al. (1995) so ably demonstrated.

The early claims from Basingstoke of single-figure local recurrence rates by TME were complemented by reports from Leeds which showed high positive predictive values of circumferential margin involvement (CMI) for local recurrence (LR) (Quirke and Dixon 1998). What has been difficult for many to comprehend is that this high predictive value applies only to series where the local recurrence rate is high; e.g. in Leeds at the time of the first CMI publication, the overall local recurrence rate was 36%, whereas CMI was a much poorer predictor in Guildford, where TME surgery was delivering a much lower LR rate (Breaching the mesorectum, Editorial 1990). Reports also appeared of wide variation in results between surgeons. The fact that three-quarters of the Leeds LRs had been predicted by CMI reflected a key reality, which went largely unnoticed; that most of these CMI cases could have been avoided by the wider circumferential clearance afforded by TME. Thus the lower the local recurrence rate in any given series the less good a predictor CMI becomes, although it remains a predictor of cancer death of one kind or another. Thus in 'bad' series CMI is largely a predictor of *preventable* local recurrence. In the future, the presence of CMI will indicate that a failure has occurred in one of the following steps; local staging, surgical technique, or the wrong choice of pre-operative therapy. It is logical that patients recognised as having an involved margin pre-operatively should receive a down-staging/down-sizing therapy. However, perhaps the greatest importance of CMI in the management of rectal cancer is that it provides a key audit tool for surgery. It is axiomatic that margins of any surgical cancer specimen must be clear of cancer: low CMI rates reflect 'better' surgery and are an end in themselves: if TME surgeons deliver lower CMI rates then this is a self-evident benefit. Modern MRI provides the basis for a whole new discipline in prediction of the relationship of the outer tentacles of cancer to the mesorectal fascia and thus to the risk of an involved margin. The development of this technique has been led by Brown et al. in the United Kingdom and Blomqvist et al. in Sweden (Brown et al. 1999). The recent completed European multicentre, multidisciplinary study (MERCURY) has assessed the feasibility and reproducibility of MRI in the staging of rectal cancer and the prediction of a clear CMI (R0 resection). This study, for the first time in rectal cancer, recruited consecutive patients of all stages of disease and assessed an attempt to optimise management of the cancers through the multidisciplinary process. Those where the mesorectal fascia appeared 'threatened' received pre-operative therapy whilst all participating surgeons were performing TME with histopathological audit.

During recent years by far the highest-profile published trial in the rectal cancer field came from Holland. Despite the initial determination to subject the actual surgical technique of TME to randomisation, the planners of the Dutch study made three very interesting decisions:

1. Firstly they recognised the impracticability of a PRCT of surgical technique and decided instead on a training protocol to *standardise* the surgery whilst *randomising* only short-course radiotherapy.
2. Secondly, they decided that the value of routine chemotherapy in *rectal* cancer was so dubious that they omitted it altogether. It should be noted that this decision was made before either Oxaliplatin or Irinotecan became available,
3. Thirdly, no standardised pre-operative imaging modality was used. Instead tumours described as mobile were included, leading to a clinically selected patient group being assessed.

The first paper to appear from Holland was in the *New England Journal of Medicine* (Kapiteijn 2001). No doubt it was ruthless editing that eliminated all but a single message—that short-course RT (Swedish style 5×5 Gy in 5 days) reduced the local recurrence rate in *standardised TME surgery* from 8% to 2%. However, there are several caveats—the mean follow-up time was only two years, and the involved margin rate on Quirke-style histopathology audit was 23%. A recent publication by Hermanek and Heald asked several questions. For mobile tumours, the margin involvement and longer-term LR rates are really far too high and suggest that not all the surgeons were performing good-quality TMEs. This underlines the great difficulty of refining a surgical technique, although the audit practice and histopathology schedule introduced by Professor Quirke were exemplary demonstrations of 'logical best practice'.

One of the authors (RJH) was the primary TME 'workshop instructor' for the 'Dutch TME Trial'. So far the paper in the NEJM, the only message is about more RT, and this is already producing a large knock-on effect in British practice and in many other countries. In many centres all patients are being given short-course RT without any attempt at pre-operative staging. Many more details of interest have emerged, and the wisdom of this rapid change in practice must be questioned. The Basingstoke data published by Simunovic et al. (2003) do show that a combination of clinical assessment and fine-slice MRI do make it possible, in a unit where precision TME is the priority, to select more than 75% of all referrals as being suitable for *no* RT and to deliver a 2.5% local recurrence rate in this group.

RT is not without its own morbidity, and it must surely be a priority for us to identify those patients where it is *not* required ...? Further analysis of the effect of RT (randomised) on a substantial number of patients with involved surgical margins will shortly be published and will still further fuel the confusion regarding short-course RT and the rationale for giving it. It is the authors' opinion that *selection* is the key to future progress within the UK. For example, the *selective* use of CRT, almost invariably given *pre*-operatively, is surely the only efficient way to cut RT waiting times? The identification of a group requiring *no* RT is really urgent in the UK for this reason alone. Although data on long-course RT leak rates are not yet available, it is safer to regard such cases as at high risk for anastomotic leakage.

Specialisation in deep pelvic surgery and the recognition that two consultants operating together is sometimes a good investment of specialist time are key steps forward. Selection of the low or ultralow anterior cancer in a difficult male for referral to such a team is a further logical step. In this most challenging malignancy, selective use of neo-adjuvants based on MRI, combined with improvements in surgery, mean that complete elimination of local disease is now a real possibility. This will also mean a substantial survival advantage and a real reduction in human suffering.

References

Brown et al (1999) Rectal carcinoma: thin-section MR imaging for staging in 28 patients. Radiol 1999:211(1):215–222

Editorial (1990) Breaching the mesorectum. The Lancet 335, 1067–1068

Heald RJ (1995) Total mesorectal excision is optimal surgery for rectal cancer: a Scandinavian consensus. Br J Surg 82:1297–1299

Heald RJ (1997) Total mesorectal excision: history and anatomy of an operation. In Soreide O, Norstein J, eds, Rectal Cancer Surgery: Optimisation—standardisation—documentation. Berlin: Springer-Verlag, pp203–219

Heald RJ, Husband EM, Ryall RDH (1982) The mesorectum is rectal cancer surgery—the clue to pelvic recurrence? Br J Surg 69:613–616

Heald RJ, Moran BJ, Ryall RDH, Sexton R, MacFarlane JK (1998) Rectal Cancer. The Basingstoke Experience of Total Mesorectal Excision, 1978–1997. Arch Surg 133:894–898

Heald RJ, Ryall RDH (1986) Recurrence and survival after total mesorectal excision for rectal cancer. The Lancet i, 1479–1482

Hermanek P, Wiebelt H, Staimmer D, Riedl S (1995) Prognostic factors of rectum carcinoma—experience of the German Multicentre Study SGCRC German Study Group Colo-Rectal Carcinoma. Tumori 8 (Suppl 3): 60–64

Isbister WH (1990) Basingstoke revisited. Aus NZ J Surg 60:243–246

Isbister WH (1998) Food for thought—Basingstoke revisited again. Australia and New Zealand Journal of Surgery (in press)
Kapiteijn E et al (2001) Preoperative radiotherapy combined with total mesorectal excision for respectable rectal cancer. NE J Med 345:638–646
Lehander Martling A, Holm T et al (2000) Effect of a surgical training programme on outcome of rectal cancer in the County of Stockholm. The Lancet 356: 93–96
Markel S et al (2001) Prognostic inhomogeneity in pT3 rectal cancer. Intl J Col Dis 16.5:298–304
Moran BJ, Docherty A, Finnis D (1994) Novel stapling technique to facilitate low anterior resection for rectal cancer. Br J Surg 81:1230
Quirke P and Dixon MF (1998) The prediction of local recurrence of rectal adenocarcinoma by histopathological examination. Intl J Col Dis 3:127–131
Silen W (1993) Mesorectal excision for rectal cancer. The Lancet 341:1279–1280
Simunovic M et al (2003). Optimal preoperativeassessment and surgery for rectal cancer may greatly limit the need for radiotherapy. Br J Surg 90:999–1003
Wibe A et al (2002) A national strategic change in treatment policy for rectal cancer implementation of total mesorectal excision as routine treatment in Norway. A national audit. Dis Col Rect 45:857–866

Teaching Efforts to Spread TME Surgery in Sweden

Lars Påhlman, Urban Karlbom

L. Påhlman (✉)
Colorectal Unit, Department of Surgery, University Hospital, 751 85 Uppsala, Sweden
e-mail: lars.pahlman@surgsci.uu.se

Introduction

Rectal cancer surgery in Sweden has changed dramatically during the last three decades. In the early to late 1970s very bad results were noted, with high local recurrence rates, and most Swedish centres reported a local failure rate above 30% [1]. It was thought that this was a matter of the complexity of the tumour growth and tumour biology. Therefore, radiotherapy was considered to be the solution to reduce the local recurrence rate. Subsequently, three large trials were conducted in Sweden during the 1980s. The Stockholm/Malmö trial compared preoperative short-course radiotherapy, 25 gray (Gy) in 1 week versus surgery alone [2]. The Uppsala trial compared preoperative short-course radiotherapy versus postoperative radiotherapy to 60 Gy in patients with a tumour at stage B or C [3], and the Swedish Rectal Cancer Trial compared the use of short-course 25 Gy in 1 week versus surgery alone [4]. The data from those three trials can be summarised as follows: preoperative radiotherapy is superior to postoperative radiotherapy, the local failure rates are reduced from around 30% to 15%, and this reduction will have an overall survival benefit. However, an interesting finding from these trials was the fact that in many hospitals, half of the patients were operated upon by a surgeon doing less than one rectal cancer per year.

During the same time period, data from single centres all around the world showed very low local recurrence rates, and surgeons started to claim that the high local recurrence rate was a matter of bad surgery and had really nothing to do with tumour biology [5–7]. The new type of surgery is the total mesorectal excision technique (TME), and it has been adopted in many centres in Sweden. Also in Sweden, several centres could prove very low local recurrence rates after having embarked on the new surgical technique [8–10].

Recent Results in Cancer Research, Vol. 165

Concentration of Surgery to Fewer Units and Auditing the Results

Due to the findings that some hospitals did worse than others and the fact that too many surgeons performed the operations, it was postulated that surgery should be concentrated to fewer hospitals. In Sweden in the early 1990s, many small hospitals were closed due to economic reasons and infrastructural changes in health care. In addition, workshops teaching TME surgery were given all around Sweden, and rectal cancer was no longer considered a procedure for general surgeons. The results from these workshops have been proven to be beneficial [11]. The auditing of the results was also highlighted and became necessary, since due to this new infrastructure and the concentration of rectal cancer surgery to fewer centres, many surgeons wanted to have some confirmation that this was the correct way to do the surgery. Therefore, by the initiative from the Swedish Board of Health and Welfare, the Swedish Rectal Cancer Register (SRCR) was started in 1995.

The Swedish Rectal Cancer Register

The SRCR has data on preoperative investigations, surgical technique, and postoperative complications [12]. It is mandatory for all units dealing with rectal cancer to fill in a specific questionnaire after patient discharge. Moreover, all patients must be reported on once a year postoperatively, where oncological end-points such as distant metastases and local recurrences are reported as well as long-term side effects and complications.

The Swedish health care system is organised into six health care regions, and in each region there is an oncological centre responsible for that specific area of the country. According to Swedish law, all cases of cancer must be reported by both the clinician and the pathology department, to this specific oncological centre. Therefore, the Swedish Cancer Register has almost 100% coverage of all cancers diagnosed and treated in our country. In the SRCR, 99.5% of all rectal cancers are registered, indicating a true population-based register. Each region has its own registration formula with slight regional differences dependent upon local interest of research. However, there is a similar mini-database, where all oncological centres report to one centre responsible for collecting all the data and performing a yearly national report. By definition a rectal cancer is 15 cm from the anal verge. Approximately 1,500 new cases per year are diagnosed, giving almost 13,000 patients recorded in our register today. Due to the large numbers it is now possible to evaluate trends in the treatment, as well as 5 years' oncological data. To summarise, 50% of all patients with a rectal cancer will have a sphincter-preserved procedure, i.e. an anterior resection, and 25% will have an abdominal perineal excision. The rest of the patients will have other procedures such as a low Hartmann, and a local excision, and approximately 5% of all patients will not be operated upon at all due to distant spread or being too old and/or fragile.

How to Use Those Data

All yearly reports are displayed on the web-site of the Swedish National Board of Health and Welfare [12]. So far the annual reports are splitting the figures into different regions of Sweden. There are data from each hospital, but those have not yet been presented due to too small numbers when divided not only into hospitals but also different treatment options. However, all hospitals will have their own specific report together with the national report, which makes it possible for each department of surgery to check whether or not their own data are within the accepted frames. Many specific end-points have been noted, such as the type of procedures presented above, the overall postoperative complications, re-operation rates, postoperative mortality, local recurrence rates, and survival figures for all Dukes' stages, among others. Having identified the median values for each relevant endpoint, it has been decided that these figures should be the guidelines for the gold standards in the treatment of rectal cancer. All units have been urged to try to fulfil the criteria for being a good unit. If a single unit has figures below the accepted range of good quality, the unit must within a short period of time (2 years) prove that they can reach those figures. Similarly, those with good results must prove that they are still producing good results [13].

Summary and Conclusion

The whole infrastructure of rectal cancer treatment in Sweden has changed dramatically due to the awareness of the local recurrence rate, good surgical technique, and selective use of radiotherapy. Surgeons have been trained in a proper way, and it has been proven that the outcome has improved enormously in our country [14]. Due to repeated reports from the SRCR to each unit, it is possible for every surgeon to follow the process. It has been shown that the outcome for not only colon cancer but also rectal cancer has improved dramatically during the last 40 years, and there is a marked improvement in survival from approximately 40% in the early 1960s to almost 60% in the late 1990s [15]. An interesting phenomenon is that the relative 5-year survival rate has, during the 5-year cohort, been better for patients with colon cancer compared to those with rectal cancer. For the last two 5-year cohorts in Sweden, 1990–1995 and 1996–2000, the results for rectal cancer patients have improved, and in the most recent cohort, rectal cancer patients are actually doing better than colon cancer patients in terms of relative survival [16]. This increase has been interpreted to be a result of much better surgery, a more selective use of radiotherapy, but most of all an awareness of the results and focus on good auditing.

This quality assurance and quality control of rectal cancer surgery is important and will be mandatory in the future for all units to not only know the results but also be able to present them in a way that patients can understand. We are facing a new generation of young patients who are familiar with the Internet and find all types of information before having surgery. It is obvious that only the best units will survive in such a competition, and the only way to be able to compete is to show good results within a good and validated population-based quality registration, as is the situation for many different diseases in Sweden today. A tremendous change has been seen in our country over the last two decades, and it is in part a result of registration and quality auditing, where the results are displayed to the surgeons.

References

1. Påhlman L, Glimelius B (1984) Local recurrence after surgical treatment for rectal carcinoma. Acta Chir Scand 150:331–335
2. Cedermark B, Johansson H, Rutqvist LE, Wilking N (1995) The Stockholm I trial of preoperative short course radiotherapy in operable rectal cancer: a prospective randomised controlled trial. Cancer 75:2269–2275
3. Påhlman L, Glimelius B (1990) Pre- or postoperative radiotherapy in rectal and rectosigmoid carcinoma—report from a randomized multicentre trial. Ann Surg 211:187–195
4. Swedish Rectal Cancer Trial (Påhlman L, Glimelius B) (1997) Improved survival with preoperative radiotherapy in resectable rectal carcinoma. N Engl J Med 336:980–987
5. Heald RJ, Karanjia ND (1992) Results of radical surgery for rectal cancer. World J Surg 16:848–57
6. Moriya Y, Hojo K, Sawada T, Koyama Y (1989) Significance of lateral node dissection for advanced rectal carcinoma at or below the peritoneal reflection. Dis Colon Rectum 32:307–315
7. Enker WE (1992) Potency, cure, and local control in the operative treatment of rectal cancer. Arch Surg 127:1396–1401
8. Dahlberg M, Glimelius B, Påhlman L (1999) Changing strategy for rectal cancer is associated with improved outcome. Br J Surg 86:379–384
9. Arbman G, Nilsson E, Hallböök O, et al (1996) Local recurrence following total mesorectal excision for rectal cancer. Br J Surg 83:375–379
10. Smedh K, Olsson L, Johansson H, Åberg C, Andersson M (2001) Reduction of postoperative morbidity and mortality in patients with rectal cancer following the introduction of a colorectal unit. Br J Surg 88:273–277
11. Bohe M, Cedermark B, Damber L, Lindmark G, Nordgren S, Påhlman L, Sjödahl R (2000) Kvalitetsregister etablerat för bättre rektalcancerbehandling. Läkartidningen (Swe) 97:3587–3591
12. Swedish Rectal Cancer Register. http://www.SOS.se/mars/kvaflik.htm (Swe).
13. Påhlman L, Sjödahl R, Dahlberg M, Öjerskog B, Bohe M, Cedermark B. (2004) How to use the outcome in The Swedish Rectal Cancer Register. Sv Kirurgi, 62: 132-134. (Swe).
14. Leander Martling A, Holm T, Rutqvist L-E, et al (2000) Effect of a surgical training programme on the outcome of rectal cancer in the County of Stockholm. Lancet 356:93–96
15. Tallbäck M, Stenbeck M, Rosén M, Barlow L, Glimelius B (2003) Cancer survival in Sweden 1960–1998 - Developments across four decades. Acta Oncologica 42:637–659
16. Birgisson H, Tallbäck M, Gunnarsson U, Påhlman L, Glimelius B (2003) Improved survival of cancer of the colon and rectum in Sweden. Colorectal Dis 5[Suppl 2]:3

Learning Curve: The Surgeon as a Prognostic Factor in Colorectal Cancer Surgery

Pietro Renzulli, Urban T. Laffer

P. Renzulli (✉)
Department of Visceral and Transplantation Surgery, Inselspital,
University of Berne, 3010 Berne, Switzerland
e-mail: pietro.renzulli@insel.ch

Abstract

The individual surgeon is an independent prognostic factor for outcome in colorectal cancer surgery. The surgeon's learning curve is therefore directly related to the patient's outcome. The exact shape of the learning curve, however, is unknown. The present study reviewed supervision, training/teaching, specialization, surgeon's caseload, and hospital's caseload as the five main surgeon- and hospital-related confounding factors for outcome, and examined their influence on the learning curve as well as their interactions and prognostic significance. All five confounding factors were related to outcome. The highest degree of evidence, however, was found for training/teaching (introduction of total mesorectal excision), specialization in colorectal surgery (special interest, board-certification, specialized colorectal cancer units), and the surgeon's caseload. Five surgeon- and hospital-related factors directly influence the surgeon's learning curve and are therefore rightly considered predictors of outcome in colorectal cancer surgery. Improvements in supervision, training/teaching, specialization, the surgeon's caseload, and the hospital's caseload will therefore translate into enhanced patient outcome.

Introduction

The individual surgeon is an independent prognostic factor for outcome in colorectal cancer surgery. The surgeon's learning curve is therefore directly related to the patient's outcome. The learning curve is a two-dimensional representation plotting the number of years of training against the outcome for any given surgical procedure and with respect to any given outcome measurement. For illustrative purposes, a learning curve has been drawn in Fig. 1. On the left-hand side we find the young and inexperienced surgeon in training, who has just graduated from university. Outcome for a patient operated on by this surgeon might be as low as 20%. With increasing years of training and accumulating experience, the young trainee will eventually become an expert surgeon with an outcome reaching almost

Recent Results in Cancer Research, Vol. 165

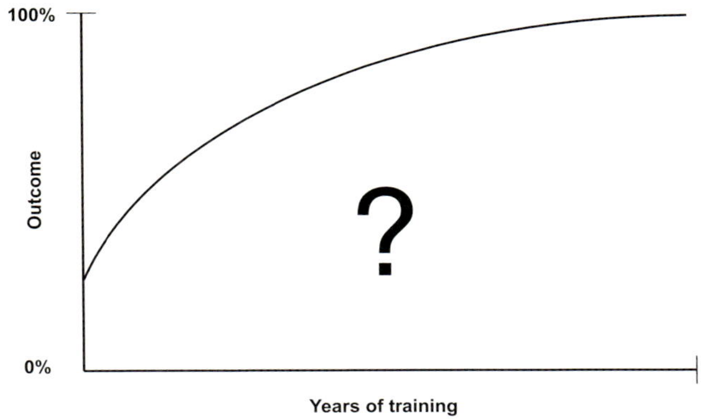

Figure 1. Learning curve

100%. Unfortunately, the exact shape of the learning curve is unknown. All factors changing the shape of the learning curve, however, will alter the patient's outcome.

Several surgeon- and hospital-related characteristics have recently been described as new prognostic factors in colorectal cancer surgery. These new predictors of outcome, in contrast to traditional prognostic factors, which are tumor- and patient-related, can be influenced positively. An improvement of these surgeon- and hospital-related factors leads to enhancement and acceleration of the surgeon's learning curve and therefore to an improvement in the patient's outcome. No attempt will therefore be made to determine the exact shape of the learning curve. The present study will focus on supervision, training/teaching, specialization, surgeon's caseload, and hospital's caseload as the five main surgeon- and hospital-related confounding factors, and will examine their influence on the learning curve as well as their interactions and prognostic significance.

Background

The surgical world was, until recently, quite simple and straightforward. A patient suffering from colorectal cancer would undergo surgery, and the only factors determining the patient's outcome would have been related to either the tumor (e.g., TNM classification, tumor grading), the patient (e.g., age, sex, co-morbidity), or the treatment (e.g., urgency of operation, type of resection, chemo-radiotherapy). The surgeon or surgeon-related factors were not part of the equation.

However, it is a long-standing and common perception of the general public as well as the medical community that there are good and not-so-good surgeons. The first reports on differences in outcome (operative mortality, anastomotic leakage, local recurrence) between individual surgeons for colorectal surgery emerged more than two decades ago (Fielding et al. 1978, 1980; Phillips et al. 1984). In 1991 McArdle and Hole published a prospective study investigating inter-surgeon variability by looking at the outcomes of individual surgeons. Thirteen consultants, none of whom had a special interest in colorectal surgery, operated on 645 patients with colorectal cancer. Outcome differed tremendously between the individual surgeons. The rate of curative resection varied from 40% to 76%, postoperative mortality from 0% to 20%, local recurrence from 0% to 21%, anastomotic leakage from 0% to 25%, and survival at 10 years from 20% to 63%. These important differences in outcome were not entirely explained by differences in patient population (case-mix, e.g., more advanced tumor stage). The existence of a significant inter-surgeon variability was hereby proven.

The individual surgeon was later identified as an independent prognostic factor for the frequency of locoregional recurrence and survival in rectal cancer patients by applying multiple logistic regression analysis adjusting for case mix differences (Hermanek et al. 1995). A great number of publications followed, investigating the prognostic role of the surgeon as well as of surgeon- and hospital-related factors (e.g., board certification, subspecialty training, annual caseload, teaching status).

Most tumor-related, patient-related, and treatment-related predictors of outcome cannot be altered. The majority of surgeon- and hospital-related factors, however, can be influenced positively. Herein lies great promise, since an enhancement of surgeon- and hospital-related factors will lead to a significant improvement in the patient's outcome.

Supervision

It is generally accepted that colorectal cancer surgery performed by young surgeons in training will be less successful and effective than such surgery performed by experienced and well-trained senior surgeons. Supervision of surgeons in training, however, may help to bridge this difference in experience and surgical expertise. Two recent publications address the issue of supervision for colorectal cancer surgery.

The first publication, from Edinburgh, UK, reviewed the results of 245 consecutive patients with colorectal cancer undergoing surgery by either a consultant (a general surgeon with colorectal interest), a supervised surgical trainee, or an independent surgical trainee (Singh and Aitken 1999). A supervised operation was one in which the consultant was scrubbed and actively assisting the surgical trainee. The study did not control for tumor and patient characteristics, and there was a clear patient selection bias which was believed to be inevitable and even desirable, as stated by the authors. Any given operation was therefore allocated to a junior or senior surgical trainee, with or without supervision by a consultant dependent on the accumulated experience of the trainee as well as the expected difficulties of the surgery. There was a comparatively high proportion of supervised operations, as 28.6% of all resections, and 51.1% of those undertaken by trainees, were consultant supervised. This proportion was higher than that reported in the Lothian and Borders Large Bowel Cancer Project (13.9% and 31.5%, respectively) as well as for recent UK colorectal cancer audits (7.6% and 17.4%) (Aitken et al. 1999). The study showed no difference between operations by the consultant, by supervised trainees, and by independent trainees in terms of 30-day mortality (6.5%, 6%, and 4%, respectively), clinical anastomotic leakage rate

(9%, 2%, and 5%), local recurrence rate (2%, 3% and 7%), and adjusted 5-year disease-related survival rate. Therefore it was concluded that, with careful patient selection and patient allocation, properly supervised trainees could resect a high proportion of colorectal cancers without compromising immediate outcome or long-term survival.

The second publication reviewed 194 rectal cancer patients (Tytherleigh et al. 2002). Six consultants operated on 126 patients, and six supervised surgical specialist registrars operated on 68 patients. Supervision always meant that the consultants were scrubbed for the operation and actively assisting. Comparing the outcome between the two groups, there were no differences in postoperative morbidity/mortality, local recurrence rates, or crude survival.

Both publications showed that supervision of surgical trainees significantly improved outcome and effectively compensated for the lack in experience. Taking into consideration the important improvement in outcome by supervision, it is likely that supervision will also improve outcomes of board-certified surgeons. Therefore, it may be desirable that even fully certified surgeons ask for the assistance of a senior specialist surgeon, at least for the critical surgical steps of a difficult operation.

Training/Teaching

The best illustration for the importance of training and teaching was the introduction of the total mesorectal excision (TME) technique for the treatment of rectal cancer, leading to an increase in the rate of sphincter preservation (Lehander Martling et al. 2000) and enhanced preservation of male genital function (Maurer et al. 2001) as well as a decrease in local recurrence and an increase in survival (Arbman et al. 1996; Kapiteijn et al. 2002; Wibe et al. 2003; Lehander Martling et al. 2000). Two Scandinavian studies and one Dutch study have documented the impact of training and teaching on the patient's outcome by the introduction of the TME technique for rectal cancer surgery.

The first study investigated the impact of a surgical training program on the outcomes of rectal cancer patients in the county of Stockholm, Sweden (Lehander Martling et al. 2000). In 1994, the TME concept was introduced and surgeons were trained in workshops through television-based demonstrations, histopathology sessions, and direct operative instruction by senior members of the Colorectal Research Unit from Basingstoke, UK. From 1995 to 1996, a total of 447 patients underwent TME. The outcomes at 2 years were compared with those from the Stockholm I (n=790) and II (n=542) trials investigating the value of preoperative radiotherapy as historical controls. There were no differences in 30-day mortality rate, anastomotic leakage rate, and overall postoperative morbidity, despite a decrease in the proportion of abdominoperineal resections from 55% and 60% (Stockholm I and II trials) to 27% (TME group). The rate of local recurrence at 2 years decreased significantly from 15% and 14% (Stockholm I and II trials) to 6% (TME group), as did the 2-year cancer-related mortality rate (15% and 16% to 9%).

The second publication reported on the introduction of the TME technique in Norway (Wibe et al. 2003). The results of rectal cancer surgery in Norway have been poor. The rate of local recurrence amounted to 28% following treatment with a curative intent. Five-year overall survival was 55% for patients younger than 75 years according to a national audit for the period 1986–1988. In 1994, the Norwegian Rectal Cancer Group was founded. The TME technique was implemented on a national level. All surgeons were taught the TME technique in courses, and pathologists were trained in both macroscopic and microscopic assessment of specimens. A rectal cancer registry was established. A total of 3,432 patients underwent rectal resection with a curative intent from November 1993 until December 1999. Of these, 9% had adjuvant radiotherapy and 2% were given chemotherapy. There was a rapid implementation of the new technique; the percentage of patients undergoing TME increased from 78% in 1994 to 96% in 1998. After 39 months' mean follow-up, the rate of local recurrence was 8%, and 5-year overall survival was 71% for patients younger than 75 years.

The third study described the introduction of the TME technique in the Netherlands by the Dutch Colorectal Cancer Group (Kapiteijn et al. 2002). Surgeons were trained in workshops and symposia. Specially trained instructor-surgeons were used for local teaching and supervision. A large trial investigating short-term preoperative radiotherapy combined with the TME technique for resectable rectal cancer was subsequently initiated (Kapiteijn et al. 2001). The outcome of patients undergoing surgery alone from the TME trial was compared to the outcome of patients from the CRAB (cancer recurrence and blood transfusion) trial. The CRAB trial (1987–1990) included 269 curatively operated patients after conventional rectal surgery, and the TME trial (1996–1999) involved 661 curatively operated patients after TME. The local recurrence rate decreased from 16% (CRAB) to 9% (TME), and the overall 2-year survival increased from 77% (CRAB) to 86% (TME). The type of operation (conventional vs. TME) remained an independent predictor of local recurrence and overall survival after adjustment for tumor and patient characteristics.

Specialization

Three different degrees of specialization in the treatment of colorectal cancer patients can be described: treatment by general surgeons with a special interest in and dedication to colorectal surgery, treatment by colorectal surgeons with subspecialty training and special board certification, and treatment by colorectal surgeons working in specialized colorectal cancer units.

Colorectal Surgery by General Surgeons

General surgeons with a special interest in colorectal surgery tend to perform a different kind of surgery.

Two publications from Glasgow, UK, studied the influence of the surgeon's specialty interest on outcome. The primary study was a pathology investigation reviewing the type of operation performed (Reinbach et al. 1994). Ten surgeons with four different specialty interests treated 116 patients for primary colorectal cancer. Surgeons with an interest in colorectal cancer resected twice as much colon (280 mm vs. 130 mm) and were more likely to perform a multivisceral resection in order to remove adjacent clinically involved organs (15% vs. 0%) for left-sided colon and rectal cancers. Distal resection margins for sigmoid cancers (55 mm vs. 20 mm) and the number of lymph nodes retrieved from the mesentery (13 nodes vs. 7.5 nodes) were significantly greater in the group of surgeons with a special interest in colorectal surgery. The subsequent study examined the long-term outcome depending on the surgeon's specialty interest (Dorrance et al. 2000). Twelve surgeons, with different specialty interests, treated 378 patients for primary colorectal cancer over a 4-year period. There were six surgeons with a vascular or transplant emphasis, four surgeons with a general background, and two surgeons with colorectal subspecialty interest. They operated on 126, 98, and 154 patients, respectively. A significant association between colorectal specialty interest and a reduced local and overall recurrence rate was found. Patients operated on by a surgeon with a general background were 3.42 times more likely to develop a local recurrence than those operated on by a surgeon with a colorectal interest. It is, however, important to notice the difference in the individual caseload for vascular/transplant, general, and colorectal surgery-interested surgeons (21, 24.5, and 77 patients/study period, respectively)—a difference that may have contributed to the differences in outcome. Surgeons with a special interest in and dedication to colorectal surgery seem to be more familiar with the guidelines for colon and rectal cancer surgery, which recently have been critically reviewed and published by the American National Cancer Institute (Nelson et al. 2001). This familiarity translates into a different kind of resection performed, resulting in enhanced radicality in accordance with the principles of surgical oncology (Reinbach et al. 1994), and eventually leads to an improvement in the patient's outcome (Dorrance et al. 2000).

The Royal College of Surgeons of England and the Association of Coloproctology of Great Britain and Ireland published recommended treatment outcomes for colorectal cancer surgery (Royal College of Surgeons and Association of Coloproctology, 1996). These criteria demand an operative mortality of less than 5% for elective surgery, an anastomotic leak rate of less than 8% after anterior resection and less than 4% for other anastomoses, a wound infection rate below 10% after elective surgery, and a local recurrence rate inferior to 10% after curative resection.

Two publications by nonspecialist surgeons reported results in accordance with the above-mentioned recommendations. The first study reviewed patients with colonic and rectal cancer treated by nonspecialist surgeons (Singh et al. 1997). Between 1987 and 1991, four general surgeons, none of whom was a specialist in colorectal surgery, operated on 267 patients and achieved a rate of intraperitoneal sepsis of 1%, a clinical anastomotic dehiscence rate of 3%, and postoperative mortality rates after elective and emergency surgery of 2% and 13%, respectively. The 5-year disease-related survival rates for curative and palliative surgery were 67%

and 9%, respectively. There were no significant differences between the surgeons. The authors concluded that nonspecialist surgeons in a district general hospital could obtain acceptable results. The need for further specialization and centralization was questioned.

The second study originated from a district general hospital before the era of surgical specialization (Saha et al. 2002). A single gastrointestinal surgeon operated on 73 consecutive rectal cancer patients over a 5-year period and reported an operative mortality of 4.1%, an anastomotic leak rate of 6.2%, a wound infection rate of 2.7%, and a pelvic recurrence rate after curative resection of 9.6%. The authors concluded that trained gastrointestinal surgeons could achieve good results with acceptable complication rates outside the setting of a specialist unit.

Both studies reported results in accordance with the recommendations mentioned above. However, it is important to notice that in both studies the surgeons can be considered as high-caseload surgeons. In the first study the individual annual caseload for colonic and rectal cancer amounted to 13.4 patients, and in the second study the individual annual caseload for rectal cancer alone amounted to an impressive 14.6 patients. Whereas the surgeons in both studies considered themselves nonspecialists, it can be assumed that the good results achieved are partly explained by the high-caseload figures.

Board Certification in Colorectal Surgery

Surgery is becoming increasingly complex, and subspecialization is therefore often considered necessary. The American Society of Colon and Rectal Surgeons was founded in 1899. Thus subspecialty training in colorectal surgery and subsequent specialist board certification has a long tradition in the United States. In contrast to the North American situation, subspecialty training in visceral surgery is just being introduced in Switzerland. Table 1 summarizes the major publications that investigated the impact of colorectal subspecialty training on outcome. Specialization in colorectal surgery led to a significant reduction in in-hospital mortality (Rosen et al. 1996; Callahan et al. 2003) and an increase in sphincter preservation (Read et al. 2002). Concerning long-term outcome, specialization led to a significant reduction in the rate of local recurrence (Porter et al. 1998; Read et al. 2002) and an increase in survival (Porter et al. 1998; Read et al. 2002; Bokey et al. 1997). There are compelling data showing that even after adjusting for case mix differences as well as caseload, subspecialty training in colorectal surgery remains an independent prognostic factor for outcome.

Specialized Colorectal Cancer Units

The formation of specialized colorectal cancer units was the next logical step in an attempt to improve the patient's outcome. Two Swedish studies and one Spanish study compared the results for rectal cancer surgery before and after the

Table 1. Specialization in colorectal surgery

Publication	Setting	Surgeons	Outcome measure
Rosen et al. 1996	1986–1994, MC, 2805 P, CRC	1565 P/6 colorectal surgeons, 1240 P/33 other surgeons	↓ In-hospital mortality
Bokey et al. 1997	1971–1994, SC, 709 P, RC	428 P/n colorectal surgeons, 281 P/n other surgeons	↑ Long-term survival
Porter et al. 1998	1983–1990, MC, 683 P, RC	109 P/5 colorectal surgeons, 574 P/47 other surgeons	↓ Local recurrence, ↑ Disease-specific survival
Read et al. 2002	1977–1995, MC, 384 P, RC	251 P/5 colorectal surgeons, 133 P/68 other surgeons	↓ Local recurrence, ↑ disease-free survival, ↑ Sphincter preservation
Callahan et al. 2003	1998–2001, MC, 48582 P, CR	4757 P/61 colorectal surgeons, 43771 P/2590 other surgeons	↓ In-hospital mortality
Smith JAE et al. 2003	1991–1994, MC, 4562 P, CRC	2100 P/12 colorectal surgeons, 2462 P/65 other surgeons	↓ 30-day mortality, ↓ Anastomotic leakage, ↑ Local recurrence-free survival, ↑ Long-term survival

MC, multicenter; SC, single-center; P, patients; RC, rectal cancer; CRC, colorectal cancer; CR, colon resection.
↓ Reduction, decrease in outcome for patients operated on by colorectal surgeons/specialists.
↑ Improvement, increase in outcome for patients operated on by colorectal surgeons/specialists.

formation of a specialized colorectal cancer unit. The common feature of these three publications was that fewer specialized surgeons treated a greater number of patients, which resulted in an increase of both the individual surgeon's caseload as well as the hospital's caseload.

The first study reviewed the results from the county of Västmanland, Sweden (Smedh et al. 2001). Between 1993 and 1996, 133 patients were operated on at four county hospitals. After centralization, 144 patients were operated on at the new colorectal unit in the county central hospital from 1996 to 1999, supervised by a colorectal surgeon. The number of operating surgeons was reduced from 26 to four. There was a significant reduction in the postoperative mortality rate (8% vs. 1%), the total postoperative complication rate (57% vs. 24%), the number of surgical complications (37% vs. 11%), the relaparotomy rate (11% vs. 4%), and the postoperative hospital stay (13 days vs. 9 days).

The second report originated from the Ersta Hospital, Sweden (Machado et al. 2000). During the first period (1990–1992), 18 general surgeons operated on 72 patients with rectal cancer. Substantial changes in the treatment strategy of rectal cancer were implemented (increased use of preoperative radiotherapy, standardized surgical technique, concentration of the surgery to a limited number of colorectal surgeons). Thereafter, 180 patients were treated in the newly created colorectal cancer unit between 1994 and 1996, and two colorectal surgeons treated more than 90% of these patients. This specialization led to a significant decrease in permanent stoma formation (52% vs. 33%) and in the rate of local recurrence (18% vs. 3%). There was no increase in the frequency of postoperative complications, reoperations or pelvic sepsis, although more extensive surgery was used and the anastomotic level decreased from 8 to 4 cm ($p<0.001$). Furthermore, cancer-specific survival at two years increased significantly.

The third study was conducted in Valencia, Spain (Garcia-Granero et al. 2001). During a first period from 1986 to 1991, fourteen general surgeons operated on 94 patients with rectal cancer. Thereafter a Colorectal Surgery Unit was established. During the second period (1992–1995), four specialized surgeons operated on 108 patients. This resulted in a reduction of the abdominoperineal resection rate (25.8% to 16.7%) and an increase in the radical resectability rate (67.7% to 82.4%). Local recurrence after low anterior resection was reduced from 30% to 9%, and cancer-specific 5-year survival increased from 61% to 87%.

Surgeon's Caseload

Surgical expertise is acquired through practice. The more operations a surgeon is able to perform, the better the outcome for the patient. A positive beneficial relationship between a higher individual surgeon's caseload and better outcome is generally assumed.

Two multicenter trials investigated the influence of the surgeon's caseload on survival by studying the outcome of 3217 colorectal cancer patients from Northern Ireland (Kee et al. 1999) and 927 from the UK (Parry et al. 1999). Both trials failed to show any influence of caseload on survival. However, the large majority of publications seem to support a positive caseload–outcome relationship in colorectal cancer surgery.

Table 2 summarizes the major publications that have investigated the influence of the surgeon's caseload on outcome. A higher surgeon's caseload was positively linked to a reduction in the anastomotic leakage rate (Consultants 1995), a reduction of in-hospital mortality (Harmon et al. 1999; Ko et al. 2002; Hannan et al. 2002), a reduction in hospital stay and cost (Harmon et al. 1999), a reduction in the local recurrence rate (Hermanek et al. 1995; Porter et al. 1998; Stocchi et al. 2001; Martling et al. 2002), and an increase in survival (Porter et al. 1998; Martling et al. 2002; Schrag et al. 2002). There is today an impressive body of evidence showing that after adjustment for case mix differences, the surgeon's caseload confidently can be considered an independent prognostic factor for both short- and long-term outcome.

Interaction of Training/Teaching and Surgeon's Caseload

Conventional blunt surgical resection of rectal cancer is linked to a high rate of local recurrence and to an important inter-surgeon variability (McArdle and Hole 1991). It was reasonable to expect that through the introduction of the standardized TME technique, the intersurgeon variability wound be substantially reduced or even eliminated. A recent study from Stockholm, Sweden, reviewed 652 patients with rectal cancer who underwent TME (Martling et al. 2002). All surgeons were trained in the TME technique in workshops. Nevertheless, high-caseload surgeons (>12 operations/year) had a reduced rate of local recurrence (4% vs. 10%) and a reduced rate of rectal cancer death (11% vs. 18%). Intersurgeon variability persisted even after the introduction of the standardized TME technique. Therefore, both training and caseload must be regarded as prognostic factors for outcome, and it is not sufficient to be only a well-trained surgeon—it is necessary to be a well-trained surgeon with a high annual caseload.

Interaction of Specialization and Surgeon's Caseload

Specialization in colorectal surgery and the surgeon's annual caseload have both been shown to positively influence outcome. A Canadian study investigated the interaction between both prognostic factors by reviewing the results of 683 rectal cancer patients (Porter et al. 1998). The risk of local recurrence was increased for those patients operated on by non-colorectal-trained surgeons (hazard ratio 2.49) as well as for patients operated on by low-caseload surgeons (hazard ratio 1.80). Patients operated on by low-caseload and non-colorectal-trained surgeons had an observed hazard ratio for local recurrence of 4.29. This figure correlated closely with the calculated hazard ratio for local recurrence of 4.48 (2.49×1.80). A corresponding calculation was valid for the hazard ratios of survival. Therefore it was concluded that both co-variables were independent prognostic factors for outcome in rectal cancer surgery. For that reason, it is not sufficient to be a good

Table 2. Surgeon's caseload in colorectal surgery

Publication	Setting	Cut-off value for caseload	Outcome measure
Consultants 1995	1990–1992, MC, 260 P, RC	131 P/2 years/5 surgeons, 129 P/2 years/23 surgeons	↓ Anastomotic leakage
Hermanek et al. 1995	1984–1986, MC, 1121 P, RC	6.4 P/year	↓ Local recurrence, ↑ 5-year survival, no effect on 5-year cancer survival and overall survival
Grabham et al. 1996	1991–1994, MC, 603 P, RC	10 P/year	↓ Anastomotic leakage
Porter et al. 1998	1983–1990, MC, 683 P, RC	2.6 P/year	↓ Local recurrence, ↑ Disease-specific survival
Parry et al. 1999	1993, MC, 927 P, CRC	$\leq$ 6, 7–12, 13–18, $\geq$ 19 P/6 months	No effect on sphincter preservation and overall survival
Kee et al. 1999	1990–1994, MC, 3217 P, CRC	$\leq$ 9.7, 9.8–12.7, 12.8–16.1, 16.2–24.9, $\geq$ 25 P/year	No effect on 2-year overall survival
Harmon et al. 1999	1992–1996, MC, 9739 P, CRC	$\leq$ 5, 5–10, $\geq$ 10 P/year	↓ In-hospital mortality, ↓ Hospital stay, ↓ Cost
Stocchi et al. 2001	1979–1992, MC, 673 P, RC	10 P/study period	↓ 5-year local recurrence
Ko et al. 2002	1996, MC, 22408 P, CC	Continuous variable, mean 10.8±7.8 P/year	↓ In-hospital mortality
Hannan et al. 2002	1994–1997, MC, 3711 P, CC	$\leq$ 11, 12–20, 21–34, $\geq$ 35 P/4 years	↓ In-hospital mortality
Martling et al. 2002	1995–1997, MC, 652 P, RC	12 P/year	↓ Local recurrence, ↓ Rectal cancer death, no effect on postoperative mortality and anastomotic leakage
Schrag et al. 2002	1992–1996, MC, 2815 P, RC	1, 2, 3–5, 6–26 P/5 years	↓ 2-year mortality, ↑ Overall survival, no effect on 30-day mortality and sphincter preservation

MC, multicenter; P, patients; RC, rectal cancer; CC, colon cancer; CRC, colorectal cancer.
↓ Reduction, decrease in outcome for patients operated on by high-caseload surgeons.
↑ Improvement, increase in outcome for patients operated on by high-caseload surgeons.

colorectal surgeon—it is necessary to be a good colorectal surgeon performing a large number of colorectal cancer surgeries.

Hospital's Caseload

The outcome for complex surgical procedures is not only dependent on the surgeon's skill and expertise but also on the experience of an interdisciplinary team. Therefore the outcome is considerably influenced by the hospital's caseload. A positive relationship between a higher hospital caseload and an improved outcome has been found for esophagectomy, pancreatic resection, resection for lung cancer, and liver transplantation (Birkmeyer et al. 2002; Bach et al. 2001; Begg et al. 1998; Edwards et al. 1999; Ho and Heslin 2003). However, it can be argued that the outcome in colorectal cancer surgery is largely dependent on the surgeon's skill and less on the hospital's infrastructure (e.g., an experienced interdisciplinary team with gastroenterologists, radiologists, oncologists, anesthesiologists, critical care specialists, specialized nursing professionals). Whereas the surgeon's caseload can confidently be considered an independent prognostic factor for outcome, the impact of the hospital's caseload is somewhat less clear. Table 3 summarizes the major publications that have investigated the influence of the hospital's caseload on outcome. Several studies were unable to find any influence of greater hospital caseload on survival for patients with colorectal cancer (Kee et al. 1999; Parry et al. 1999; Simunovic et al. 2000). Evidence, however, is slowly increasing that the caseload of an individual hospital might be an independent prognostic factor. Investigators found a reduction of in-hospital mortality (Hannan et al. 2002; Schrag et al. 2000; Ko et al. 2002; Marusch et al. 2001b; Hodgson et al. 2003), an increase in sphincter preservation (Simons et al. 1997; Marusch et al. 2001a; Hodgson et al. 2003), an increase in survival (Simons et al. 1997; Schrag et al. 2000; Hodgson et al. 2003), and a borderline nonsignificant reduction in local recurrence (Holm et al. 1997) for hospitals with higher colorectal cancer caseloads.

Interaction of Surgeon's Caseload and Hospital's Caseload

A study from The Johns Hopkins Hospital, Baltimore, Maryland, drew attention to the interaction between the individual surgeon's caseload and the hospital's caseload (Harmon et al. 1999). During a 5-year period, 812 surgeons at 50 hospitals performed 9739 resections for colorectal carcinoma. The annual surgeon's caseload was stratified into low (≤ 5), medium (5–10), and high (>10). Hospitals were stratified into low (<40), medium (40–70), and high (>70) caseload institutions. A higher surgeon's caseload was associated with a significant improvement in all three outcome measurements (in-hospital death, length of stay, cost) after multivariate analysis and adjustment for variations in type of resections performed, cancer stage, patient co-morbidities, urgency of admission, and patient demographics. Interestingly, medium-caseload surgeons achieved excellent outcomes similar to high-caseload surgeons when operating in medium-caseload or high-

Table 3. Hospital's caseload in colorectal surgery

Publication	Setting	Cut-off value for caseload	Outcome measure
Holm et al. 1997	1980–1993, 1399 P, RC	≤ 5, 6–10, ≥ 10 P/year	↓ Local recurrence (borderline significance $p = 0.06$)
Simons et al. 1997	1988–1992, 2006 P, RC	≤ 5, ≥ 5 P/year	↑ Spincter preservation, ↑ Survival
Kee et al. 1999	1990–1994, 3217 P, CRC	≤ 23, 24–32, 33–46, 47–54, ≥ 55 P/year	No effect on 2-year overall survival
Parry et al. 1999	1993, 927 P, CRC	≤ 30, 31–44, 45–55, ≥ 56 P/6 months	No effect on sphincter preservation or overall survival
Khuri et al. 1999	1991–1993, 13310 P, CR	≤ 13, 13–22, 23–30, 31–52 P/year	No effect on 30-day mortality
Schrag et al. 2000	1991–1996, 27986 P, CC	≤ 57, 58–112, 113–165, 166–383 P/6 years	↓ 30-day mortality, ↑ Overall and cancer-specific long-term survival
Simunovic et al. 2000	1990, 1072 P, RC	≤ 11, 12–17, ≥ 18 P/year	No effect on operative mortality and long-term overall survival
Marusch et al. 2001a	1999, 1463 P, RC	≤ 20, 20–40, ≥ 40 P/year	↓ Postoperative morbidity, ↓ Permanent stoma formation, no effect on complications that required reoperation (afterbleeds, burst abdomen, ileus, anastomotic leakage)
Marusch et al. 2001b	1999, 2293 P, CC	≤ 30, 31–60, ≥ 60 P/year	↓ General postoperative complications, no effect on resection rate, intraoperative complications, in-hospital mortality
Ko et al. 2002	1995, 22408 P, CC	Continuous variable, mean 60 ± 41 P/year	↓ In-hospital mortality
Hannan et al. 2002	1994–1997, 3711 P, CC	≤ 83, 84–144, 145–253, ≥ 254 P/4 years	↓ In-hospital mortality
Birkmeyer et al. 2002	1994–1999, 304285 P, CR	≤ 33, 33–56, 57–84, 85–124, ≥ 124 P/year	↓ In-hospital mortality
Hodgson et al. 2003	1994–1997, 7257 P, RC	≤ 7, 7–13, 14–20, ≥ 20 P/year	↓ Permanent colostomy formation, ↓ 30-day mortality, ↑ 2-year survival

P: patients, RC: rectal cancer, CC: colon cancer, CRC: colorectal cancer, CR: colon resection
↓ reduction, decrease in outcome for patients operated on in high-caseload hospitals
↑ improvement, increase in outcome for patients operated on in high-caseload hospitals

caseload hospitals, but not in low-caseload hospitals. The results of low-caseload surgeons improved with increasing hospital caseload but never equaled those of the high-caseload surgeons.

A second study investigated the relative importance of surgeons' and hospitals' caseloads on short- and long-term outcome following rectal cancer resection (Schrag et al. 2000). The outcomes of 2,815 rectal cancer patients were reviewed. Neither hospital-specific nor surgeon-specific caseload was significantly associated with 30-day postoperative mortality or rates of sphincter-sparing surgery. Although an association between hospital caseload and mortality at 2 years was evident, this finding was no longer significant once the surgeon's caseload was controlled for. In contrast, a higher surgeon's caseload was associated with a reduced 2-year mortality, and the surgeon's caseload remained an important predictor of outcome even after adjustment for the hospital's caseload. The surgeon's caseload proved to be superior to the hospital's caseload in predicting long-term survival. The authors concluded that in order to improve outcome following rectal cancer resection, greater emphasis should be placed on understanding surgeon-specific rather than hospital-specific practice patterns.

The Relative Importance of Caseload on Outcome

Relying on the data of the Healthcare Cost and Utilization Program, a large study from the United States reviewed 22,408 patients with colon cancer for in-hospital mortality (Ko et al. 2002). A multivariate logistic regression model was applied, adjusting for more than 30 different independent variables, including demographic factors (e.g., age, gender, race, ethnicity, socio-economic status), burden of morbid and co-morbid disease (prevalence and severity), and provider variables (e.g., hospital size, location, teaching status, surgeon's and hospital's caseload). The baseline probability analysis showed a mortality rate for the baseline colon cancer patient of 12 in 1,000. Being operated on by a high-caseload surgeon or in a high-caseload hospital reduced the mortality to 10 in 1,000 and 11 in 1,000, respectively. However, if this baseline colon cancer patient had coexistent liver disease or required an emergency operation, mortality increased to 44 in 1,000 and 45 in 1,000, respectively. The authors concluded that although both surgeon and hospital caseloads were independent prognostic factors for in-hospital mortality, their relative impact on outcome was rather small as compared to other confounding factors such as co-morbidity and emergency operation.

Defining Caseload Threshold Values

The Leapfrog Group, a consortium of more than 100 large employers in the United States, has set up arbitrary caseload thresholds for hospitals performing coronary artery bypass grafts (500 patients/year), coronary angioplasties (400 patients/year), abdominal aortic aneurysm repairs (30 patients/year), carotid endarterectomies (100 patients/year), and esophagectomies (seven patients/year). These threshold recommendations were recently critically reviewed (Christian et al. 2003). As for colorectal cancer, threshold values have not yet been established, either for the surgeon's or for the hospital's caseload. The vast majority of publications listed in Tables 2 and 3 describe a gradual improvement in outcome with increasing caseload. Caseload thresholds, however, were not defined.

Discussion

The individual surgeon is an independent prognostic factor in colorectal cancer surgery. The surgeon's learning curve is therefore directly related to the patient's outcome. The exact shape of the learning curve is unknown. Several surgeon- and hospital-related factors, however, might positively influence the learning curve and therefore enhance the patient's outcome. A beneficial relationship between supervision, teaching/training, specialization in colorectal surgery, higher surgeon caseload, higher hospital caseload, and improvements in different outcome measurements has been established. The whole issue, which is extremely policy-relevant, has generated huge interest even beyond the medical community. An impressive number of excellent publications have appeared in the most prestigious medical journals. The evidence seems to be overwhelming.

However, several potential shortcomings of the cited publications deserve to be mentioned. The majority of publications included only patients with rectal cancer; some, however, extended their analyses to patients with colon cancer or to patients undergoing colon resection for whatever reason. Most studies were retrospective, and an important number of studies were based on large but rather unsophisticated administrative databases. Elaborate adjustments for differences in case mix by multivariate logistic regression models were not always performed. End-point measurements were often limited to short-term outcome (e.g., in-hospital mortality) or crude survival (e.g., overall survival instead of cancer-specific disease-free survival). The definitions of surgeons with colorectal interest as well as specialist surgeons were not always precise. Cut-off values defining low- and high-caseload surgeons as well as low- and high-caseload hospitals showed an important and somewhat disturbing diversity. Several studies considered only one surgeon- or hospital-related factor without adjustment for the other potential confounding factors (e.g., only hospital's caseload investigated, but not surgeon's caseload or specialization).

Despite these limitations, all five surgeon- and hospital-related confounding factors can today be considered as significant and mostly independent predictors of outcome in colorectal cancer surgery.

The prognosis of colorectal cancer is largely determined by factors related to the tumor (e.g., TNM classification, tumor grading) and the patient (e.g., age, sex, co-morbidity). These factors cannot significantly be influenced. The relative prognostic importance of surgeon- and hospital-related factors might be rather small (Ko et al. 2002). However, these surgeon- and hospital-related characteristics are the only predictors of outcome that can be influenced in a way benefiting the patient.

Policy makers and surgical leaders will have to decide which prognostic factors they would like to promote in order to improve the outcomes of their patients. They may enhance the supervision of trainees and even extend the supervision to board-certified surgeons. They may invest in teaching and training by organizing colorectal cancer workshops, video-conferencing, and expert-surgeon instruction, or by promoting colorectal fellowships at centers of excellence. Furthermore, they may choose to introduce a certain degree of specialization. The establishment of subspecialty training in visceral surgery may be a first step. Some countries may even proceed further and launch colorectal subspecialty training. Eventually, specialized colorectal cancer units may be founded. However, policymakers and surgical leaders won't be able to completely elude the caseload–outcome relationship for the individual surgeon as well as for a specific hospital. since the most convincing evidence so far has been produced for this association. A low surgeon or hospital caseload may be compensated for by intensified supervision or by improved training and teaching. However, most surgeon- and hospital-related factors are, at least on a practical level, interdependent, and neither supervision nor training/teaching nor specialization is possible without an adequate caseload. The caseload–outcome relationship has been discussed in a recent editorial commenting on a publication linking the hospital's caseload to the rate of permanent stoma formation and survival (Hodgson et al. 2003). The authors (Smith TJ et al. 2003) stressed the importance of the caseload–outcome relationship, and wrote that "it is time for us to take our heads out of the colostomy bag, and take some action."

Therefore, the surgeon's learning curve in colorectal cancer can and should be effectively altered and accelerated by promoting improvements in all five surgeon- and hospital-related characteristics.

Conclusion

Five surgeon- and hospital-related factors directly influence the surgeon's learning curve and are therefore rightly considered predictors of outcome in colorectal cancer surgery. Improvements in supervision, training/teaching, specialization, the surgeon's caseload, and the hospital's caseload will therefore translate into enhanced patient outcome.

References

Aitken RJ, Thompson MR, Smith JAE, Radcliffe AG, Stamatakis J, Steele RJC (1999) Training in large bowel cancer surgery: observations from three prospective regional United Kingdom audits. BMJ 318:702–703

Arbman G, Nilsson E, Hallböök O, Sjödahl R (1996) Local recurrence following total mesorectal excision for rectal cancer. Br J Surg 83:375–379

Bach PB, Cramer LD, Schrag D, Downey RJ, Gelfand SE, Begg CB (2001) The influence of hospital volume on survival after resection for lung cancer. N Engl J Med 345:181–188

Begg CB, Cramer LD, Hoskins WJ, Brennan MF (1998) Impact of hospital volume on operative mortality for major cancer surgery. JAMA 280:1747–1751

Birkmeyer JD, Siewers AE, Finlayson EVA, Stukel TA, Lucas FL, Batista I, Welch HG, Wennberg DE (2002) Hospital volume and surgical mortality in the United States. N Engl J Med 346:1128–1137

Bokey EL, Chapuis PH, Dent OF, Newland RC, Koorey SG, Zelas PJ, Stewart PJ (1997) Factors affecting survival after excision of the rectum for cancer: a multivariate analysis. Dis Colon Rectum 40:3–10

Callahan MA, Christos PJ, Gold HT, Mushlin AI, Daly JM (2003) Influence of surgical subspeciality training on in-hospital mortality for gastrectomy and colectomy patients. Ann Surg 238:629–639

Christian CK, Gustafson ML, Betensky RA, Daley J, Zinner MJ (2003) The Leapfrog volume criteria may fall short in identifying high-quality surgical centers. Ann Surg 238;447–457

Dorrance HR, Docherty GM, O'Dwyer PJ (2000) Effect of surgeon specialty interest on patient outcome after potentially curative colorectal cancer surgery. Dis Colon Rectum 43:492–498

Edwards EB, Roberts JP, McBride MA, Schulak JA, Hunsicker LG (1999) The effect of the volume of procedures at transplantation centers on mortality after liver transplantation. N Engl J Med 341:2049–2053

Fielding LP, Stewart-Brown S, Dudley HAF (1978) Surgeon-related variables and the clinical trial. Lancet 2:778–779

Fielding LP, Stewart-Brown S, Blesovsky L, Kearney G (1980) Anastomotic integrity after operations for large-bowel cancer: A multicentre study. Br Med J 281:411–414

Garcia-Granero E, Marti-Obiol R, Gomez-Barbadillo J, Garcia-Armengol J, Esclapez P, Espi A, Jiménez E, Millan M, Lledo S (2001) Impact of surgeon organization and specialization in rectal cancer outcome. Colorectal Disease 3:179–184

Grabham JA, Coleman MG, Moss S, Thompson MR (1996) Wessex colorectal cancer audit: anastomotic leakage following elective anterior resection. Br J Surg 83:Suppl.1, 22–23

Hannan EL, Radzyner M, Rubin D, Dougherty J, Brennan MF (2002) The influence of hospital and surgeon volume on in-hospital mortality for colectomy, gastrectomy, and lung lobectomy in patients with cancer. Surgery 131:6–15

Harmon JW, Tang DG, Gordon TA, Bowman HM; Choti MA, Kaufman HS, Bender JS, Duncan MD, Magnuson TH, Lillemoe KD, Cameron JL (1999) Hospital volume can serve as a surrogate for surgeon volume for achieving excellent outcomes in colorectal resection. Ann Surg 230:404–411; discussion 411–413

Hermanek P, Wiebelt H, Staimmer D, Riedl S, German Study Group Colo-Rectal Carcinoma (SGCRC) (1995) Prognostic factors of rectum carcinoma—experience of the German multicentre study SGCRC. Tumori 81:Suppl. 60–64

Ho V, Heslin MJ (2003) Effect of hospital volume and experience on in-hospital mortality for pancreaticoduodenectomy. Ann Surg 237:509–514

Hodgson DC, Zhang W, Zaslavsky AM, Fuchs CS, Wright WE, Ayanian JZ (2003) Relation of hospital volume to colostomy rates and survival for patients with rectal cancer. J Natl Cancer Inst 95:708–716

Holm T, Johansson H, Cedermark B, Ekelund G, Rutqvist LE (1997) Influence of hospital- and surgeon-related factors on outcome after treatment of rectal cancer with or without preoperative radiotherapy. Br J Surg 84:657–663

Kapiteijn E, Marijnen CA, Nagtegaal ID, Putter H, Steup WH, Wiggers T, Rutten HJ, Pahlman L, Glimelius B, van Krieken JH, Leer JW, van de Velde CJ, Dutch Colorectal Cancer Group (2001) Preoperative radiotherapy combined with total mesorectal excision for resectable rectal cancer. N Engl J Med 345:638–646

Kapiteijn E, Putter H, van de Velde CJH (2002) Impact of the introduction and training of total mesorectal excision on recurrence and survival in rectal cancer in The Netherlands. Br J Surg 89:1142–1149

Kee F, Wilson RH, Harper C, Patterson CC, McCallion K, Houston RF, Moorehead RJ, Sloan JM, Rowlands BJ (1999) Influence of hospital and clinician workload on survival from colorectal cancer: cohort study. BMJ 318:1381–1386

Khuri SF, Daley J, Henderson W, Hur K, Hossain M, Soybel D, Kizer KW, Aust JB, Bell RH, Chong V, Demakis J, Fabri PJ, Gibbs JO, Grover F, Hammermeister K, McDonald G, Passaro E, Phillips L, Scamman F, Spencer J, Stremple JF and the participants in the VA National Surgical Quality Improvement Program (1999) Relation of surgical volume to outcome in eight common operations. Results from the VA National Surgical Quality Improvement Program. Ann Surg 230;414–432

Ko CY, Chang JT, Chaudhry S, Kominski G (2002) Are high-volume surgeons and hospitals the most important predictors of in-hospital outcome for colon cancer resection ? Surgery 132:268–273

Lehander Martling A, Holm T, Rutqvist LE, Moran RJ, Heald RJ, Cedermark B (2000) Effect of a surgical training programme on outcome of rectal cancer in the county of Stockholm. Lancet 356:93–96

Machado M, Goldman S, Järhult J (2000) Improved results in rectal cancer surgery—an effect of specialization ? Colorectal Disease 2:264–269

Martling A, Cedermark B, Johansson H, Rutqvist LE, Holm T (2002) The surgeon as a prognostic factor after the introduction of total mesorectal excision in the treatment of rectal cancer. Br J Surg 89:1008–1013

Marusch F, Koch A, Schmidt U, Pross M, Gastinger I, Lippert H (2001a) Hospital caseload and the results achieved in patients with rectal cancer. Br J Surg 88:1397–1402

Marusch F, Koch A, Schmidt U, Zippel R, Lehmann M, Czarnetzki HD, Knoop M, Pross M, Gastinger I, Lippert H (2001b) Effect of caseload on the short-term outcome of colon surgery: results of a multicenter study. Int J Colorectal Dis 16:362–369

Maurer CA, Z'graggen K, Renzulli P, Schilling MK, Netzer P, Büchler MW (2001) Total mesorectal excision preserves male genital function compared to conventional rectal cancer surgery. Br J Surg 88:1501–1505

McArdle CS, Hole D (1991) Impact of variability among surgeons on postoperative morbidity and mortality and ultimate survival. BMJ 302:1501–1505

Nelson H, Petrelli N, Carlin A, Couture J, Fleshman J, Guillem J, Miedema B, Ota D, Sargent D (2001) Guidelines for colon and rectal cancer surgery. J Natl Cancer Inst 93:583–596

Parry JM, Collins S, Mathers J, Scott NA, Woodman CBJ (1999) Influence of volume of work on the outcome of treatment for patients with colorectal cancer. Br J Surg 86:475–481

Phillips RKS, Hittinger R, Blesovsky L, Fry JS, Fielding LP (1984) Local recurrence following 'curative' surgery for large bowel cancer: I. The overall picture. Br J Surg 71:12–16

Porter GA, Soskolne CL, Yakimets WW, Newman SC (1998) Surgeon-related factors and outcome in rectal cancer. Ann Surg 227:157–167

Read TE, Myerson RJ, Fleshman JW, Fry RD, Birnbaum EH, Walz BJ, Kodner IJ (2002) Surgeon specialty is associated with outcome in rectal cancer treatment. Dis Colon Rectum 45:904–914

Reinbach DH, McGregor JR, Murray GD, O'Dwyer PJ (1994) Effect of the surgeon's specialty interest on the type of resection performed for colorectal cancer. Dis Colon Rectum 37:1020–1023

Rosen L, Stasik JJ Jr, Reed JF III, Olenwine JA, Aronoff JS, Sherman D (1996) Variations in colon and rectal surgical mortality: comparison of specialties with a state-legislated database. Dis Colon Rectum 39:129–135

Royal College of Surgeons and Association of Coloproctology (1996) Guidelines for the management of colorectal cancer. Royal College of Surgeons, London

Saha S, Booth MI, Dehn TCB (2002) The results of total mesorectal excision for rectal carcinoma in a district general hospital before the era of surgical specialization. Colorectal Disease 4:36–40

Schrag D, Cramer LD, Bach PB, Cohen AM, Warren JL, Begg CB (2000) Influence of hospital procedure volume on outcomes following surgery for colon cancer. JAMA 284:3028–3035

Schrag D, Panageas KS, Riedel E, Cramer LD, Guillem JG, Bach PB, Begg CB (2002) Hospital and surgeon procedure volume as predictors of outcome following rectal cancer resection. Ann Surg 236:583–592

Simons AJ, Ker R, Groshen S, Gee C, Anthone GJ, Ortega AE, Vukasin P, Ross RK, Beart RW Jr (1997) Variations in treatment of rectal cancer: the influence of hospital type and caseload. Dis Colon Rectum 40:641–646

Simunovic M, To T, Baxter N, Balshem A, Ross E, Cohen Z, McLeod R, Engstrom P, Sigurdson E (2000) Hospital procedure volume and teaching status do not influence treatment and outcome measures of rectal cancer surgery in a large general population. J Gastrointest Surg 4:324–330

Singh KK, Aitken RJ (1999) Outcome in patients with colorectal cancer managed by surgical trainees. Br J Surg 86:1332–1336

Singh KK, Barry MK, Ralston P, Henderson MA, McCormick JSC, Walls ADF, Auld CD (1997) Audit of colorectal cancer surgery by non-specialist surgeons. Br J Surg 84:343–347

Smedh K, Olsson L, Johansson H, Åberg C, Andersson M (2001) Reduction of postoperative morbidity and mortality in patients with rectal cancer following the introduction of a colorectal unit. Br J Surg 88:273–277

Smith JAE, King PM, Lane RHS, Thompson MR (2003) Evidence of the effect of 'specialization' on the management, surgical outcome and survival from colorectal cancer in Wessex. Br J Surg 90:583–592

Smith TJ, Hillner BE, Bear HD (2003) Taking action on the volume-quality relationship: how long can we hide our heads in the colostomy bag ? J Natl Cancer Inst 95:695–697

Stocchi L, Nelson H, Sargent DJ, O'Connell MJ, Tepper JE, Krook JE, Beart R Jr, North Central Cancer Treatment Group (2001) Impact of surgical and pathological variables in rectal cancer: a United States community and cooperative group report. J Clin Oncol 19:3895–3902

The consultant surgeons and pathologists of the Lothian and Borders health boards (1995) Lothian and Borders large bowel cancer project: immediate outcome after surgery. Br J Surg 82:888–890

Tytherleigh M, Wheeler J, Birks M, Farouk R (2002) Surgical specialist registrars can safely perform resections for carcinoma of the rectum. Ann R Coll Surg Engl 84:389–392

Wibe A, Eriksen MT, Syse A, Myrvold HE, Soreide O on behalf of The Norwegian Rectal Cancer Group (2003) Total mesorectal excision for rectal cancer – what can be achieved by a national audit ? Colorectal Disease 5:471–477

Surgical Results of Total Mesorectal Excision for Rectal Cancer in a Specialised Colorectal Unit

KokSun Ho, Francis Seow-Choen

F. Seow-Choen (✉)
Department of Colorectal Surgery, Singapore General Hospital, Singapore, Singapore
e-mail: seowchoen@colorectalcentre.com

Abstract

Our aim was to review the results of total mesorectal excision (TME) in a specialised colorectal unit. Perioperative and follow-up data were prospectively collected in a computerised database. A review of all the records was made. The morbidity rate was about 14%, and was higher in patients with coloplasty due to a higher anastomotic leak rate. The local recurrence rate was 2%, the distant metastasis rate was 11%, and both local and distant metastasis occurred in 4%. About 95% of recurrence occurred within 3 years. There was better bowel function in patients with a colonic J-pouch in the first 2 years after surgery, but the advantage disappeared thereafter. There were no differences in function between descending and sigmoid colonic J-pouches. TME in a specialised colorectal unit has low morbidity and mortality. Our procedure of choice is that of a sigmoid colon J-pouch anal anastomosis.

Introduction

Total mesorectal excision (TME) was first introduced by Heald [1] in 1982, and it is now the accepted standard of care for mid- and low rectal cancer surgery [2, 3]. However, despite the initial claims of a lower locoregional recurrence rate associated with TME, the actual recurrence rate varies from below 10% to up to 25%–35% [4–7]. This may be due to variations in surgical technique. In this chapter, we review the results of TME in a specialised colorectal unit.

Recent Results in Cancer Research, Vol. 165

Procedure

Total mesorectal excision has been the procedure of choice used in our unit for low rectal cancer. In the patient population described herein, the left colon, and if necessary, the splenic flexure was mobilised to allow a tension-free anastomosis. In all cases, the inferior mesenteric artery was ligated proximal to the left colic artery. The rectum was dissected down to the anorectal junction at the pelvic floor, with total clearance of the mesorectum. Special care was taken not to breach the mesorectal fascia during sharp dissection. After mobilisation of the rectum, a clamp was applied below the tumour and the rectum irrigated with chlorhexidine solution. A TLC 30 transverse stapler (Ethicon Endo-Surgery, Cincinnati, Ohio, USA) was applied at the anorectal junction, and the rectum was removed. The proximal colon or pouch was then anastomosed to the anorectal stump using a CDH 29 intraluminal stapler (Ethicon Endo-Surgery). All patients had a defunctioning ileostomy that was closed 3–6 weeks later.

All of the patients were followed up at 3-month intervals for the first 2–3 years after surgery. Patients with Dukes' C lesion were offered adjuvant chemotherapy and radiotherapy.

Operative Morbidity and Mortality

In a study comparing the use of descending versus sigmoid colon pouch function after TME in 92 patients [8], the overall morbidity was 14%. The complications were as follows: anastomotic leak (three patients), rectovaginal fistula (one patient), pelvic abscess (one), chest infection (one), anastomotic bleeding (one), cardiovascular accident (one), wound infection (three), prolonged ileus (one), and myocardial infarction (one). None of the patients required a repeat laparotomy. There were no operative mortality in any of these patients.

In another study comparing the use of a colonic pouch versus a coloplasty pouch [9] after TME in 88 patients, the complication rate of 20.5% was higher, due mainly to a higher anastomotic leak with the coloplasty pouch (7 of 44; 15.9%). One patient required laparotomy for peritonitis, while another two required transrectal drainage for well-localised abscesses. The other four patients had subclinical leaks that were detected on contrast studies prior to closure of the ileostomy. All of the leaks occurred at the anterior of the coloanal anastomosis, below the site of the coloplasty. Anastomotic leaks were not significantly associated with postoperative chemotherapy or radiotherapy. This is comparable to a leak rate of 13.2% in another study [10], though there were no statistical differences in leak rate in that study. Other complications include chest infection (five patients), wound infection (five), and rectovaginal fistula (one). There was one mortality from chest infection in the coloplasty group in this series.

Oncologic Results

Perioperative and follow-up data of all patients managed in our department were collected prospectively into a customized database as soon as an event (e.g. surgery, follow-up) occurred. A review of the records of all patients operated with a curative intent was done [11]. Over a 10-year period from April 1989 to March 1999, curative operations were performed on a total of 1,731 primary colorectal cancers (including 910 cases of rectal cancer) and 357 recurrent colorectal cancers (including 193 cases of rectal cancer). Patients with disseminated carcinoma and palliative surgery, as well as patients with disseminated disease or distant metastasis within 3 months of primary surgery were excluded, as were cases lost to follow-up or incomplete documentation.

There were a total of 1,103 patients with rectal cancer who were operated with curative intent. In this paper, we did not distinguish between patients who had TME or wide mesorectal excision (WME). Local recurrence alone occurred in 47 (2%) patients, and distant metastasis alone occurred in 236 patients (11%). Seventy-four (4%) patients had both local and distant tumour recurrence. The median time to diagnosis of local recurrence was 15 months, and that to diagnosis of distant metastases was 14 months. Within 2 years after operation, 70.5% of local recurrence and 68.5% of distant metastases were detected. At 3 years, the percentages were 94.5% and 94.8%, respectively.

Others have reported that the tumour site affects the site and rate of recurrence [12, 13]. However, in our series of 2,088 patients, the tumour site does not affect the rates of local or distant recurrence. There were also no differences in the pattern of recurrence, as noted in other studies [12, 14–18].

Univariate analysis of risk factors showed invasion of and fixation to adjacent tissues to be significant. Poorly differentiated tumours also have a higher risk of recurrence.

In another study [19], we found that localised tumour perforation, either spontaneous or iatrogenic, does not affect local recurrence nor survival when compared with non-perforated tumours of the same stage.

Distant recurrence is related mainly to the inability of staging investigations to detect such metastasis at the time of surgery. On the other hand, local recurrence in a potentially curable patient is related directly to surgical technique, and local recurrence may be regarded as a failure in surgical technique [20]. While it has been stated in other studies that the splenic flexure or rectal carcinoma has greater risk of recurrence, our results at these sites are equal with the rest of the colon [11]. It may be that radical surgery performed in a specialised unit for these technically more difficult sites can achieve equal results with the "easier" parts of the colon, while in a non-specialised unit, these problematic areas might result in a higher recurrence rate because of inadequate oncologic clearance. In particular, although all surgeons would claim to do TME or WME for rectal cancer, the surgical quality of TME and WME varies greatly among surgeons [21]. It is thus not surprising that the local recurrence rate for rectal cancer varies widely from 2.6% to 32.0% [5–7].

Functional Results

Bowel Function

It is well established that direct end-to-end straight anastomosis of proximal colon to the anorectal junction results in poorer functional results in the earlier postoperative period [22–25]. Even though most studies showed that pouch and straight coloanal anastomosis function becomes comparable after 1–2 years [26], the better function in the early postoperative period is especially important in the elderly who have impaired sphincter function, as well as those with a limited life expectancy due to advanced disease [27].

Our unit has looked at the function of different types of pouches. We initially used a 6-cm descending colon pouch [28]. Twenty-one patients with colonic pouch were compared with 26 straight coloanal anastomosis patients. All Dukes' C patients were offered radiotherapy, and there were no differences in the proportion of patients with radiotherapy. There were no anastomotic leaks in either group. At 1 year after primary surgery, patients with straight anastomosis had a higher stool frequency and clustering of stools. However, more patients in the pouch group had some evacuation difficulty, though this did not reach statistical significance in our group. There were also no differences in the postoperative bowel function score. Ambulatory manometry in the patients showed a lower anorectal pressure gradient in the straight anastomosis patients at 1 year.

In another study of 42 patients performed at 6 months and 2 years after primary surgery [26], we again showed that stool frequency was higher in the straight group, as well as the inability to release gas without soiling. However, by 2 years after surgery, there was no significant difference in stool frequency between the two groups, though there was still a higher proportion of patients in the straight group with more than four stools per day.

We also looked at the role of using sigmoid colon versus descending colon for the construction of the colonic J pouch [8]. Eighty-eight patients were followed up for a median of 12 months. There were no differences in the morbidity or mortality between the groups. Functional results at 6 weeks after ileostomy closure, 6 months and 1 year after surgery showed no significant differences. We also found that splenic flexure mobilisation was not routinely required in constructing a sigmoid J pouch, and this resulted in the slightly shorter though statistically insignificant operation time for the sigmoid pouch group. We recommend that sigmoid colon be used for pouch construction after TME if it is viable and grossly free from diverticulosis.

Z'graggen [29, 30] first introduced the idea of a coloplasty pouch in 1999 in pigs, and this was later performed in human patients [31, 32]. We thus performed a randomized controlled trial to compare bowel function between coloplasty and colonic J-pouch [9]. For coloplasty patients, a 7-cm longitudinal incision was made between the tenia along the antimesenteric side of the descending colon, starting 4 cm above the distal end of the colon. The incision was closed transversely using a single layer of seromuscular absorbable suture. The pouch was then anastomosed to the anorectal stump by means of a double stapling technique.

In the J-pouch group, all the colonic pouches were constructed using descending colon.

We looked at the functional results at 4 months and 12 months after primary surgery. Patients with the coloplasty pouch had a longer stool deferment time and less nocturnal leak, but had worse stool fragmentation at 4 months. However, there were no differences between the groups at 12 months follow-up. These results were also similar to those of another randomised trial [33].

Bladder Function

Bladder dysfunction has been reported in up to 54% of patients after surgical resection of the rectum [34]. TME involves dissection in the tissue plane outside the mesorectal fascial envelope, and should avoid damage to the sympathetic and parasympathetic nerves that run along the pelvic side wall. However, these can still be damaged by excessive traction or lateral dissection outside the correct planes. In a study of 170 patients comparing bladder function after open and laparoscopic rectal resection, we found that the median I-PSS score [35] did not deteriorate after open or laparoscopic surgery.

Sexual Function

Rectal resection is also associated with sexual dysfunction in up to 59% of patients [36–39]. In our series of 96 male patients who had rectal resection, six became impotent while another three had impaired erection. A total of seven patients had ejaculatory problems. Laparoscopic resection was significantly associated with more sexual problems. Of the 76 female patients who were studied, only 12 were sexually active before surgery, and 11 remained sexually after surgery. Only one patient reported dyspareunia, but she remained sexually active.

Conclusion

We have shown that TME performed in a specialised colorectal unit can result in low morbidity and low mortality. Our procedure of choice is that of an open sigmoid J pouch–anal anastomosis for its lower complication rate and similar functional results.

References

1. Heald RJ, Husband EM, Ryall RD (1982) The mesorectum in rectal cancer surgery–the clue to pelvic recurrence? Br J Surg 69(10):613–616
2. Nelson H, Petrelli N, Carlin A, Couture J, Fleshman J, Guillem J et al (2001) Guidelines 2000 for colon and rectal cancer surgery. J Natl Cancer Inst 93(8):583–596

3. Becouarn Y, Blanc-Vincent MP, Ducreux M, Lasser P, Dubois JB, Giovannini M et al (2001) Cancer of the rectum. Br J Cancer 84 Suppl 2:69–73
4. Wiig JN, Carlsen E, Soreide O (1998) Mesorectal excision for rectal cancer: a view from Europe. Semin Surg Oncol 15(2):78–86
5. Kapiteijn E, Marijnen CA, Nagtegaal ID, Putter H, Steup WH, Wiggers T et al (2001) Preoperative radiotherapy combined with total mesorectal excision for resectable rectal cancer. N Engl J Med 345(9):638–46
6. MacFarlane JK, Ryall RD, Heald RJ (1993) Mesorectal excision for rectal cancer. Lancet 341(8843):457–460
7. Gunderson LL, Sosin H (1974) Areas of failure found at reoperation (second or symptomatic look) following "curative surgery" for adenocarcinoma of the rectum. Clinicopathologic correlation and implications for adjuvant therapy. Cancer 34(4):1278–1292
8. Heah SM, Seow-Choen F, Eu KW, Ho YH, Tang CL (2002) Prospective, randomized trial comparing sigmoid vs. descending colonic J-pouch after total rectal excision. Dis Colon Rectum 45(3):322–328
9. Ho YH, Brown S, Heah SM, Tsang C, Seow-Choen F, Eu KW et al (2002) Comparison of J-pouch and coloplasty pouch for low rectal cancers: a randomized, controlled trial investigating functional results and comparative anastomotic leak rates. Ann Surg 236(1):49–55
10. Pimentel JM, Duarte A, Gregorio C, Souto P, Patricio J (2003) Transverse coloplasty pouch and colonic J-pouch for rectal cancer–a comparative study. Colorectal Dis (5):465–470
11. Kraemer M, Wiratkapun S, Seow-Choen F, Ho YH, Eu KW, Nyam D (2001) Stratifying risk factors for follow-up: a comparison of recurrent and nonrecurrent colorectal cancer. Dis Colon Rectum 44(6):815–821
12. Galandiuk S, Wieand HS, Moertel CG, Cha SS, Fitzgibbons RJ, Jr., Pemberton JH et al (1992) Patterns of recurrence after curative resection of carcinoma of the colon and rectum. Surg Gynecol Obstet 174(1):27–32
13. Phillips RK, Hittinger R, Blesovsky L, Fry JS, Fielding LP (1984) Local recurrence following 'curative' surgery for large bowel cancer: I. The overall picture. Br J Surg 71(1):12–16
14. Adloff M, Arnaud JP, Schloegel M, Thibaud D (1985) Factors influencing local recurrence after abdominoperineal resection for cancer of the rectum. Dis Colon Rectum 28(6):413–415
15. Obrand DI, Gordon PH (1997) Incidence and patterns of recurrence following curative resection for colorectal carcinoma. Dis Colon Rectum 40(1):15–24
16. Halvorsen TB, Seim E (1987) Tumour site: a prognostic factor in colorectal cancer? A multivariate analysis. Scand J Gastroenterol 22(1):124–128
17. Pilipshen SJ, Heilweil M, Quan SH, Sternberg SS, Enker WE (1984) Patterns of pelvic recurrence following definitive resections of rectal cancer. Cancer 53(6):1354–1362
18. Takahashi T, Kato T, Kodaira S, Koyama Y, Sakabe T, Tominaga T et al (1996) Prognostic factors of colorectal cancer. Results of multivariate analysis of curative resection cases with or without adjuvant chemotherapy. Am J Clin Oncol 19(4):408–415
19. Kagda FH, Nyam DC, Ho YH, Eu KW, Leong AF, Seow-Choen F (1999) Surgery may be curative for patients with a localized perforation of rectal carcinoma. Br J Surg 86(11):1448–1450
20. Seow-Choen F (2002) Adjuvant therapy for rectal cancer cannot be based on the results of other surgeons. Br J Surg 89(8):946–947
21. Hermanek P, Hohenberger W, Klimpfinger M, Kockerling F, Papadopoulos T (2003) The pathological assessment of mesorectal excision: implications for further treatment and quality management. Int J Colorectal Dis 18(4):335–341
22. Seow-Choen F, Goh HS (1995) Prospective randomized trial comparing J colonic pouch-anal anastomosis and straight coloanal reconstruction. Br J Surg 82(5):608–610
23. Ho YH, Tan M, Seow-Choen F (1996) Prospective randomized controlled study of clinical function and anorectal physiology after low anterior resection: comparison of straight and colonic J pouch anastomoses. Br J Surg 83(7):978–980
24. Hallbook O, Pahlman L, Krog M, Wexner SD, Sjodahl R (1996) Randomized comparison of straight and colonic J pouch anastomosis after low anterior resection. Ann Surg 224(1):58–65
25. Lazorthes F, Chiotasso P, Gamagami RA, Istvan G, Chevreau P (1997) Late clinical outcome in a randomized prospective comparison of colonic J pouch and straight coloanal anastomosis. Br J Surg 84(10):1449–1451
26. Ho YH, Seow-Choen F, Tan M (2001) Colonic J-pouch function at six months versus straight coloanal anastomosis at two years: randomized controlled trial. World J Surg 25(7):876–881

27. Williams N, Seow-Choen F (1998) Physiological and functional outcome following ultra-low anterior resection with colon pouch-anal anastomosis. Br J Surg 85(8):1029–1035
28. Ho YH, Tan M, Leong AF, Seow-Choen F(2000) Ambulatory manometry in patients with colonic J-pouch and straight coloanal anastomoses: randomized, controlled trial. Dis Colon Rectum 43(6):793–799
29. Maurer CA, Z'Graggen K, Zimmermann W, Hani HJ, Mettler D, Buchler MW (1999) Experimental study of neorectal physiology after formation of a transverse coloplasty pouch. Br J Surg 86(11):1451–1458
30. Z'Graggen K, Maurer CA, Mettler D, Stoupis C, Wildi S, Buchler MW (1999) A novel colon pouch and its comparison with a straight coloanal and colon J-pouch–anal anastomosis: preliminary results in pigs. Surgery 125(1):105–112
31. Mantyh CR, Hull TL, Fazio VW (2001) Coloplasty in low colorectal anastomosis: manometric and functional comparison with straight and colonic J-pouch anastomosis. Dis Colon Rectum 44(1):37–42
32. Fazio VW, Mantyh CR, Hull TL (2000) Colonic "coloplasty": novel technique to enhance low colorectal or coloanal anastomosis. Dis Colon Rectum 43(10):1448–1450
33. Furst A, Suttner S, Agha A, Beham A, Jauch KW (2003) Colonic J-pouch vs. coloplasty following resection of distal rectal cancer: early results of a prospective, randomized, pilot study. Dis Colon Rectum 46(9):1161–1166
34. Quah HM, Jayne DG, Eu KW, Seow-Choen F (2002) Bladder and sexual dysfunction following laparoscopically assisted and conventional open mesorectal resection for cancer. Br J Surg 89(12):1551–1556
35. Barry MJ, Fowler FJ, Jr., O'Leary MP, Bruskewitz RC, Holtgrewe HL, Mebust WK et al (1992) The American Urological Association symptom index for benign prostatic hyperplasia. The Measurement Committee of the American Urological Association. J Urol 148(5):1549–1557; discussion 1564
36. Cosimelli M, Mannella E, Giannarelli D, Casaldi V, Wappner G, Cavaliere F et al (1994) Nerve-sparing surgery in 302 resectable rectosigmoid cancer patients: genitourinary morbidity and 10-year survival. Dis Colon Rectum 37(2 Suppl):42–46
37. Cunsolo A, Bragaglia RB, Manara G, Poggioli G, Gozzetti G (1990) Urogenital dysfunction after abdominoperineal resection for carcinoma of the rectum. Dis Colon Rectum 33(11):918–922
38. Danzi M, Ferulano GP, Abate S, Califano G (1983) Male sexual function after abdominoperineal resection for rectal cancer. Dis Colon Rectum 26(10):665–668
39. Havenga K, Enker WE, McDermott K, Cohen AM, Minsky BD, Guillem J (1996) Male and female sexual and urinary function after total mesorectal excision with autonomic nerve preservation for carcinoma of the rectum. J Am Coll Surg 182(6):495–502

Total Mesorectal Excision: The Heidelberg Results after TME

Alexis Ulrich, Jan Schmidt, Jürgen Weitz, Markus W. Büchler

A. Ulrich (✉)
Department of General, Visceral and Trauma Surgery,
Ruprecht-Karls-University Heidelberg, Im Neuenheimer Feld 110,
69120 Heidelberg, Germany
e-mail: alexis.ulrich@med.uni-heidelberg.de

Abstract

The introduction of the total mesorectal excision (TME) has changed the treatment of rectal cancer dramatically by reducing the local recurrence rate. We report the results of 208 patients undergoing a low anterior resection (LAR, n=180) or abdominoperineal resection (APR, n=28) with TME between 1 October 2001 and 30 September 2003. No adjuvant therapy was administered to any patient; however, 108 patients received neoadjuvant radiotherapy or radiochemotherapy. Since February 2002, 51 patients underwent a short-course radiotherapy with 5×5 Gy prior to surgery in cases of a T3 tumor or positive lymph node in the preoperative CT-scan or endoanal ultrasound. Patients with a T4 tumor or T3 tumor close to the sphincter received radiochemotherapy. We discuss the results for mortality, morbidity, functional outcome, and overall survival between the LAR and APR groups. The mortality rate was 3% in the LAR and 0% in the APR group, whereas the morbidity was higher in the APR group. Anastomotic leakages occurred in eight patients (7%), and reoperations had to be performed in14 LAR and four APR patients. After a median follow-up of 11 months, the overall survival was 93% for LAR and 89% for APR. To assess the functional outcome after TME, questionnaires were sent to all patients undergoing LAR and APR. In conclusion, the TME has become the gold standard for rectal cancer surgery. Neoadjuvant treatment modalities such as preoperative short term radiotherapy (5×5 Gy) or combined radiochemotherapy will most likely replace the adjuvant combined radiochemotherapy.

Introduction

The treatment of rectal cancer patients has changed dramatically within the last two decades. This is mainly due to the introduction of the total mesorectal excision (TME) by Heald in 1980, allowing the reduction of the local recurrence rate to 4%–10% even without neo- or adjuvant therapy [4, 9, 10, 16]. In comparison, Hermanek

Recent Results in Cancer Research, Vol. 165

Table 1. Comparison of local recurrence rates after surgery alone [classic technique (OP) and TME] and combination with radio- (RT) or radiochemotherapy (RCT), respectively

Trial	GITSG [6]		NCCTG [18]		Tveit [25]	
	OP	OP+RCT	OP+RT	OP+RCT	OP	OP+RCT
LR (%)	24	11	25	14	30	12

Trial	Heald [10]	DCRCG [13]		CAO / ARO / AIO-94 [24]	
	TME	TME	TME+nRT	TME+nRCT	TME+RCT
LR (%)	3.9	8.2	2.4	7	11

LR, local recurrence rate; nRT, neoadjuvant radiotherapy; nRCT, neoadjuvant radiochemotherapy.

et al. reported local recurrence rates of 4%–55%, with a median of 20%, as the results of a German multicenter trial including TME and classical surgery in 1995 [11]. Even comparing the local recurrence rates of TME and classical surgery combined with neo- or adjuvant therapy—as proposed in the consensus guidelines of the German Cancer Society and the National Institutes of Health—shows a superior outcome after TME alone (Table 1).

What is so special about the total mesorectal excision? By respecting the integrity of the fascia pelvis, a separation plane between the mesorectum and the pelvine structures, called "the holy plane" by Heald, the mesorectum can be removed completely. This is so important as the mesorectum surrounds the vessels and lymphatic system of the rectum, reducing the risk of local recurrence. Additionally, the risk of damaging the inferior hypogastric plexus is reduced, resulting in less functional impairment of the genitourinary system [9].

Therefore, the total mesorectal excision is regarded as the "gold standard" for rectal cancer surgery and routinely performed at the surgical department of the University of Heidelberg.

We discuss our results obtained with TME between 1 October 2001 and 30 September 2003 in Heidelberg.

Results

TME in Heidelberg

Within the above-mentioned time span, 1,084 colorectal operations were performed in total, 563 for colorectal cancer, comprising 322 colon cancer and 241 rectal cancer patients. The 241 patients with rectal cancer underwent a low anterior or anterior resection (LAR) in 180 cases (75%), in 28 cases an abdominoperineal resection (APR) (12%), in 11 cases a pelvic exenteration (4%), and in 22 cases other procedures as local excision, explorative laparotomy with creation of an ileostomy,

Table 2. Data of 208 patients undergoing low anterior resection or abdominoperineal resection for rectal cancer between 1 October 2001 and 30 September 2003

	LAR (*n*=180)	APR (*n*=28)
Average age (range)	62 (37–89)	60 (15–74)
Male:female	133:47	16:12
Tumor level (cm from anal verge)	8	4
Preoperative radiotherapy (5×5 Gy)	51	3
Preoperative radiochemotherapy	42	12

etc. (9%). Seventeen of the patients had a local recurrence at the time of their operation (7%).

In the following, we focus on the 208 patients with LAR and APR. The patient data are shown in Tables 2 and 3. The tumor level of the 180 patients with sphincter preservation was (median) 8 cm above the anal verge, for the 28 patients with APR 4 cm. The high percentage of sphincter-preserving procedures (87%) is explained by the widespread opinion that a 1-cm safety margin to the distal border of the tumor is sufficient for curative resection [3, 14, 21]. Looking at the histological tumor stage, 70 of the180 patients with LAR were UICC stage I, a stage not seen in any patient undergoing APR; 44 and 40 patients were stage II and III in the LAR group, respectively. Stage III was the most often diagnosed stage in patients undergoing APR, seen in 12 patients (43%). Stage IV accounted for 9% in the LAR and 25% in the APR group (Table 3). Although 10 of the 180 patients with LAR had a recurrent tumor at the time of surgery, the R0-resection rate was 97% (176 of 180 patients). Seven of the 28 patients with APR had recurrent disease, and R0-resection could be achieved in 20 patients (71%) (Table 3).

No adjuvant radiotherapy was administered to any patient; however, a total of 108 patients underwent neoadjuvant radiotherapy or radiochemotherapy.

Fifty-one patients had a short-course preoperative radiotherapy with 5×5 Gy (5 Gy each day for 5 consecutive days, surgery within 2 days after completion of the radiotherapy) prior to LAR, three patients prior to APR. The short-course radiotherapy was introduced in Heidelberg in February 2002 for patients with a T3

Table 3. Data of 208 patients undergoing low anterior resection or abdominoperineal resection for rectal cancer between 1 October 2001 and 30 September 2003

	LAR (*n*=180)	APR (*n*=28)
UICC I	70	0
UICC II	44	7
UICC III	40	12
UICC IV	16	6
Recurrent tumor	10	7
R0-resection	176	20

Table 4. Operative results of 208 patients undergoing low anterior resection or abdominoperineal resection for rectal cancer between 1 October 2001 and 30 September 2003

LAR (*n*=180)
APR (*n*=28)
Operating time (median, min)
260 (120–420)
290 (150–480)
Blood loss (median, ml)
650 (200–2500)
800 (200–4000)
Blood transfusions (median, *n*)
0 (0–12)
0 (0–9)
Hospital stay (days)
12 (7–48)
14 (9–46)

tumor or positive lymph nodes in the preoperative CT scan or endoanal ultrasound. Before February 2002 these patients received preoperative radiochemotherapy (50 Gy, combined with 5-FU chemotherapy), as did patients with T4 tumors or T3 tumors close to the sphincter.

The operative and postoperative results are shown in Tables 4 and 5. The mean operating time was slightly higher for the APR than the LAR (290 min vs. 260 min) as was the median blood loss (650 ml vs. 800 ml). However, no differences were seen in the median number of blood transfusions. The hospital stay was a slightly shorter for LAR than APR patients (Table 4).

Five patients with LAR (3%) died within the first 60 days after the operation, two patients from aspiration pneumonia, one from pulmonary embolism, one from a heart attack, and one from sepsis due to an anastomotic leakage with peritonitis. None of the patients undergoing APR died within the above-mentioned period. The morbidity was higher in the APR than the LAR group (36% vs. 26%). Anastomotic leakages occurred in 12 patients (7%), wound infections and abscesses in 8% of the patients with LAR. In the APR group, the latter were the most common complications with 25%. Voiding problems (*n*=13) and bleeding (*n*=2) were other surgical complications seen. Cardiopulmonary complications occurred in seven patients with LAR; four of these patients died during their hospital stay. Re-operations had to be performed in 14 LAR and four APR patients (8% vs. 14%) (Table 5). Eight of these re-operations in the LAR group and all four in the APR group were due to anastomotic leakages or abscesses; the remainder of the relaparotomies were performed due to wound dehiscence and bleeding.

After a median follow-up of 11 months, local recurrences occurred in three patients (1.5%) after LAR and none after APR. In one of the three patients with local recurrence, the LAR was performed for a locally recurrent tumor. The overall

Table 5. Postoperative results of 208 patients undergoing low anterior resection or abdominoperineal resection for rectal cancer between 1 October 2001 and 30 September 2003

	LAR (*n*=180)	APR (*n*=28)
Mortality (*n*)	5 (3%)	0
Morbidity (*n*)	50 (28%)	10 (36%)
Anastomotic leakage (*n*)	12 (7%)	
Wound infection / abscess (*n*)	14 (8%)	7 (25%)
Bleeding (*n*)	2 (1%)	
Voiding problems (*n*)	10 (5%)	3 (11%)
Cardio/pulmonary (*n*)	7 (4%)	
Others (*n*)	5 (3%)	
Re-operation (*n*)	14 (8%)	4 (14%)

Table 6. Outcome of 208 patients undergoing low anterior resection or abdominoperineal resection for rectal cancer between 1 October 2001 and 30 September 2003

	LAR (*n*=180)	APR (*n*=28)
Median follow-up (months)	11	11
Local recurrence (*n*)	3 (1.5%)	0
Hepatic metastases (*n*)	11 (6%)	2 (7%)
Pulmonary metastases (*n*)	2 (1%)	0
Overall survival (*n*)	168 (93%)	25 (89%)

survival after 11 months' median follow-up was 93% for LAR and 89% for APR. Hepatic metastases have been diagnosed in 11 LAR (6%) and two APR (7%) patients, pulmonary metastases in two patients (LAR) (Table 6).

Rectal Reservoir Reconstruction

Of the 180 patients with LAR, 128 received a pouch reconstruction; the remaining 51 patients a straight anastomosis. In 106 cases, the reconstruction was created as a transverse coloplasty pouch (TCP) (59%), in 22 cases as a colon J pouch (CJP). All 22 CJPs and 24 TCPs were performed as part of a randomized controlled trial comparing the two techniques. The trial started in October 2002 and will be closed when a total of 130 patients have been enrolled.

Genitourinary Function

To assess the functional outcome after TME, we send questionnaires to all patients undergoing LAR or APR concerning bladder and genital function. One hundred-twenty-three patients with LAR (68%) and 20 patients with APR (71%) answered the questionnaire regarding the questions on bladder function. However, for the genital function, these figures were much lower; 72 patients (LAR, 40%) and nine patients (APR, 32%), all male. Questions on erection and ejaculations disorders were answered by only 40 patients with LAR.

Bladder dysfunction (voiding problems, urge, or incontinence) was seen in 25% of the patients, which is in line with the literature, reporting a range of 5%–32% for the TME [7, 8, 19]. With the classical surgical technique, bladder dysfunction was seen even in up to 60% [12, 15]. The data concerning the genital function must be interpreted more carefully due to the low response (the answers were voluntary). Thirteen of the 40 answering patients (33%) reported erection problems and 12 patients (30%) ejaculation problems. Based on the literature, erection disorders range between 13% and 24% after TME and 32% to 80% after classical operation. Ejaculation disorders occurred in 11%–45% after TME and 30%–81% after classical operation, respectively [12, 15, 17, 19, 20, 22].

Discussion

The total mesorectal excision has become the gold standard for rectal cancer surgery. The Heidelberg results document the safety of the procedure with low mortality and morbidity rates. Especially the local recurrence rate could be reduced significantly with the new technique. Reported rates range between 4% and 11% after TME, compared with 4–55% (median 20%) with the classical technique (Tumori). The Dutch Colorectal Cancer Group was the first to prove that the local recurrence rate can be further reduced by neoadjuvant therapy as it dropped from 8.2% to 2.6% due to short-term preoperative radiotherapy with 5×5 Gy [13]. A superiority compared to the postoperative radiochemotherapy, still recommended by the consensus guidelines of the National Institutes of Health and the German Cancer Society, was seen for the preoperative radiochemotherapy in a randomized controlled trial, as the local recurrence rate was lower in the neoadjuvant treatment group (7% vs. 11%) [23,24]. In Heidelberg we have the following treatment concept: Patients with T3- or node-positive rectal cancer receive a preoperative short-term radiotherapy (5×5 Gy). The benefits are the low costs and the short delay of surgery, as the operation should be performed within 2 days after completion of the radiotherapy. Randomized controlled trials as well as meta-analyses have shown that the short-term radiotherapy can significantly reduce the local recurrence rate and increase the overall survival [1, 2, 5, 13, 26]. Furthermore, the acute toxicity is lower compared to preoperative radiochemotherapy. In cases of a T4 tumor or lesion close to the sphincter, radiochemotherapy is preferred preoperatively to achieve a downsizing of the tumor and possible preservation of the sphincter. Postoperative radiotherapy is not performed anymore. With this concept, we report a very low local recurrence rate of 1.5% in our series, so far, which could be in part explained by the short follow-up of 11 months, though it is known that 80% of the local recurrences occur within the first 2 years after the operation.

Additionally, the functional outcome after low anterior resection could be improved significantly by respecting the integrity of the fascia pelvis. Damage to the nerves responsible for bladder and genital function can be avoided, reducing the incidence of voiding problems, impotence, and retrograde ejaculation. With the classical surgical technique, bladder dysfunction was seen in 50%–60% of the patients; after introduction of the TME only in 3%–33% [7, 8, 12, 15, 19]. Similar improvements were reported for the genital function with impotence of 30%–81% of the patients after classical surgery compared to 11%–24% after TME [12, 15, 17, 19, 20, 22].

To reconstruct the rectum we prefer the transverse coloplasty pouch over the colon J-pouch as it can be done safely and easily, saves operating time, and has functional results comparable to those of the J-pouch [27], but as to avoiding late evacuation problems, however, we still await the results of our randomized trial.

Conclusion

Total mesorectal excision represents the gold standard for rectal cancer surgery. Neoadjuvant treatment modalities such as preoperative short-term radiotherapy (5×5 Gy) or combined radiochemotherapy will most likely replace the adjuvant combined radiochemotherapy.

References

1. Swedish Rectal Cancer Trial (1997) Improved survival with preoperative radiotherapy in resectable rectal cancer. N Engl J Med 336:980–987
2. Colorectal Cancer Collaborative Group (2001) Adjuvant radiotherapy for rectal cancer: a systematic overview of 8,507 patients from 22 randomised trials. Lancet 358:1291–1304
3. Bruch HP, Schwandner O, Farke S, Nolde J (2003) Pouch reconstruction in the pelvis. Langenbecks Arch Surg 388:60–75
4. Buchler MW, Heald RJ, Maurer CA, and Ulrich BC (1998) Rektumkarzinom: Das Konzept der Totalen Mesorektalen Exzision. Basel, Karger.
5. Dahlberg M, Glimelius B, Pahlman L (1999) Improved survival and reduction in local failure rates after preoperative radiotherapy: evidence for the generalizability of the results of Swedish Rectal Cancer Trial. Ann Surg 229:493–497
6. Douglass HO, Jr, Moertel CG, Mayer RJ, Thomas PR, Lindblad AS, Mittleman A, Stablein DM, Bruckner HW (1986) Survival after postoperative combination treatment of rectal cancer. N Engl J Med 315:1294–1295
7. Enker WE (1992) Potency, cure, and local control in the operative treatment of rectal cancer. Arch Surg 127:1396–1401
8. Havenga K, Enker WE, McDermott K, Cohen AM, Minsky BD, Guillem J (1996) Male and female sexual and urinary function after total mesorectal excision with autonomic nerve preservation for carcinoma of the rectum. J Am Coll Surg 182:495–502
9. Heald RJ, Husband EM, Ryall RD (1982) The mesorectum in rectal cancer surgery—the clue to pelvic recurrence? Br J Surg 69:613–616
10. Heald RJ, Ryall RD (1986) Recurrence and survival after total mesorectal excision for rectal cancer. Lancet 1:1479–1482
11. Hermanek P, Wiebelt H, Staimmer D, Riedl S (1995) Prognostic factors of rectum carcinoma—experience of the German Multicentre Study SGCRC. German Study Group Colo-Rectal Carcinoma. Tumori 81:60–64

12. Hojo K, Vernava AM, III, Sugihara K, Katumata K (1991) Preservation of urine voiding and sexual function after rectal cancer surgery. Dis Colon Rectum 34:532–539
13. Kapiteijn E, Marijnen CA, Nagtegaal ID, Putter H, Steup WH, Wiggers T, Rutten HJ, Pahlman L, Glimelius B, van Krieken JH, Leer JW, van de Velde CJ (2001) Preoperative radiotherapy combined with total mesorectal excision for resectable rectal cancer. N Engl J Med 345:638–646
14. Kapiteijn E, van de Velde CJ (2002) Developments and quality assurance in rectal cancer surgery. Eur J Cancer 38:919–936
15. Kinn AC, Ohman U (1986) Bladder and sexual function after surgery for rectal cancer. Dis Colon Rectum 29:43–48
16. Kockerling F, Reymond MA, Altendorf-Hofmann A, Dworak O, Hohenberger W (1998) Influence of surgery on metachronous distant metastases and survival in rectal cancer. J Clin Oncol 16:324–329
17. Koukouras D, Spiliotis J, Scopa CD, Dragotis K, Kalfarentzos F, Tzoracoleftherakis E, Androulakis J (1991) Radical consequence in the sexuality of male patients operated for colorectal carcinoma. Eur J Surg Oncol 17:285–288
18. Krook JE, Moertel CG, Gunderson LL, Wieand HS, Collins RT, Beart RW, Kubista TP, Poon MA, Meyers WC, Mailliard JA (1991) Effective surgical adjuvant therapy for high-risk rectal carcinoma. N Engl J Med 324:709–715
19. Maurer CA, Z'Graggen K, Renzulli P, Schilling MK, Netzer P, Buchler MW (2001) Total mesorectal excision preserves male genital function compared with conventional rectal cancer surgery. Br J Surg 88:1501–1505
20. Nesbakken A, Nygaard K, Bull-Njaa T, Carlsen E, Eri LM (2000) Bladder and sexual dysfunction after mesorectal excision for rectal cancer. Br J Surg 87:206–210
21. Ruo L, Guillem JG (1999) Major 20th-century advancements in the management of rectal cancer. Dis Colon Rectum 42:563–578
22. Saito N, Sarashina H, Nunomura M, Koda K, Takiguchi N, Nakajima N (1998) Clinical evaluation of nerve-sparing surgery combined with preoperative radiotherapy in advanced rectal cancer patients. Am J Surg 175:277–282
23. Sauer R (2003) Adjuvant versus neoadjuvant combined modality treatment for locally advanced rectal cancer: first results of the German rectal cancer study (CAO/ARO/AIO-94). Int J Radiat Oncol Biol Phys 57:124–125
24. Sauer R, Fietkau R, Wittekind C, Rodel C, Martus P, Hohenberger W, Tschmelitsch J, Sabitzer H, Karstens JH, Becker H, Hess C, Raab R (2003) Adjuvant vs. neoadjuvant radiochemotherapy for locally advanced rectal cancer: the German trial CAO/ARO/AIO-94. Colorectal Dis 5:406–415
25. Tveit KM, Guldvog I, Hagen S, Trondsen E, Harbitz T, Nygaard K, Nilsen JB, Wist E, Hannisdal E (1997) Randomized controlled trial of postoperative radiotherapy and short-term time-scheduled 5-fluorouracil against surgery alone in the treatment of Dukes B and C rectal cancer. Norwegian Adjuvant Rectal Cancer Project Group. Br J Surg 84:1130–1135
26. Ulrich A, Hartel M, Weitz J, Friess H, Buchler M (2004) [The value of (neo-) adjuvant therapy in rectal carcinoma]. Dtsch Med Wochenschr 129:957–962
27. Ulrich A, Z'graggen K, Schmied B, Weitz J, Buchler MW (2004) [The transverse coloplasty pouch after low anterior resection: early postoperative results]. Chirurg 75:430–435

Is Local Excision of T2/T3 Rectal Cancers Adequate?

D. L. Beral, J. R. T. Monson

J.R.T. Monson (✉)
Academic Surgical Unit, Castle Hill Hospital, Cottingham HU16 5JQ, UK
e-mail: J.R.Monson@hull.ac.uk

Abstract

In selected patients, local excision of rectal cancer may be an alternative to radical surgery such as abdominoperineal excision of the rectum or anterior resection. Local excision carries lower mortality and morbidity, without the functional disturbance or alteration in body image that can be associated with radical surgery. There are several techniques of local therapy for rectal cancer, with most experience being available in transanal excision. Transanal endoscopic microsurgery is also used but experience with this newer technique is limited. Patient selection is the most important factor in successful local excision; however, specific criteria for selecting patients have not been universally accepted. Review of the published literature is difficult because of the variation in adjuvant therapy regimes and follow-up strategies, as well as results reported in terms of local recurrence and survival rates. There is increasing evidence to suggest that local excision should be restricted to patients with T1-stage rectal cancer without high-risk factors. The place for local excision in patients with T2 or high-risk T1 tumours requires prospective, randomised multicentre trials comparing radical surgery with local excision, with or without adjuvant therapy. Local excision for T3 tumours should be restricted to the palliative setting or patients unfit for radical surgery.

Introduction

In the UK, colorectal cancer (CRC) is the third most common cancer behind lung and prostate cancer in males and is second only to breast cancer in females. In 1996 the UK incidence of CRC was 17,500 men and 16,800 women. In 1998, there were 17,110 deaths due to CRC. The lifetime risk of developing CRC is 5.7% and 4.9% for males and females respectively, or in terms of odds, 1 in 18 men and 1 in 20 women (National Statistics Online 2003).

Recent Results in Cancer Research, Vol. 165

Table 1. Variation in 5-year survival rates with TNM tumour stage

Stage	5-Year survival rate
T1/T2–N0	80%–90%
T3/T4–N0	60%–70%
T1/T2/T3/T4–N1/N2	25%–40%

Modern therapy of rectal cancer is multidisciplinary but centres around surgery, which offers the only hope of cure. Radiotherapy and chemotherapy are used alone or in combination in an adjuvant, neo-adjuvant, or palliative setting. Success of surgical treatment depends upon four variables: surgeon, operative technique, tumour biology, and patient-related features. The principal goals in the management of any patient with rectal cancer are to provide the optimum chance for cure while maintaining quality of life and pelvic autonomic nerve function and avoiding a stoma (Spencer 2001). The standard surgical therapy for rectal cancers has been radical resection, either with an abdominoperineal resection (APR) or an anterior resection (AR). Unfortunately, resection of the rectum is a major surgical procedure associated with significant morbidity (7%–68%), mortality (0%–6.5%), alteration in body image, and sometimes distressing functional consequences for the patient (Mellgren et al. 2000). Local excision of low rectal cancers has long been used as an alternative surgical option in patients thought to be unfit for major abdominal resection or who are unwilling to countenance a stoma (Sengupta and Tjandra 2001). Therefore local excision of distal rectal cancers has been explored as an option for selected patients with early-stage rectal cancer (Mellgren et al. 2000).

The stage of disease at the time of diagnosis is the main prognostic factor in rectal cancer. The extent of invasion of the tumour through the bowel wall and nodal status govern the stage of disease and therefore the chances of survival. The node-bearing areas are not removed by local excision techniques, rendering these procedures inadequate for node-positive tumours. However, even in node-negative tumours, extension beyond the muscularis mucosa (T3) reduces the 5-year survival probability by approximately 20%–30%, making the T-stage of critical importance in local excision (Wexner and Rotholtz 2000) (Table 1).

Many authors agree that local excision of properly selected rectal cancers is an acceptable alternative to radical surgery which may provide long-term survival, with minimal morbidity, negligible mortality, and excellent functional results, as well as avoiding a colostomy (Balani et al. 1999; Rothenberger and Garcia-Aguilar 2000; Visser et al. 2001). The main issue is appropriate patient selection. However, there is little consensus about the specific criteria for local excision and the indications for adjuvant therapy in those patients.

Historical Background

At the turn of the century, perineal excision was the accepted approach for nearly all rectal cancers, but inconsistent surgical outcomes and high local recurrence rates promoted the search for alternative treatment. In 1908 Sir Ernest Miles described abdomino-perineal resection (APR) in *The Lancet* (Miles 1908). Although not the first description, this report led to the establishment of the operation in the UK and North America (Goligher 1984). The acceptance of APR reduced recurrence and improved long-term survival but resulted in body image alteration due to the permanent stoma created. The introduction of circular staplers in the mid-1970s (Goligher et al. 1979) and the concept of the low anterior resection (AR) with total mesorectal excision, as championed by Heald in the early 1980s (Heald et al. 1982), allowed survival and tumour recurrence rates comparable to APR without the need for permanent stoma formation (Camilleri-Brennan and Steele 1998). Unfortunately, low anterior resection is not without significant morbidity, with sexual and urinary dysfunction being common (Table 2). Operative mortality rates following the two approaches are broadly similar at around 4%–6% (Sengupta and Tjandra 2001).

In recent years there have been remarkable advances in the treatment of rectal cancer, stimulated by a greater understanding of tumour biology and aided by the development of diagnostic tools that allow the surgeon to select the most suitable tumours for the various treatment strategies available. The role of local excision has evolved during the latter part of the twentieth century. As abdominal surgery became safer, local excision was usually considered only in the palliative setting or for patients considered a high anaesthetic risk. More recently, as preoperative tumour staging methods have improved, local excision has been performed with curative intent in selected patients (Rothenberger and Garcia-Aguilar 2000).

Table 2. Morbidity following anterior resection

Urinary dysfunction	7%–68%
Sexual impotence	15%–100%
Absent ejaculation	3%–39%
Dyspareunia	18%–90%
Anastomotic leak	5%–10%
Mortality	4%

Tumour Staging

Rectal cancer is staged preoperatively using the Dukes' or TNM classifications in order to predict the likelihood of a curative resection, based upon the depth of rectal wall penetration and the presence of lymphatic and distant metastases. The presence of lymph node metastasis, confirmed postoperatively by histopathological examination, mandates radical surgery if the intention is for a curative resection, and will usually lead to the administration of adjuvant chemotherapy. Methods of staging comprise the following:

Digital Rectal Examination

Digital rectal examination is the simplest method of preoperative staging, but is highly surgeon-dependent. Nicholls et al. reported the accuracy rate amongst colorectal specialists and trainees as 44%–83% for the assessment of the depth of invasion (T-stage), and 57%–67% for the assessment of lymph node involvement (N-stage) (Nicholls et al. 1982) (Table 3).

Endorectal Ultrasound

Endorectal ultrasonography (ERUS) is the most useful preoperative method to stage the depth of invasion of rectal lesions; in fact the T-stage can be measured accurately in 82%–93%, although overstaging has been reported. The assessment of lymph node involvement by ERUS is less reliable, with difficulty in distinguishing between malignant deposits and reactive changes. Accuracy for this varies between 65% and 81% (Table 3). Previous biopsies or irradiation may reduce the accuracy of assessment, and a stenosing lesion may limit access of the ultrasound probe. Newer three-dimensional imaging technology may improve the accuracy of ERUS staging and overcome some of the difficulties associated with stenotic lesions (Sengupta and Tjandra 2001).

Computed Tomography

Computed tomography (CT) scanning for rectal cancer, which lies within the bony pelvis, is not as accurate as ERUS for the assessment of either local invasion (66%–88% accuracy) or nodal spread (60% accuracy) (Table 3). The main value of CT imaging is in the excellent definition of regional and distant spread (Sengupta and Tjandra 2001).

Table 3. Diagnostic accuracy of pre-operative staging modalities

Staging modality	T-Stage	N-Stage
Digital rectal examination	44%–83%	57%–67%
Endorectal ultrasound	82%–93%	65%–81%
Computed tomography	66%–88%	60%
Magnetic resonance imaging	68%–90%	62%

Magnetic Resonance Imaging

Magnetic resonance imaging (MRI) has accuracy rates comparable to CT scanning (Table 3), and in some centres MRI is used in preference to CT for rectal cancer. Some evidence suggests MRI is superior to both CT and ERUS (Gualdi et al. 2000). Endorectal MRI coils may improve accuracy, but their use depends on operator expertise which is not yet widely available (Sengupta and Tjandra 2001). Endorectal coil MRI and ERUS have shown similar results, so the use of endorectal coils would seem to be justified only in patients where ERUS has yielded doubtful results (Gualdi et al. 2000).

Case Selection

The need for appropriate patient selection is the main issue in local excision of rectal cancers. The high local recurrence rates and compromised survival reported in some series has convinced many surgeons to restrict the use of local excision in otherwise healthy patients to only the most favourable rectal cancers (Rothenberger and Garcia-Aguilar 2000). Several retrospective studies have demonstrated that tumour control in properly selected patients treated with local excision is comparable to that which is anticipated after radical surgery. However, the case mix within these series is variable, and results after local excision differ greatly between centres (Garcia-Aguilar et al. 2000).

Pre-operative Staging

Local excision does not remove the draining lymph nodes, so the surgeon needs to be confident of the absence of nodal spread before undertaking such a procedure. The staging modalities described above have limits to their accuracy, particularly with regard to the assessment of lymph node involvement. However, the depth of wall invasion has been shown to be related to lymph node metastasis and a higher risk of local recurrence (Brodsky et al. 1992; Lezoche et al. 2000; Mellgren et al. 2000; Zenni et al 1998) (Table 4), as well as survival (Table 1). As such, wall invasion as classified by the TNM T-stage during pre-operative assessment provides a good estimate of the probability of nodal involvement and thus the feasibility of local excision. Overstaging of the tumour may lead to suitable patients not being offered local excision. The major concern however, is the risk of understaging by the

Table 4. Risk of nodal involvement and recurrence by TNM tumour stage

	T1	T2	T3	T4
Nodal involvement	0%–12%	12%–28%	36%–66%	53%–79%
Risk of recurrence	9.7%	25%	–	–

currently available imaging modalities leading to inappropriate selection for local excision.

There is general consensus that the use of local therapy with curative intent should not be considered for tumours that are advanced (T3 or T4) due to the high risk of lymph node involvement. However, clear suggestion of nodal involvement on the pre-operative imaging, whatever the T-stage, will also necessitate radical surgery.

Clinicopathologic Variables

These other variables contribute towards the assessment of the suitability of the tumour for local excision by determining whether the patient is at higher risk of relapse than another patient with a tumour of the same stage. For example, the histologic grade of the tumour, based upon the degree of cytologic differentiation of the tumour cells, reflects its aggressiveness. The probability of lymph node metastases for a T1-G1 (well-differentiated) tumour is 0% with recurrence rates of only 0%-3%, compared with 12% nodal metastases and 10%–63% recurrence for a T1-G3 (poorly-differentiated) tumour (Sengupta and Tjandra 2001).

Lymphovascular invasion is believed to be a premetastatic event carrying a greater risk of nodal spread and increasing local recurrence by more than 25% (Sengupta and Tjandra 2001). Mucinous and ulcerated tumours are often excluded from local excision because they are believed to behave in a more aggressive manner (Sengupta and Tjandra 2001).

Tumour size may also be of relevance, with several studies suggesting that recurrence is higher following local excision of tumours greater than either 3 cm or 4 cm (Balani et al. 2000; Blair and Ellenhorn 2000; Sengupta and Tjandra 2001; Willett et al. 1994; Zenni et al. 1998). Tumours that occupy over 40% of the circumference of the rectal wall may also be excluded from local excision, based upon the possibility of technical difficulties in closure of the defect (although it is not always necessary to close the defect).

Age has not been shown to be an important criterion for patient selection (Mellgren et al. 2000). However, clearly we wish to balance the risk of local recurrence against a patient's anticipated lifespan, based upon their co-morbidities. Thus we would be more aggressive in younger, fitter patients, judging each case on its individual merits. Other factors such as chromosomal ploidy and genetic markers (e.g. p53, bcl2, c-myc, k-ras) may influence prognosis within each pathologic stage and are being actively investigated. If shown to be significant with respect to prognosis, recurrence, or the likelihood of nodal metastasis, they will prove particularly useful in selecting low-risk rectal cancer patients suitable for local excision.

Currently therefore, commonly utilised criteria for local excision of rectal cancer are: TNM stage T1-T2, N0, M0, histological grading G1 or G2, and tumours up to 3–4cm in size which are technically accessible (Balani et al. 2000).

Methods of Local Excision

There are several techniques used for local therapy of rectal cancer. These include: transanal excision, dorsal approaches (York-Mason or Kraske procedures), transanal endoscopic microsurgery (TEM), endocavity radiation, and transanal fulguration (Visser et al. 2001). For most groups, conventional transanal excision is favoured for its low rate of complications, promising outcomes, and the ability to secure tissue for pathological examination (Rothenberger and Garcia-Aguilar 2000). In recent years TEM, following good results in the excision of rectal adenomas, has become more widely accepted as a technique for local excision of rectal cancer; however, experience is still limited (Sengupta and Tjandra 2001).

Transanal Excision

For transanal excision the patient is best positioned prone for anterior wall tumours or in the lithotomy position if the tumour is posterior. Bowel preparation and preoperative antibiotics are given in all patients. Anaesthesia may be general or regional (e.g. pudendal nerve block). Retractors, preferably with a fibre-optic light source, are used to visualize the lesion, and adrenaline may be injected around the lesion to prevent bleeding. Traction sutures are conventionally placed around the lesion and the line of excision marked using diathermy, aiming for a margin of at least 1–2 cm. Full-thickness excision is performed taking care to protect the vagina or prostate. After haemostasis, the defect may be closed with transverse absorbable sutures or, if below the peritoneal reflection, left open with the perirectal fat exposed. Fibrin gauze may be positioned in the rectum, depending on the surgeon's preference, following checking by proctoscopy. Postoperative analgesia requirements are minimal, and antibiotics may be continued for 24 h. Normal diet may be taken by the next day, and in-patient stay is often as little as 2 days. The complication rate is very low (0%–22%) with the most commonly occurring being: bleeding, local sepsis, urinary infection or retention, faecal incontinence, and rectovaginal fistula (Sengupta and Tjandra 2001). Transanal excision is not usually performed for lesions beyond 10 cm from the dentate line, due to technical difficulties.

Transanal Endoscopic Microsurgery

Transanal endoscopic microsurgery (TEM) is a relatively new technique first described in 1985 (Buess et al. 1985). It is performed through a 40-mm operating rectoscope with carbon dioxide insufflation to obtain vision. Operating instruments are introduced through sleeves in the same manner as laparoscopic surgery, and the tumour is excised using bipolar diathermy. The preparation and positioning of the patient are the same as for transanal excision. Disadvantages of TEM include costly equipment, a long learning curve, and difficulty in haemostasis of large vessels. Although, in theory, lesions up to 25 cm from the anal verge may be excised by TEM, it is usually reserved for tumours in the extraperitoneal rectum due to the risk of perforation and formation of pneumoperitoneum, as well as technical difficulties. This limits the technique to lesions up to 20 cm on the posterior wall, 15 cm laterally and 12 cm on the anterior wall. Also, the most distal lesions are often unsuitable for TEM excision, as it is difficult to maintain an adequate seal around the rectoscope and insufflation pressure is lost. To date, experience with TEM excision of rectal cancers is limited. However, TEM gives a magnified view of the operative field which enables precise excision of the tumour whilst maintaining a constant view of the margin, which may facilitate a more accurate and oncologically sound excision. Complications are infrequent but include bleeding, intraperitoneal perforation, fistula formation, incontinence, and wound breakdown.

Posterior Approaches

The posterior approaches for local excision of rectal cancers via a trans-sacral (Kraske) or trans-sphincteric (York-Mason) approach have been largely abandoned. These techniques had an advantage over conventional transanal excision in that the perirectal nodes could be removed for histopathological examination. However, they are associated with a significant rate of faecal fistula formation, wound breakdown and incontinence (Sengupta and Tjandra 2001).

Palliative Procedures

Other methods for local control include electrocoagulation, endocavitary irradiation, photodynamic therapy, cryosurgery, and laser ablation, but they have been abandoned in the potentially curative setting as they are unable to obtain a pathological specimen for staging and give poor results in terms of survival. These are ablative procedures largely limited to palliation in modern colorectal surgical practice.

Results

The results of local excision of rectal cancer vary widely between centres. Most of the data derive from single-institution retrospective case series, and the different techniques of local excision have never been subjected to analysis in a randomised controlled trial.

Local Excision Alone

A review conducted by Sengupta and Tjandra published in 2001 found reported local recurrence rates following local excision ranging from 0% to 32%. The wide

Table 5. Recurrence following local excision of rectal cancer

T-Stage	Local recurrence % (range)
Overall	13.7
T1	9.7 (0–24)
T2	25 (0–50)
T3	38 (0–100)

variation is easily explained by differences in patient selection, surgical technique, duration, and frequency of follow-up. In addition the histopathological criteria used to assess the adequacy of surgical excision vary between institutions, as do the policies for re-operation following an inadequate resection. The review included 958 patients in 22 studies; the stage-related local recurrence rates are shown in Table 5 (Sengupta and Tjandra 2001).

The favourable results reported by Blair and Ellenhorn (not included in the review by Sengupta and Tjandra) demonstrate the importance of patient selection. In 20 patients with Tis or T1 lesions and favourable histology, they achieved 0% recurrence and 0% cancer-related mortality at 60 months follow-up following trans-anal excision (Blair and Ellenhorn 2000).

In contrast, Garcia-Aguilar et al. (also not included in the review) reported on 82 patients with T1 or T2 tumours following transanal excision. After 54 months' follow-up, they reported 18% recurrence in T1 tumours and 37% in T2 tumours (Garcia-Aguilar et al. 2000). The same researchers also compared their results following local excision to those after radical surgery in a retrospective review, which is the only large study of its kind. Patients with tumours that were pathologically identified as T1 or T2 and who did not receive adjuvant chemoradiation were selected from a database covering a 10-year period. Those with positive resection margins were excluded, which amounted to 19 out of a total of 133 patients who had local excision. There were 108 local excisions (T1=69, T2=39) with 4.4 years follow-up, and 153 radical resections (T1=30, T2=123) with 4.8 years follow-up. There were significant differences between the two groups in the distance of the lesions from the anal verge (average 3 cm lower in local excision patients, as might be expected as higher lesions would not be accessible for local excision), the size of the tumours (smaller in local excision), as well as the stage bias shown above. Bearing in mind these inequalities, the results show a high rate of local recurrence after local excision (T1=18%, T2=47%) compared to radical surgery (T1=0%, T2=6%). There was also a higher rate of overall recurrence, including distant metastases, in the local excision group (T1=21%, T2=47%) compared to radical surgery (T1=9%, T2=16%), which was statistically significant for T2 lesions. The 5-year cancer-specific mortality was similar between the two groups, but there was a significantly lower 5-year overall survival rate in the local excision group for T2 lesions (65% vs. 81%, p=0.03) (Mellgren et al. 2000).

This study would seem to point towards two key conclusions: firstly, when judged on overall survival, patients with T2 tumours are disadvantaged by local excision alone. Secondly, local and overall recurrence is significantly higher following local excision in T2 tumours. There is a clear implication that T2 lesions in particular are not suitable for local resection. Histopathological characteristics such as differentiation, lymphovascular invasion, and mucinous tumours do not form part of the selection criteria in this study, only positive resection margins, which are not available to the surgeon pre-operatively. The authors state that the rate of local recurrence remained comparatively high even after the exclusion of patients with unfavourable histology, but the methodology and data for this are not included. This and the other limits to this study in terms of the control group chosen, as discussed above, make it difficult to draw definitive conclusions. As the authors acknowledge, debate in this area is likely to continue until there is a prospective, randomised clinical trial comparing radical surgery to local excision (Mellgren et al. 2000).

Local Excision with Adjuvant Therapy

The use of radiotherapy and chemotherapy represents an additional variable in any assessment of local excision for rectal carcinoma. The indications for neoadjuvant (pre-operative) or adjuvant therapy and local excision vary between centres, but such treatments are increasingly being offered for T2 tumours and T1 tumours with poor histopathologic characteristics, due to the poor results achieved by local excision alone. Adjuvant or neoadjuvant chemoradiotherapy regimes do appear to improve results following local excision when compared to historical series of surgery alone, but there is a lack of good, controlled data. Variations in the results from single-institution studies that include these therapies are partly due to differences in the timing and dose/fractionation of the therapy utilized. Overall, these uncontrolled studies suggest that adjuvant chemotherapy reduces local recurrence and improves survival in high-risk tumours (Benson et al. 2001; Bleday et al. 1997; Chakravarti et al. 1999; Coco et al. 1992; Fortunato et al. 1995; Frazee et al. 1995; Graham et al. 1999; Le Voyer et al. 1999; Ota et al. 1992; Taylor et al. 1998; Valentini et al. 1996; Varma et al. 1999; Wagman et al. 1999).

The Cancer and Leukaemia Group B (CALGB) researchers report a multi-institutional phase 2 trial with local excision alone for T1 tumours and local excision followed by chemoradiotherapy for T2 tumours. The median follow-up period was 4 years (range 1.8–7.7 years). Fifty-nine patients with T1 lesions underwent local excision alone, and their estimated 6-year overall survival rate was 87% with disease-free survival of 83%. Fifty-one patients with T2 tumours were treated with local excision followed by chemoradiotherapy, with 85% 6-year overall survival and 71% disease-free survival. Disease-free survival is continuing to decline after 5 years, and long-term follow-up is awaited (Steele et al. 1999).

The Radiation Therapy Oncology Group report a phase 2 trial of local excision in 65 patients selected on the basis of T1–3 lesions, less than 4 cm and less than 40% of the diameter of the rectal wall. Those patients identified with high-risk lesions following local excision (T2, T3, high grade, lymphovascular invasion, size >3 cm, or elevated CEA) were treated with adjuvant chemoradiotherapy (with higher-dose radiotherapy in the case of doubtful margins). Overall recurrence was 4% for T1, 16% for T2, and 23% for T3 cancers (Russell et al. 2000).

There have also been reports of the use of neo-adjuvant therapy to downstage tumours before local excision. The earliest study, in 1989, used pre-operative radiotherapy (35 Gy over 3 weeks) in 25 patients, over half of whom were considered unfit for radical surgery. The study protocol included postoperative interstitial radiotherapy (20 Gy for T1 and 25 Gy for T2–3 lesions), and pre-operative staging was based upon EUA rather than radiologic imaging. However, 92% of patients showed a reduction in tumour diameter, and two patients showed a complete response with a pathologic stage of pT0. Local recurrence rates were 0% for T1, 25% for T2, and 30% for T3 lesions (Otmezguine et al. 1989).

Mohiuddin et al. reported on 48 patients with T1–3 lesions, 15 of which were large T3 cancers that underwent local excision due to contraindications to radical surgery. In this study staging included ERUS and in some cases endorectal-coil MRI. The total radiation dose was 40–45 Gy with a boost given in fixed tumours. After a median follow-up of 40 months the local recurrence rates were 11%, 0%, and 67% for T0–1, T2, and T3 lesions, respectively. The 5-year survival rate was 90% for T0–1, 89% for T2, and 50% for T3 lesions (Mohiuddin et al. 1994). A second report from the same department specifically analysed patients with tumours in the distal 2 cm of the rectum, with the intention of establishing that pre-operative high-dose radiotherapy enhances the options for sphincter-preserving surgery. All patients received pre-operative radiotherapy as in the first study, and were then restaged clinically and, as appropriate, with ERUS or MRI. No mention is made of any criteria used in deciding between the several different surgical approaches, both radical and local, that were included in the study. It is stated that local excision was initially considered only in patients with cardiorespiratory problems who were unsuitable for radical resection, but the criteria were subsequently expanded to healthy patients with tumours of <1.5 cm, confined to the rectal wall. Twenty-two out of 70 patients had full-thickness local excision. Two of these (9%) developed local recurrence after a median follow-up of 4 years, and actuarial 5-year survival was 95% (Mohiuddin et al. 1998). It is difficult to interpret these results with any degree of certainty, as they are not sufficiently separated from the results of the other surgical techniques included in the study, and there is likely to have been bias in the selection of patients for local excision.

Kim et al. reported a series of patients who received neo-adjuvant chemoradiotherapy before local excision. This is a retrospective review which included 26 patients with T2–3 lesions, all but one of whom were staged with ERUS. They received 45 Gy in 25 fractions with continuous-infusion 5FU 5 days a week, followed by re-assessment for clinical response with sigmoidoscopy and digital rectal examination. Twelve patients also had a further ERUS examination, but the authors comment that the accuracy of T-staging post-chemoradiotherapy by this technique was only 30%. Only lesions that had complete clinical response (defined as no evidence of residual disease) were initially considered for local excision, although patients with partial response (decrease in size of at least 50%) who refused or were unfit for radical surgery were also included. Pre-therapy staging was T2N0=5, T3N0=13, and T3N1=7. Four were deemed partial and 22 complete responders clinically. Following histopathological examination, the number of complete responders was reduced to 17, and one patient had a positive margin. Median follow-up was 19 months, and one patient had both local (intramural) and regional (inguinal lymph node) recurrence. This patient was a partial responder who initially refused the radical surgery recommended to all partial responders, but later underwent salvage APER and inguinal lymph node dissection (Kim et al. 2001).

Clearly, the data are limited with respect to neo-adjuvant therapy prior to local excision, but they do suggest that it may have a role to play. For both neo-adjuvant and adjuvant therapy, the data are usually retrospective, single-institutional experiences in which there are few defined selection criteria and limited standardisation of surgical technique, with variation in chemotherapeutic regimes.

Transanal Endoscopic Microsurgery

Results for this new technique are usually reported separately from conventional methods of local excision, and frequently include results for benign rectal lesions. A full review of this emerging technology lies beyond the scope of this article. It is generally accepted that TEM preserves anorectal function with limited morbidity and mortality, but in terms of recurrence and survival, results vary too greatly between centres for it to be fully accepted at this time. Again, differences in patient selection, adjuvant therapy, and follow-up policies will account for some of the variation. As the technique is simply an alternative method of providing full-thickness rectal excision it would seem unlikely, all other things being equal, that results will prove to be significantly different to conventional local excision techniques.

Sengupta and Tjandra included in their review 11 TEM series from 1992 to 1998 including 314 patients, and found local recurrence rates varying from 4.2% to 25% and overall survival rates from 62% to 100% at an average follow-up of 35 to 60 months. As alluded to above, these studies included some T3 patients, variably administered adjuvant radiotherapy and with variable follow-up duration, making overall evaluation of the technique difficult (Sengupta and Tjandra 2001).

Analysis of these initial results leads most authors to conclude that TEM has a useful place in the management of adenomas of the rectum, in particular if they are sessile and are located in the mid and upper thirds of the rectum, as well as for carefully selected patients with carcinoma. It has the potential for greater precision of resection than other techniques, low morbidity and mortality, and a short hospitalization period. However, the results of larger series of rectal cancer treated by TEM is required, with appropriate patient selection and complete follow-up, before the technique will be fully accepted. Even then, the cost of the equipment and the specialised surgical expertise required may limit the procedure to tertiary referral centres.

Recurrence Following Local Excision

The ability to successfully perform salvage surgery in patients with local recurrence following local excision is important. It is thought that these recurrences may be biologically different to recurrences after radical surgery. This may be due to the greater proportion of recurrences occurring within the rectal wall, rather than extraluminal pelvic recurrence. For example Mellgren et al. reported 17 (68%) rectal wall recurrences and eight (32%) exclusively extrarectal recurrences (Mellgren et al. 2000). However, the number of attempted salvage procedures following local excision reported in the literature is low, and disease-free survival ranges from 20% to 100% with variable follow-up duration (Sengupta and Tjandra 2001). A further variable to take into account is the salvage procedure undertaken. Some rectal wall recurrences may be dealt with by repeat local excision rather than proceeding directly to radical surgery. Patient-related factors as well as the type of recurrence will play a role in this decision. A recent report by Friel et al. included 29 patients who underwent salvage surgery (APR, low AR, or pelvic exenteration) following local excision of T1 or T2 rectal cancer. Of these, 90% involved the rectal wall with only 10% being purely extrarectal. They found the stage of the recurrence to be more advanced than the original primary in 93% despite the use of preoperative radiotherapy in 12 (44%) of patients. The disease-free survival was 59% following salvage surgery at a mean follow-up of 39 months; however, six (21%) of the operations were noncurative due to positive margins or unresectable liver metastases. Eleven patients developed further recurrences after salvage surgery, only two of which occurred in the noncurative group. Interestingly, they found that the disease-free survival following salvage surgery for those with primary tumours that had favourable histology (68%) was higher than for those with unfavourable histology of the locally excised primary (29%) (Friel et al. 2002). These results indicate that delayed radical surgery for recurrence after local excision may not provide the same chance of cure as a radical resection performed as the initial treatment, and emphasise the importance of careful patient selection. Whether locally excised tumours found to display high-risk characteristics should have immediate radical surgery is a question that has not yet been answered. Early detection of recurrence is essential to allow surgical salvage. As extrarectal recurrences occur in a significant proportion of patients, ERUS or MRI must be a key component of follow-up following local excision.

Conclusions

The published literature leaves several unanswered questions regarding local excision for rectal cancer. The ongoing concerns regarding the morbidity, mortality, and quality of life issues associated with radical resection have led the surgical community to revisit local therapy as a means of managing selected patients with rectal cancers. It is clear that accurate staging of rectal cancer will, in the long term, be the key to the success of local excision, as it will allow appropriate selection of patients. ERUS is currently the most effective method of assessing the depth of wall invasion by the tumour, but it is less reliable at predicting lymph node involvement, which is a crucial factor. CT and MRI have similar limitations. Improved imaging with 3D-ERUS or endorectal coil MRI may improve accuracy, but neither technology is at present widely available.

Appropriate patient selection is the critical requirement for local excision of rectal cancer. Currently, with less than perfect pre-operative prediction of nodal involvement, tumour stage is the most useful discriminatory factor. Only T1 or T2 lesions without evidence of nodal or distant spread should be considered for local excision in otherwise fit patients. Local excision of T3 tumours results in high rates of local recurrence, which should restrict its usage to those patients unable to withstand radical surgery or where the procedure is being performed for palliative reasons. In addition, large tumours (>3–4 cm) occupying >40% of the rectal circumference, or with poor prognostic factors such as mucinous tumours, high histological grade, lymphovascular invasion, or ulceration should also be excluded from local excision alone due to higher than acceptable recurrence rates. We await, as in radical surgery, the emergence of other biological factors which are predictive of stage, recurrence, and survival.

Current data suggest that T1 tumours with no high-risk factors may be suitable for local excision alone with good results, although data comparing local excision to radical surgery in a randomised, controlled fashion do not exist. T2 tumours or T1 tumours with high-risk factors do less well following local excision alone and may benefit from adjuvant therapy. The data supporting this approach are limited and suffer from variability in patient selection and treatment regimes. There are two phase 2 trials, but long-term data for these are not yet available. The data supporting neo-adjuvant therapy in local excision are even more limited and require further evaluation.

The best method of local excision is also open to question. Trans-anal excision produces good results with minimal complications. It is possible that TEM excision will allow a more oncologically sound full-thickness excision with equally minimal complications, but this has yet to be proven. Whatever surgical approach is chosen, postoperative follow-up should be the same as that which follows radical surgery and should include radiologic imaging of the pelvis and liver as well as endoscopic examination of the rectum.

In summary, there is a clear need for well designed and controlled randomised controlled trials to answer the questions surrounding local excision of rectal cancer. Local excision alone is not adequate surgery for T2 or T3 rectal cancer, as it leads to unacceptably high local recurrence rates. The available evidence suggests that low-risk T1 tumours may be treated by local excision alone, and T2 or high-risk T1 tumours will benefit from adjuvant chemoradiotherapy following local excision. Local excision of T3 tumours should be restricted to patients unfit for radical surgery and the palliative setting.

References

Ambacher T, Kasperk R, Schumpelick V (1999) Effect of transanal excision on rate of recurrence of stage I rectal carcinoma in comparison with radical resection methods. Chirurg 70:1469–1474

Balani A, Turoldo, A, Braini A, Scaramucci M (1999) Role of curative local excision in rectal cancer. Annali Italiani di Chirurgia 70:713–720

Balani A, Turoldo A, Braini A, Scaramucci M, Roseano M, Leggeri A (2000) Local excision for rectal cancer. J Surg Oncol 74:158–162

Benson R, Wong CS, Cummings BJ, Brierley J, Catton P, Ringash J, Abdolell M (2001) Local excision and postoperative radiotherapy for distal rectal cancer. Intl J Radiat Oncol Biol Phys 50:1309–1316

Blair S, Ellenhorn JD (2000) Transanal excision for low rectal cancers is curative in early-stage disease with favorable histology. Am Surg 66:817–820

Bleday R, Breen E, Jessup JM, Burgess A, Sentovich SM, Steele G Jr. (1997) Prospective evaluation of local excision for small rectal cancers. Dis Col Rectum 40:388–392

Brodsky JT, Richard GK, Cohen AM, Minsky BD (1992) Variables correlated with the risk of lymph node metastasis in early rectal cancer. Cancer 69:322–326

Buess G, Theiss R, Gunther M, Hutterer F, Pichlmaier H (1985) Endoscopic surgery in the rectum. Endoscopy 17:31–35

Camilleri-Brennan J, Steele RJ (1998) Quality of life after treatment for rectal cancer. Br J Surg 85:1036–1043

Chakravarti A, Compton CC, Shellito PC, Wood WC, Landry J, Machuta SR, Kaufman D, Ancukiewicz M, Willett CG (1999) Long-term follow-up of patients with rectal cancer managed by local excision with and without adjuvant irradiation. Ann Surg 230:49–54

Coco C, Magistrelli P, Granone P, Roncolini G, Picciocchi A (1992) Conservative surgery for early cancer of the distal rectum. Dis Col Rectum 35:131–136

Fortunato L, Ahmad NR, Yeung RS, Coia LR, Eisenberg BL, Sigurdson ER, Yeh K, Weese JL, Hoffman JP (1995) Long-term follow-up of local excision and radiation therapy for invasive rectal cancer. Dis Col Rectum 38:1193–1199

Frazee R, Patel R, Belew M, Roberts J, Hendricks J (1995) Transanal excision of rectal carcinoma. Am Surg 61:714–717

Friel CM, Cromwell JW, Marra C, Madoff RD, Rothenberger DA, Garcia-Aguilar J (2002) Salvage radical surgery after failed local excision for early rectal cancer. Dis Col Rectum 45:875–879

Garcia-Aguilar J, Mellgren A, Sirivongs P, Buie D, Madoff RD, Rothenberger DA (2000) Local excision of rectal cancer without adjuvant therapy: a word of caution. Ann Surg 231:345–351

Goligher J (1984) Surgery of the anus, colon and rectum. Bailliere Tindall, London.

Goligher JC, Lee PW, MacFie J, Simkins KC, Lintott DJ (1979) Experience with the Russian model 249 suture gun for anastomosis of the rectum. Surg, Gynecol Obstet 148:516–524

Graham RA, Hackford AW, Wazer DE (1999) Local excision of rectal carcinoma: a safe alternative for more advanced tumors? J Surg Oncol 70:235–238

Gualdi GF, Casciani E, Guadalaxara A, d'Orta C, Polettini E, Pappalardo G (2000) Local staging of rectal cancer with transrectal ultrasound and endorectal magnetic resonance imaging. Dis Col Rectum 43:338–345

Hager T, Gall FP, Hermanek P (1983) Local excision of cancer of the rectum. Dis Col Rectum 26:149–151

Hainsworth P, Egan M, Cunliffe W (1997) Evaluation of a policy of total mesorectal excision for rectal and rectosigmoid cancers. Br J Surg 84:652–656

Heald RJ, Husband EM, Ryall RD (1982) The mesorectum in rectal cancer surgery—the clue to pelvic recurrence? B J Surg 69:613–616

Kim CJ, Yeatman TJ, Coppola D, Trotti A, Williams B, Barthel JS, Dinwoodie W, Karl RC, Marcet J (2001) Local excision of T2 and T3 rectal cancers after downstaging chemoradiation. Ann Surg 234:352–358

Le Voyer TE, Hoffman JP, Cooper H, Ross E, Sigurdson E, Eisenberg B (1999) Local excision and chemoradiation for low rectal T1 and T2 cancers is an effective treatment. Am Surg 65:625–630

Mellgren A, Sirivongs P, Rothenberger DA, Madoff RD, Garcia-Aguilar J (2000) Is local excision adequate therapy for early rectal cancer? Dis Col Rectum 43:1064–1071

Miles W (1908) A method of performing abdominoperineal excision for carcinoma of the rectum and of the terminal portion of the pelvic colon. Lancet 2:1812
Minsky BD, Rich T, Recht A, Harvey W, Mies C (1989) Selection criteria for local excision with or without adjuvant radiation therapy for rectal cancer. Cancer 63:1421–1429
Mohiuddin M, Marks G, Bannon J (1994) High-dose preoperative radiation and full thickness local excision: a new option for selected T3 distal rectal cancers. Intl J Radiat Oncol Biol Phys 30:845–849
Mohiuddin M, Regine WF, Marks GJ, Marks JW (1998) High-dose preoperative radiation and the challenge of sphincter-preservation surgery for cancer of the distal 2 cm of the rectum. Intl J Radiat Oncol Biol Phys 40:569–574
National Statistics Online (2003) Cancer Trends. National Statistics website: www.statistics.gov.uk
Nicholls RJ, Mason AY, Morson BC, Dixon AK, Fry LK (1982) The clinical staging of rectal cancer. Br J Surg 69:404–409
Ota DM, Skibber J, Rich T (1992) M.D. Anderson Cancer Center experience with local excision and multimodality therapy for rectal cancer. Surg Oncol Clin North Am 1:147–152
Otmezguine Y, Grimard L, Calitchi E, Despretz J, Mazeron JJ, Le Bourgeois JP, Pierquin B, Julien M (1989) A new combined approach in the conservative management of rectal cancer. Intl J Radiat Oncol Biol Phys 17:539–545
Pricolo V, Potenti F (2001) Modern management of rectal cancer. Dig Surg 18:1–20
Rothenberger DA, Garcia-Aguilar J (2000) Role of local excision in the treatment of rectal cancer. Seminars Surg Oncol 19:367–375
Russell A, Harris J, Rosenberg P et al (2000) Anal sphincter conservation for patients with adenocarcinoma of the distal rectum: long term results of radiation therapy oncology group protocol 89–02. Intl J Radiat Oncol Biol Phys 46:313–322
Sengupta S, Tjandra JJ (2001) Local excision of rectal cancer: what is the evidence? Dis Col Rectum 44:1345–1361
Sitzler P, Seow-Choen F, Ho Y, Leong A (1997) Lymph node involvement and tumour depth in rectal cancers: an analysis of 805 patients. Dis Col Rectum 40:1472–1476
Spencer MP (2001) Transanal excision for T1 and T2 rectal cancer–efficacy of local resection vs. adjuvant therapy. Extended abstract. Swiss Surg 7:275–277
Steele GD Jr, Herndon JE, Bleday R, Russell A, Benson A III, Hussain M, Burgess A, Tepper JE, Mayer RJ (1999) Sphincter-sparing treatment for distal rectal adenocarcinoma. Ann Surg Oncol 6:433–441
Taylor RH, Hay JH, Larsson SN (1998) Transanal local excision of selected low rectal cancers. Am J Surg 175:360–363
Tobaruela E, Arribas D, Mortensen N (1999) Is endosonography useful to select patients for endoscopic treatment of rectal cancer? Revista Espanola de Enfermedades Digestivas 91:614–621
Valentini V, Morganti AG, De Santis M, Vecchio FM, Coco C, Picciocchi A, Cellini N (1996) Local excision and external beam radiotherapy in early rectal cancer. Intl J Radiat Oncol Biol Phys 35:759–764
Varma MG, Rogers SJ, Schrock TR, Welton ML (1999) Local excision of rectal carcinoma. Arch Surg 134:863–867
Visser BC, Varma MG, Welton ML (2001) Local therapy for rectal cancer. Surg Oncol 10:61–69
Wagman R, Minsky, BD, Cohen, AM, Saltz, L, Paty, PB, Guillem, JG (1999) Conservative management of rectal cancer with local excision and postoperative adjuvant therapy. Intl J Radiat Oncol Biol Phys 44:841–846
Wexner SD, Rotholtz NA (2000) Surgeon influenced variables in resectional rectal cancer surgery. Dis Col Rectum 43:1606–1627
Willett CG, Compton CC, Shellito PC, Efird JT (1994) Selection factors for local excision or abdominoperineal resection of early stage rectal cancer. Cancer 73:2716–2720
Zenni GC, Abraham K, Harford FJ et al (1998) Characteristics of rectal carcinomas that predict the presence of lymph node metastases: implications for patient selection for local therapy. J Surg Oncol 67:99–103

Operative Treatment of Locally Recurrent Rectal Cancer

Johan N. Wiig, Stein G. Larsen, Karl-Erik Giercksky

J.N. Wiig (✉)
Department of Surgery, The Norwegian Radium Hospital, 0310 Oslo, Norway
e-mail: joniwii@online.no

Abstract

Few centres with varying regimens have published studies including more than 100 patients on the treatment of locally recurrent rectal cancer. The results vary considerably. Thus there seems to be a need for more studies to establish the potential benefit of a more widespread treatment of these cancers. In total, 193 patients had surgery for locally recurrent rectal cancers after preoperative irradiation 46–50 Gy in 2 Gy fractions. The patients were followed up and the data prospectively entered in a database. In 88 patients with primary low anterior resection, 3% had lower end of tumour located more than 2 cm above the anastomosis, 5% more than 2 cm below the anastomosis; 13% had exploratory laparotomy, 8% low anterior resections, the rest equally frequent abdomino-perineal resections, Hartmann's operations, and tumour resections. Nearly half had resection of part of the pelvic wall. Hysterectomy was performed in 15% and cystoprostatectomy in 9%. Three patients had en bloc prostatectomy. R0 resections were achieved in 39%, R1 in 36%, and R2 or no resection in 25%. R0 stage was twice as often achieved after a primary low anterior resection as after abdomino-perineal resections. The 30-days postoperative mortality was 1%. Postoperative morbidity was 48%, most frequently pelvic abscesses. Estimated 5-year survival was 18% for the total group. There was a statistically significant difference in survival and local re-recurrences between R0 / R1 and R2 stages. The results are discussed relative to recent studies. Patients in whom R0 resections can be achieved will benefit from the treatment, and probably patients with R1 resections would also benefit. Such operations should possibly be performed in specialised centres as joint ventures between various surgical subspecialities.

Recent Results in Cancer Research, Vol. 165

Introduction

With the introduction of total mesorectal excision (TME) (Heald et al. 1982) the frequency of local recurrence after operation for rectal cancer has dramatically decreased in many centres (Wibe et al. 2002a). Still, as rectal cancer is very common, a 5%–10% local recurrence rate means that a substantial number of patients will need treatment for this condition. Untreated the local recurrence may cause local or irradiating pain, fistulas to the vagina, bladder, or small bowel, or in a patient with a previous low anterior resection (LAR) fistula, rectal stenosis, tenesmus, and bleeding. In 20%–50% of the patients, the local recurrence starts without any concomitant disseminated metastases (Gunderson and Sosin 1974) that may cause the death of the patient before the local recurrence will cause distressing symptoms. In such cases, successful treatment of the local recurrence may cure the patients. Whether chemotherapy, which can delay the development of distant metastases, will have a similar effect on local recurrence has so far not been established. Thus both from a curative and a palliative view there is a need to invest a considerable effort in the treatment of local recurrences.

Definition of Local Recurrence

Local recurrence is usually defined as any recurrence within the true pelvis.

After abdomino-perineal excision (APR), local recurrences may develop in the perineal scar or in females on the wall of the vagina. In quite a few of these cases, the recurrence may also grow into the presacral space.

Materials and Methods

The Norwegian Radium Hospital is a tertiary referral hospital for surgical treatment of locally advanced and locally recurrent rectal cancer combined with preoperative radiotherapy.

From September 1990 until June 2002, 193 patients with recurrent rectal cancer were treated with preoperative external radiotherapy and surgery, 72 females and 121 males. The mean age was 65 years (34–82), and 19% had simultaneous metastases. During a 5-year period we operated 75% of the patients admitted with local recurrence.

All except two patients had biopsy verification of the recurrence before irradiation. If necessary, transrectal fine-needle aspiration cytology or fine-needle core biopsy was performed. In our hands cytology was more accurate than biopsy (Wiig et al. 1996). Routine examinations before inclusion were digital recto-vaginal exploration, sigmoidoscopy with rigid instrument, CT of the pelvis (in recent years often MRI), ultrasound of the liver, chest X-ray, and blood tests including CEA. If necessary, cystoscopy was performed, and in later years transrectal ultrasound if the prostate was possibly involved. Four weeks after the end of radiotherapy, the same examinations were repeated before surgery was decided upon.

Follow-up was every 3 months the first 2 years, thereafter twice a year until 5 years. The same examinations were repeated at follow-up except that MRI scans were not included. If the patient died later, this could be retrieved from The Norwegian Death Registry.

Details of the radiotherapy have been described (Wiig et al. 2002). In brief, patients were given 46 Gy in 2 Gy fractions, in later years with a 4-Gy boost to the tumour. Photon energies of 10–16 MV were used. Sensitising chemotherapy was given to a few patients as part of a randomised study. Intra-operative radiotherapy (IORT) was given to selected patients until December 1999 (Wiig et al. 2002). It was interrupted as we were not able to identify any effect of it.

Surgery was performed at a median time interval of 8 weeks, ranging from 4–14 weeks. It was performed by five surgeons, the majority of operations being performed by the same surgeon. Frozen sections were taken at the discretion of the surgeon. It was often difficult to identify the exact border of the tumour fixation due to fibrosis from previous surgery and irradiation.

The R-stage of the operation was always recorded (R0=microscopically free circumferential and distal margin, R1=microscopically involved margin, and R2=locally macroscopically residual cancer or nonresection).

Patient data were prospectively entered in a database.

Curves of actuarial survival and local control were calculated with the Kaplan-Meier product-limit method, and statistical differences between curves were calculated with the log rank test. Calculations were performed with SPSS statistical software.

Results

In summary, 56% of the patients had symptoms at the time of diagnosis despite a nationwide follow-up program. Operations on the rectum are described in Table 1. No resection was done in 23 patients (12%). We were reluctant to perform LAR when we considered the possibility of a local re-recurrence or anal incontinence relatively high. Also, quite a number of our patients had a well functioning deviating stoma and were therefore not interested in an anastomosis with its potential problems. When the cancer was not on the pelvic floor, we therefore frequently performed Hartmann's procedures.

Table 1. Rectal cancer operations performed on 193 patients

Operation	Number
Exploratory laparotomy	23
LAR	16
APR	51
Hartmann's operation	50
Tumour resections	53

Table 2. Additional resections

Organs	Number
Pelvic wall	81
Hysterectomy	27
Vaginal resection	30
Cystoprostatectomy	18
Cystectomy	4
Prostatectomy	3
Sacrum	3

Table 3. R-stage achievement relative to primary operation. Total number and percentage within each operation

Primary operation	Total no.	R-0	R-1	R-2
Total number	193	39	36	25
LAR	97	47	33	20
APR	59	24	42	34

Table 4. Postoperative complications (% of all patients)

Organs involved	%
30 Days mortality	1
Gut leakage	3
Urinary leakage	9
Pelvic abscess	25
Septicaemia	4
Pneumonia	10
Wound infections	15
DVT	3
PE	2
Patients with morbidity	48

A number of additional resections were performed (Table 2). Most often this was resection of a part of the pelvic wall. Vagina and uterus were also frequently resected. Cystoprostatectomy was performed in 18 patients, while three patients had their prostate removed en bloc with the rectum or recurrent tumour. Cystectomy was also performed in four females with a previous hysterectomy. In three cases we resected part of the sacrum.

Generally these procedures were joint ventures with a gastro-intestinal surgeon, urologist, gynaecologist, orthopaedic, and plastic surgeons involved.

Overall we achieved 75% R0/R1 resections (Table 3). The frequency of R0 resections was twice as high after a primary LAR as following an APR.

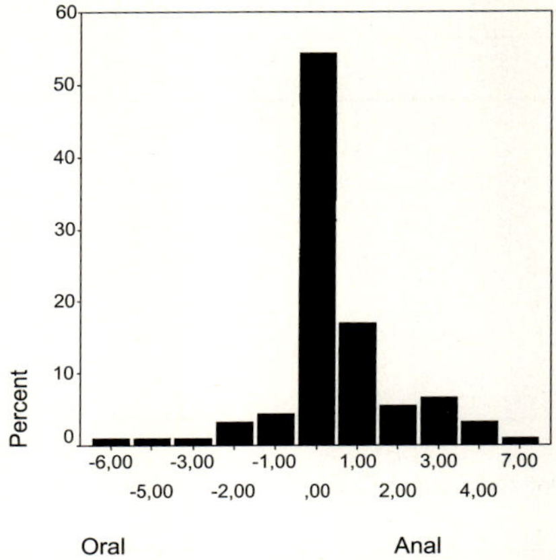

Figure 1. Location of recurrence relative to anastomosis in 88 patients with primary anterior resections

Thirty days' postoperative mortality was 1% (Table 4). One patient died the first postoperative day from pulmonary embolus, and one after 3 weeks from intra-abdominal abscess and pulmonary embolus. There was a considerable post-operative morbidity involving 48% of the patients, the most frequent being pelvic abscess with or without delayed healing of a perineal incision.

After a previous LAR the recurrence may develop in the anastomosis (Wiig et al. 1999), but in the majority of cases the recurrence develops outside the rectum and subsequently grows into the anastomosis. In the majority of cases, local recurrence (LR) seemed to be located from the anastomosis and cranially. In 88 patients with a primary LAR, we found LR with its lowest border more than 2 cm above the anastomosis in only 2% and more than 2 cm below the anastomosis in 5% (Fig. 1).

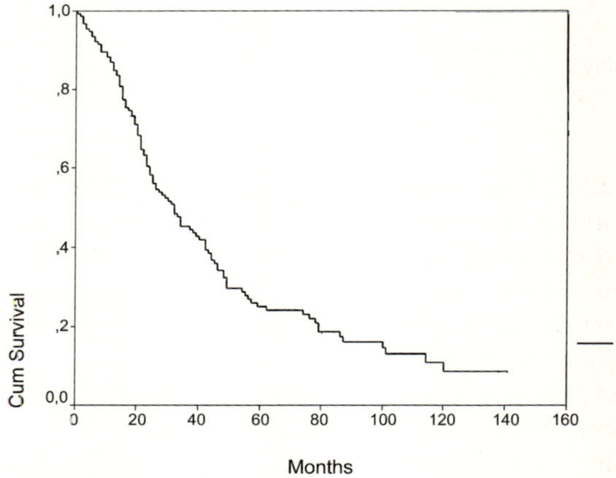

Figure 2. Estimated survival of 193 patients operated for local recurrence

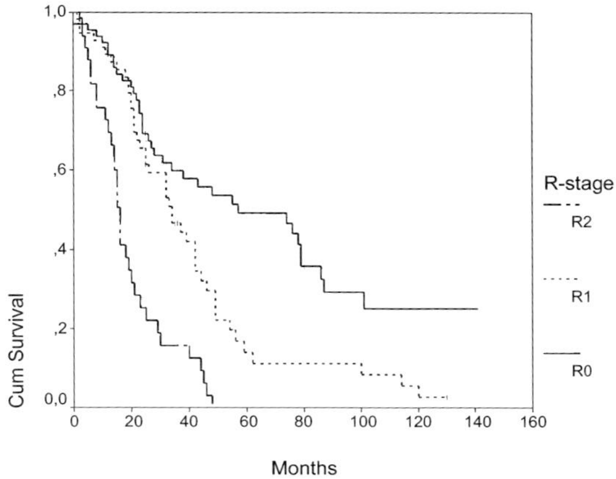

Figure 3. Estimated survival of related to R-stage in 154 patients stage M0 at operation

Thus if the anastomosis could be reached by the finger, the LR could then nearly always be reached as well.

Kaplan–Meier curves suggested 18% 5-year survival in the 193 patients, including those with simultaneous metastases (Fig. 2). In the 154 patients without distant metastases at operation, the 5-year survival differed between the various R-stages with 45% for R0, 18% for R1, and no 4-year survivors in the R2 group (Fig. 3). These differences were statistically significant ($p = 0.02$ and $p < 0.000$).

Not unexpectedly, local re-recurrence also depended on the R-stage. In R1 resections, the Kaplan–Meier curve suggested 67% local re-recurrence. Even in R0 resections, this was as high as 30% (Fig. 4).

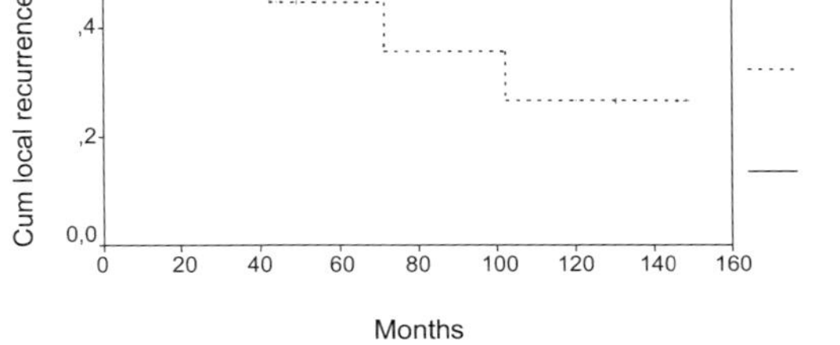

Figure 4. Estimated freedom of local re-recurrence in 144 R0/R1 patients

Discussion

Surgery with complete removal of the cancer is the only possibility for cure in patients without distant metastases.

In recurrent cancer the tumour usually grows outside the natural envelope of the mesorectum, and the cancer will possibly infiltrate further out from the macroscopic border. As it is not possible to obtain wide margins on the pelvic wall, it therefore seems reasonable to try to shrink the periphery of the cancer before surgery.

Irradiation

It has been convincingly shown that many rectal cancers are sensitive to irradiation. This radiation effect is dose-dependent (Knol et al. 1997). After preoperative irradiation, sometimes the cancer disappears even microscopically (Garcia-Aguilar et al. 2003). Generally the cancer recurs and very few patients survive 5 years (Wong et al. 1998).

As it may be difficult to identify the true borders of a recurrent cancer, our policy has been to give preoperative irradiation to patients with LR because they do not have a small and well demarcated cancer.

It has been suggested that IORT with electron beams can enhance the effect of irradiation on the cancer without prohibitively increasing the effect on the normal tissue. Many studies have claimed to show an effect. Most of the studies include a small number of patients, and the results are partly contradictory with regard to the effect on R0-R1 and R2 stages. There seems to be one common conclusion from all studies: Obtaining an R0 resection is the main prognostic factor. IORT cannot improve an R1 resection to the survival level of an R0 resection. In other words, IORT cannot compensate for an R1 resection. Recently two studies have suggested the need for a randomised study on IORT in rectal cancer treatment (Shoup et al. 2002; Wiig et al. 2002).

Chemotherapy

Several regimens with 5FU as a sensitising agent during radiotherapy have been applied (Gunderson et al. 1996). Complete pathological responses have been reported from 5% to 25% (Lowy et al. 1996), although a randomised study has not been performed to show a clinical benefit. Recently regimens with newer, potentially more effective and also more toxic drugs are being tried.

Patients with Previous Pelvic Irradiation

An increasing number of patients have in various countries been given pre- or postoperative irradiation for their primary cancer. When LR develops, some centres will give another 30 Gy external irradiation (Mohiuddin et al. 1997), while other centres give 15–20 Gy external irradiation and 15–20 Gy IORT (Haddock et al. 2001). Such doses are in the opinion of many radiotherapists too small to have a lethal effect on the cancers, and there is a great chance for complications from the normal tissues. From a theoretical point of view, LR may require higher doses of radiotherapy than primary cancers because recurrences often develop in fibrous, sparsely vascularised and therefore more hypoxic tissue which is less sensitive to the effect of irradiation. In view of this, some centres operate without further irradiation (Cunningham et al. 1997).

Special Problems During Operation for Local Recurrence

As mentioned, LR seldom develops in remnants of the mesorectum distal to the anastomosis. There are therefore usually no natural borders for the recurrent cancer. While we are accustomed to a 2-mm distance from the cancer to the CRM as adequate in a mobile cancer growing within the mesorectum (Quirke and Dixon 1988;Wibe et al. 2002b), we do not know what will be adequate margins when the cancer grows outside the mesorectum. Another problem is that it may be impossible to differentiate fibrous scar from infiltrating cancer. The true border of the LR and the proper areas from where to take the frozen sections can therefore be difficult to identify. And it may be difficult to decide whether nearby organs such as nerves, vessels, or prostate may have to be resected in order to completely remove the cancer.

Irradiation will cause an immediate acute inflammation in the tissues with oedema and brittle tissues. Eight weeks after the end of irradiation, a fibrous reaction most often has taken place. This can cause a condensation of the fasciae, and the interfascial spaces may be even easier to open. On the other hand, where the spaces are closed by inflammation the opening become even more difficult. The fasciae can also stick harder to the underlying tissues. The planes on the pelvic wall will therefore be more difficult to identify, and it is often difficult to isolate the vessels on the pelvic wall, especially the veins. Of course these problems can also have been caused by the previous operation. In some cases the thickened, oedematous mesorectum is voluminous and reduces the view in the pelvis during the dissection. The magnitude and duration of the inflammatory reaction caused by the irradiation vary considerably between patients.

Previous Studies

Surgery for LR is usually performed at referral centres. The percentage of referred patients who actually undergo surgery is seldom reported. The low numbers of patients published in the studies suggest that they represent a highly selected population.

A number of studies on the treatment of recurrent rectal cancer have been published. However, we have only been able to identify three recent papers that include more than 100 patients or centres operating on more than eight patients per year. A mixture of various treatment regimens has been applied. Most centres will give preoperative radiation therapy of 46–50 Gy when radiation was not part of their primary treatment. Patients with a previous radiotherapy (RT) will either receive no additional RT (Cunningham et al. 1997) or 10–30 Gy external beam (Mohiuddin et al. 1997; Haddock et al. 2001). IORT may be given to both groups either by an accelerator (Gunderson et al. 1996) or as high-dose-rate brachytherapy (Shoup et al. 2002). In addition to the variation in RT, there is a wide variation of chemotherapy regimens within each centre. Also adding to the difficulty in comparing the results is the fact that many centres report their recurrences at a median follow-up time and not as Kaplan-Meier curves.

Of ten recent papers, five presented less than 60 patients (Bergamaschi et al. 2001; Esnaola et al. 2003; Kuehne et al. 2003; Law et al. 2000; Lopez-Kostner et al. 2001), only three presented 100 or more (Shoup et al. 2002; Miner et al. 2003; Hahnloser et al. 2003), and the rest in between (Cunningham et al. 1997; Garcia-Aguilar et al. 2001). The results vary widely. This can be due to differences in surgical aggressiveness or patient selection. In the smaller studies, a variation in biology of operated tumour can also influence the results.

The R0 resection rate varies from 34% to 64%. As it can be difficult to identify the cancer from the fibrous scar tissue, differences in number of histological sections studied can possibly also explain part of the differences.

In the total group of reported patients, 5-year survival varied from 21% to 64%, mostly around 25%. Differences in surgical aggressiveness with differences in R0 / R1 resections achieved are probably of major importance, as the studies consistently found better survival for R0 resections. For this group, 5-year survival varied from 35% to 90%, mostly around 45%. The majority of studies find that patients with R2 resections do worse than R1 resected patients. In one centre they obtained 18% 5-year survival in the R2 group, which they considered was due to the IORT treatment (Gunderson et al. 1996).

There seems to be a correlation between survival and local control. Local control at 5 years varied from 27% to 87%. Once again it is difficult to tell whether the difference in surgical aggressiveness, oncological treatment, or patient selection is the reason for the wide variation in results.

There are no randomised studies comparing various treatment regimens for locally recurrent rectal cancer. From literature studies we have not found any particular treatment regimen consistently giving better results. Still, we consider it reasonable to give high doses of external beam radiation preoperatively.

All studies report low mortality rates varying from 0% to 3%. On the other hand, there is quite a difference in postoperative morbidity, varying from 14% to 49%, mostly around 25%.

Contraindications to Surgical Treatment

Operations for local recurrence may be time-consuming and require more blood transfusions than ordinary rectal cancer operations. The general medical condition of the patient should therefore be meticulously considered.

Local inoperability criteria will vary from centre to centre. Generally involvement of the somatic nerves to the lower extremities are considered contraindications to operation, at least when S1 and often S2 nerves are involved as indicated by irradiating pain. This may be the case when the tumour is located on the piriformis muscle. When the cancer is located near the ischial spine, it may involve the sciatic nerve and is therefore considered inoperable. It is generally agreed that total sacrectomy is hardly indicated for recurrent rectal cancer, where the possibility for cure by such a mutilating surgical procedure will be relatively low. Some studies report a relatively high number of resections between S2/S3 (Magrini et al. 1996; Yamada et al. 2002).

Resection of the common or external iliac veins does not seem to be performed in this context. Thus a DVT in these vessels does seem to be a contraindication. On the other hand, in some cases where there is a lack of plane between tumour and vein wall, the cancer can still be dissected off the vessel. In a similar situation, arteries can most often be isolated from the cancer. If the primary operation revealed the naked vessel wall, it can be difficult to tell in a secondary dissection whether the adherences are due to scar tissue only and not the local recurrence.

Hydronephrosis has been suggested to be an absolute contraindication to surgery (Cheng et al. 2001). In our experience, unilateral hydronephrosis suggests that the possibility of obtaining an R0 resection is reduced. The Mayo Clinic experience revealed that if the cancer is fixed in two or more quadrants, the possibility of a successful operation is small (Hahnloser et al. 2003).

As the majority of studies shows that 70%–80% of the patients will die within 5 years, the palliative aspect of the operation is of considerable importance. Only a few have reported on this. The largest one studied 81 nonpalliatively treated patients versus 24 palliated ones (Miner et al. 2003). Improvement in symptoms was found in 78% of the nonpalliative group versus 42% in the palliative one. This improvement lasted for 24 months in the nonpalliative versus only 4 months for the palliatively treated group. In another study it was found that less palliation was obtained with the treatment in female patients, after total pelvic exenteration or sacrum resection or when symptoms were present at the diagnosis of the LR (Esnaola et al. 2003). From our hospital we have found that total pelvic exenteration can be compatible with an acceptable quality of life (Guren et al. 2001)

Conclusions

It seems that after careful selection, R0 resections can be achieved in a substantial number of patients with local recurrence after operation for rectal cancer. This can possibly best be achieved by multimodal treatment. Also, R1 resected patients can benefit from longer survival, and local recurrence can be avoided. It seems less clear whether patients in whom a macroscopic resection cannot be achieved will benefit from operation. The diagnosis and treatment of local recurrences can be technically demanding and should probably be performed in specialised centres.

References

Bergamaschi R, Pessaux P, Burtin P, Arnaud JP (2001) Abdominoperineal resection for locally recurrent rectal cancer. Tech Coloproctol 5:97–102

Cheng C, Rodriguez-Bigas MA, Petrelli N (2001) Is there a role for curative surgery for pelvic recurrence from rectal carcinoma in the presence of hydronephrosis? Am J Surg 182:274–277

Cunningham JD, Enker W, Cohen A (1997) Salvage therapy for pelvic recurrence following curative rectal cancer resection. Dis Colon Rectum 40:393–400

Esnaola NF, Cantor S, Johnson ML, Mirza AN, Miller AR, Curley SA, Crane CH, Cleeland CS, Janjan NA, and Skibber JM (2003) Pain and quality of life after treatment in patients with locally recurrent rectal cancer. J Clin Oncol 20:4361–4367

Garcia-Aguilar J, Cromwell JW, Marra C, Lee SH, Madoff RD, Rothenberger DA (2001) Treatment of locally recurrent rectal cancer. Dis Colon Rectum 44:1743–1748

Garcia-Aguilar J, Hernandez dA, Sirivongs P, Lee SH, Madoff RD, Rothenberger DA (2003) A pathologic complete response to preoperative chemoradiation is associated with lower local recurrence and improved survival in rectal cancer patients treated by mesorectal excision. Dis Colon Rectum 46:298–304

Gunderson LL, Nelson H, Martenson JA, Cha S, Haddock M, Devine R, Fieck JM, Wolff B, Dozois R, O'Connell MJ (1996) Intraoperative electron and external beam irradiation with or without 5-fluorouracil and maximum surgical resection for previously unirradiated, locally recurrent colorectal cancer. Dis Colon Rectum 39:1379–1395

Gunderson LL, Sosin H (1974) Areas of failure found at reoperation (second or symptomatic look) following "curative surgery" for adenocarcinoma of the rectum. Clinicopathologic correlation and implications for adjuvant therapy. Cancer 34:1278–1292

Guren MG, Wiig JN, Dueland S, Tveit KM, Fosså SF, Waehre H, Giercksky K-E (2001) Quality of life in patients with urinary diversion after operation for locally advanced rectal cancer. Eur J Surg Onco 27:645–651

Haddock MG, Gunderson LL, Nelson H, Cha SS, Devine RM, Dozzois RR Wolff BG (2001) Intraoperative irradiation for locally recurrent colorectal cancer in previously irradiated patients. Int J Radiat Oncol Biol Phys 49:1267–1274

Hahnloser D, Nelson H, Gunderson LL, Hassan I, Haddock MG, O'Connell MJ, Cha S, Sargent DJ, Horgan A (2003) Curative potential of multimodality therapy for locally recurrent rectal cancer. Ann Surg 237:502–508

Heald RJ, Husband EM, Ryall RD (1982) The mesorectum in rectal cancer surgery—the clue to pelvic recurrence? Br J Surg 69:613–616

Knol HP, Hanssens PE, Rutten HJ, Wiggers T (1997) Effect of radiation therapy alone or in combination with surgery and/or chemotherapy on tumor and symptom control of recurrent rectal cancer. Strahlenther Onkol 173:43–49

Kuehne J, Kleisli T, Biernacki P, Girvigian M, Streeter O, Corman ML, Ortega AE, Vukasin P, Essani R, Beart RW (2003) Use of high-dose-rate brachytherapy in the management of locally recurrent rectal cancer. Dis Colon Rectum 46:895–899

Law WL, Chu KW, Choi HK (2000) Total pelvic exenteration for locally advanced rectal cancer. J Am Coll Surg 190:78–83

Lopez-Kostner F, Fazio VW, Vignali A, Rybicki LA, Lavery IC (2001) Locally recurrent rectal cancer: predictors and success of salvage surgery. Dis Colon Rectum 44:173–178

Lowy AM, Rich TA, Skibber JM, Dubrow RA, Curley SA (1996) Preoperative infusional chemoradiation, selective intraoperative radiation, and resection for locally advanced pelvic recurrence of colorectal adenocarcinoma. Ann Surg 223:177–185

Magrini S, Nelson H, Gunderson LL, Sim FH (1996) Sacropelvic resection and intraoperative electron irradiation in the management of recurrent anorectal cancer. Dis Colon Rectum 39:1-9

Miner TJ, Jaques DP, Paty PB, Guillem JG, and Wong WD (2003) Symptom control in patients with locally recurrent rectal cancer. Ann Surg Oncol 10:72–79

Mohiuddin M, Marks GM, Lingareddy V, Marks J (1997) Curative surgical resection following reirradiation for recurrent rectal cancer. Int J Radiat Oncol Biol Phys 39:643–649

Quirke P, Dixon MF (1988) The prediction of local recurrence in rectal adenocarcinoma by histopathological examination. Int J Colorect Dis 3:127–131

Shoup M, Guillem JG, Alektiar KM, Liau K, Paty PB, Cohen AM, Wong WD, Minsky BD (2002) Predictors of survival in recurrent rectal cancer after resection and intraoperative radiotherapy. Dis Colon Rectum 45:585–592

Wibe A, Moller B, Norstein J, Carlsen E, Wiig JN, Heald RJ, Langmark F, Myrvold HE, Soreide O (2002a) A national strategic change in treatment policy for rectal cancer—implementation of total mesorectal excision as routine treatment in Norway. A national audit. Dis Colon Rectum 45:857–866

Wibe A, Rendedal PR, Svensson E, Norstein J, Eide TJ, Myrvold HE and Soreide O (2002b) Prognostic significance of the circumferential margin following total mesorectal excision for rectal cancer. Br J Surg 89:327–334.

Wiig JN, Berner A, Tveit KM, Giercksky KE (1996) Evaluation of digitally guided fine needle aspiration cytology versus fine needle core biopsy for the diagnosis of recurrent rectal cancer. Int J Colorect Dis 11:272–275

Wiig JN, Tveit KM, Poulsen JP, Olsen DR, Giercksky K-E (2002) Preoperative irradiation and surgery for recurrent rectal cancer. Will intraoperative irradiation (IORT) be of additional benefit? A prospective study. Radiother Oncol 62:207–213

Wiig JN, Wolff PA, Tveit KM, Giercksky KE (1999) Location of pelvic recurrence after 'curative' low anterior resection for rectal cancer. Eur J Surg Oncol 25:590–594

Wong CS, Cummings BJ, Brierley JD, Catton CN, McLean M, Catton P, Hao Y (1998) Treatment of locally recurrent rectal carcinoma—results and prognostic factors. Int J Radiat Oncol Biol Phys 40:427–435

Yamada K, Ishizawa T, Niwa K, Chuman Y, Aikou T (2002) Pelvic exenteration and sacral resection for locally advanced primary and recurrent rectal cancer. Dis Colon Rectum 45:1078–1084

Laparoscopic TME: Better Vision, Better Results?

T. H. K. Schiedeck, F. Fischer, C. Gondeck, U. J. Roblick, H. P. Bruch

T.H.K. Schiedeck (✉)
Department of General and Visceral Surgery, Clinic Ludwigsburg, Posilipostr. 4, 71631 Ludwigsburg, Germany
e-mail: info-chirurgie@onlinehome.de

Abstract

One of the most controversial discussions on laparoscopic surgery deals with the question of whether to apply this technique to malignant disease and specifically to rectal cancer. The four major issues are the adequacy of oncologic resection, recurrence rates and patterns, long-term survival and quality of life. There is evidence, from nonrandomized studies, suggesting that margins of excision and lymph node harvest achieved laparoscopically reached comparable results to those known from conventional open resection. Our own experience of laparoscopic surgery on rectal cancer is based on 52 patients treated with curative intent. Focusing on the postoperative long-term run, we gained the following results: The median age of patients was 66.7 years and ranged from 42–88. Anastomotic leakage was seen in 6.1% of cases. In a median follow-up of 48 months (36–136), we reached an overall 3-year survival rate of 93% and a 5-year survival rate of 62%. Local recurrence was 1.9%, distant metastasis occurred in 11.5% of cases. We saw no port-site metastasis. To evaluate functional results following laparoscopic surgery a matched pair analysis was carried out. Matching of patients after laparoscopic and conventional open surgery was performed according to sex, age, type of resection, time period of surgery, and stage of disease classified by UICC. Regarding bladder and sexual dysfunction, using the EORTC QLQ CR38 score we found no statistical significant difference between the examined groups. As far as can be seen, laparoscopic surgery in rectal carcinoma may achieve the same or, in selected patients, even better results than open surgery. However, at present no published study has shown much evidence. Many more studies are necessary to define the place of laparoscopic technique in rectal cancer surgery, regarding appropriate selection of patients and evaluating adjuvant or neoadjuvant treatment in combination with the laparoscopic approach.

Recent Results in Cancer Research, Vol. 165

Introduction

The concept of total mesorectal excision (TME) was first developed by Westhues and Stelzner [54, 61] and later popularized worldwide by Heald in 1982 [21]. With this technique, the local recurrence rate after 5 years is less than 5% and 5-year survival reaches 70%–80%. These results represent a great improvement over traditional surgical techniques, even compared to studies where adjuvant treatment was additionally administered. Thus, TME became the gold standard for curative resection of cancer located in the middle and lower rectum.

The technique consists of a precise sharp dissection along the wall of the small pelvis to resect the entire mesentery of the hindgut with its draining lymphatics. The second goal is the preservation of the hypogastric nerve plexus by exact dissection in the tissue plane that separates the mesorectal fascia covering the mesorectum from the presacral fascia. Indeed, when these nerves are preserved, 80% of male patients below 60 years of age may retain potency [20]. On the other hand, the incidence of bladder and sexual dysfunction varies immensely, with reported percentages between 8–54 (bladder dysfunction) and 18–59 (sexual dysfunction), respectively [39].

One main concern regarding TME is the possible increase in the rate of anastomotic dehiscences. Heald [22] reported in his own series 11% clinically apparent anastomotic leaks and an additional 6.4% which where detected by contrast enema. To overcome the adverse clinical effect, many surgeons employ routine fecal diversion by loop ileostomy.

The Laparoscopic Approach to TME

The laparoscopic approach offers several potential advantages over laparotomy. Its technical feasibility, safety, and learning curve-related issues have been well documented for a variety of indications in the field of colon and rectum surgery [4, 6–8, 11, 15, 16, 23, 24, 26, 28, 29, 31, 40, 43, 45, 46, 48–50, 59, 65]. Benefits such as reduced postoperative pain, reduced need for postoperative analgesia, less ileus, shorter hospital stay, and better cosmesis are well known. There has been major controversy about the application of this approach to colorectal malignancy. In this context, questions regarding cancer clearance, local recurrence, and overall survival had to be answered. Although several studies [1, 5, 9, 13, 17, 18, 27, 34, 38, 42, 44, 47, 52, 53, 62, 63] have shown no adverse oncologic outcome, the situation remains unclear due to the fact that large randomized multicenter trials are still pending. Moreover, these larger trials, such as the NCI trial, COST Study, COLOR trial or LAPKON-II study, focus on colon cancer and explicitly exclude rectal carcinoma.

Port-site recurrence was a major drawback when laparoscopy was introduced into clinical routine for the treatment of malignancy. Whereas tumor recurrence to the abdominal wall following conventional laparotomy is rare (1%) as reported in the literature for laparoscopic resection, the frequency of port-site metastasis is reported to be between 0%–21%. Various theories have been suggested to explain this problem. Beside experimental models, routine clinical practice has shown the importance of wound protection, which became standard practice for the majority of surgeons. Nevertheless, currently there is no final explanation for port-site recurrence and abdominal wall metastasis. However, it has been demonstrated by a lot of clinical studies that port-site metastasis is not a complication induced by the laparoscopic approach itself but should be considered a technical complication following incorrect handling during the procedure [25, 57].

The number of yielded lymph nodes in the specimen is often used to demonstrate the adequacy of TME. For correct staging a minimal number of 12 nodes within the specimen is recommended. However, we have to keep in mind that the number of nodes always reflects both a precise surgical technique and the accurate work of the pathologist. In 1994 Decanini [14] and colleagues demonstrated with their experimental work on several cadavers that laparoscopic surgery is a viable option for performing TME.

Laparoscopy provides excellent exposure, particularly in the small pelvis, which may enable the surgeon to perform a more meticulous dissection under direct vision. On the other hand, inadequate excision and increased morbidity are potential risks of the laparoscopic approach. Due to the complexity of the procedure, especially in cases of anterior resection, only a few studies concerning laparoscopic rectal excision done by experts have been published [2, 3, 19, 47, 60].

In these studies the data provided regarding short-term results like hospital stay, blood loss, postoperative pain, number of harvested lymph nodes and leakage rate showed the same or even better results for the laparoscopic technique compared to standard open procedures. To date, three larger studies have been published evaluating the laparoscopic approach for the treatment of rectal cancer [35, 36, 41].

The data of those trials were collected prospectively. None of them was randomized.

Morino and Patankar in particular were able to show convincing results when the laparoscopic technique was applied to rectal cancer (Table 1).

Rullier and his group did an excellent study evaluating the completeness of the mesorectum after laparoscopic resection [41]. Again, it was demonstrated that the laparoscopic technique fulfilled all the criteria of total mesorectal excision.

Furthermore, they analyzed the rate of identification and the incidence of injury to the hypogastric nerves and evaluated the postoperative sexual and bladder functions. Identification of hypogastric nerves was possible in 24 out of 32 patients and this resulted in preservation of sexual function in about 45% and normal bladder function in 92% of patients.

Performing a retrospective analysis, the Singapore group found that despite better visualization the results of laparoscopic surgery regarding bladder and sexual function showed a worse outcome when compared to conventionally treated patients in the same time period. The noted difference in sexual dysfunction was significant especially in male patients with 7 of 15 sexually active men reporting impotence or impaired ejaculation compared with only 1 out of 22 having an open resection [39]. Additionally, two of the laparoscopic-treated patients were forced to use self-catheterization in the long term.

Table 1. Long-term results following laparoscopic surgery of rectal cancer reported in the literature

Author	*n*	Follow-up (months)	LR (%)	DM (%)	PM (*n*)	LN (*n*)	5-Year survival (%)
Poulin 2002 Surg Endosc	73	30.3	3.8	N/A	0	N/A	UICC I: 92 UICC II: 86 UICC III: 53
Patankar 2002 DCR	66	52	3.5	N/A	1	N/A	UICC I: 74 UICC II: 70 UICC III: 60
Morino 2003 Ann Surg	70	45.7	4.2	22.6	1	12.8	UICC I: 92 UICC II: 79 UICC III: 67
Own results 2003	52	48	1.9	11.5	0	14.2	UICC I: 92 UICC II: 87 UICC III: 58

Listed are only published studies dealing with rectal cancer and stating 5-year follow-up data.
LR, local recurrence; DM, distant metastasis; PM, port-site metastasis; LN, lymph nodes in specimen; N/A, not applicable.

The Luebeck Experience

Our own experience of laparoscopic surgery on rectal cancer is based on 52 patients treated with a curative intent between September 1992 and July 2003. Surgical and pathological data were recorded prospectively in an anonymous registry database. Data supplied for each patient included age, gender, indication, procedure, morbidity, mortality, duration of surgery, preoperative and postoperative hemoglobin levels, perioperative blood transfusion, data on intraoperative period and postoperative recovery, hospitalization, pathology according to UICC stage, type of resection, yield of lymph nodes, and other tumor characteristics. Follow-up information included disease-free survival, incidence of local, distant and port-site recurrence, and morbidity.

Indication and Selection for Surgery

Informed consent was obtained, addressing the laparoscopic technique in particular and specifically the undefined long-term results. Perioperative single-injection antibiotics (cefotaxime, metronidazole) and thrombosis prophylaxis were administered.

A carcinoma was considered as primary rectal carcinoma if it was located in the lower third (0–6 cm from anal verge), middle third (7–12 cm), or upper third of the rectum (12–15 cm).

Methods

Surgical Procedure

In all patients with cancer located in the middle or lower third of the rectum, a total mesorectal excision was performed. If a sphincter-preserving resection was not possible due to oncological reasons in carcinomas located directly at the anal verge or due to infiltration of the anal sphincter, an abdominoperineal resection of the rectum with permanent colostomy was carried out. In general, a standardized oncological technique was used including high ligation of the inferior mesenteric artery 2 cm distal to the aorta but proximal to the origin of the left colic artery. The inferior mesenteric vein was divided at the lower edge of the pancreas. Restoration of continuity was reached by the double-stapling technique. Left splenic flexure was routinely mobilized. For retrieval of the specimen, a wound protection device was used in each procedure.

Bladder and Sexual Dysfunction

To evaluate functional results following laparoscopic surgery a matched pair analysis was carried out. Matching of patients after laparoscopic and conventional open surgery was performed according to sex, age, type of resection (anterior resection, abdominoperineal resection), time period of surgery, and stage of disease classified according to the UICC. For evaluation the EORTC QLQ-CR-38 score system was used. For matching, 12 male and 10 female patients in each group were selected.

Statistical Analysis

Survival was calculated according to Kaplan-Meier. To determine significant differences between laparoscopically and conventional open surgery-treated patients within the matched pairs, the Mann-Whitney *U* test and the Wilcoxon W test were used (SPSS soft ware package, SPSS, Chicago, Ill., USA). $P<0.05$ was defined to be statistically significant.

Results

Our short-term results such as blood loss, hospital stay, 30-day morbidity and time to recovery are published elsewhere and not for interest in this context [10, 44, 47]. Focusing on the long-term follow-up, we gained the following results: The median age of patients was 66.7 years and ranged from 42–88. Anastomotic leakage was seen in 6.1% of cases. In a median follow-up of 48 months (36–136), we reached an overall 3-year survival rate of 93% and a 5-year survival rate of 62% (follow-up rate 100%). Local recurrence was 1.9% ($n=1$ in UICC III with T3N2M0 stage), distant

Table 2. Own results following laparoscopic rectal cancer surgery

Stages	Pat (*n*)	5-Year survival (%)	LR (*n*)	LR (%)	DM (*n*)	DM (%)
UICC I	28	92	0	0	0	0
UICC II	9	87	0	0	0	0
UICC III	15	58	1	6.6	6	11.1

Laparoscopic surgery for rectal carcinoma with TME revealed a very low local recurrence rate within a follow-up period of 48 months. Local recurrence occurred in one single patient with T3N2M0 rectal carcinoma.
LR, local recurrence; DM, distant metastasis.

metastasis occurred in 11.5%. We saw no port-site metastasis. For differentiation within the several stages, see Table 2.

Regarding bladder and sexual dysfunction using the EORTC QLQ CR38 score, we found no statistically significant difference between the examined groups. For urinary function, the overall score in the open group was 67.6 and in the laparoscopically treated group 72.7 (0=poor, 100=excellent). For sexual function, the overall score for males was 56.6 in the open as well as in the laparoscopic group, and for females 66.6 in the open and 70 in the laparoscopic group. Erectile disorder was seen in 1 out of 5 sexually active patients, and was the same for the laparoscopic group. Ejaculation disorder was recognized in both groups with the same incidence (1/5).

Discussion

One of the most controversial ongoing discussions on laparoscopic surgery deals with the question of whether or not to apply this technique to malignant disease and specifically to rectal cancer. The four major issues are the adequacy of oncologic resection, recurrence rates and patterns, and long-term survival with quality of life. Nonrandomized studies show evidence that margins of excision and lymph node harvest achieved laparoscopically reached comparable results to those seen after conventional open resection [2, 3, 12, 30, 32, 33, 35–38, 47, 51, 58, 64].

Rullier and colleagues are the first to demonstrate the adequacy of laparoscopic TME on specimens. With their examination, they gave a pathological basis to clinically achieved results. It is worth mentioning that open performed TME is also connected with the risk of injuring the mesorectal fascia. As suggested by Sterk and colleagues, it is therefore advisable to inject blue ink into the resected specimen through the inferior mesenteric artery (IMA) thereby testing the integrity of the mesorectal fascia [55, 56].

Our own results regarding trocar-site recurrence are in accordance with others (Table 1). In our series of 52 patients treated by laparoscopy we saw no incidence of trocar-site recurrence, others reporting rates below 2% [36].

Local recurrence (1.9–4.2%) following laparoscopic surgery for rectal cancer in all cited studies (Table 1) was as low as that seen in conventional open surgery performed by experts. The same has to be mentioned for long-term survival. At present, no difference can be seen between laparoscopic and open rectal surgery.

Of course, we face the inherent limitations that exist in a nonrandomized study. It has to be realized that there is a bias in all published data dealing with laparoscopic surgery for rectal cancer regarding surgeon, center and patient selection. But we should not forget that TME itself was advocated by Heald [22] and later adopted by others without any randomized trial, simply accepting the convincing rates of local recurrence and survival.

Every surgeon would agree that long-term survival and recurrence rate are the most important issues in treatment of colorectal malignancy. Seen from the patient's point of view, questions regarding quality of life, especially postoperative urinary and sexual function, may gain more and more relevance. In this context, the results of bladder and sexual dysfunction following laparoscopic TME reported by Quah [39] and colleagues were very disappointing. Our own results are not in accordance with their findings. Unfortunately, there is very little information in the literature dealing with functional results after laparoscopic and even open rectal resection. As suggested by Quah and his group, one of the reasons for this may be the fact that in all of their patients with disturbed urogenital function, very low situated and advanced tumors were resected. Bearing in mind that the reported rate of bladder denervation was low, the nerve damage must have occurred after the nerve to the bladder has branched off. Furthermore, the authors report that not only specimen delivery but also completion of rectal dissection was performed via a small suprapubic wound incision. Thus it may be concluded that injury of the hypogastric nerve plexus occurred not during the laparoscopic procedure itself but during preparation in the small pelvis of the male, where precise visualization and dissection through the small suprapubic incision may be more difficult.

However, as far as can be seen, laparoscopic surgery in rectal carcinoma may achieve the same or, in selected patients, even better results than open surgery. However, at present no published study has shown much evidence. Many more studies are necessary to define the place of the laparoscopic technique in rectal cancer surgery, regarding appropriate selection of patients and evaluating adjuvant or neoadjuvant treatment in combination with the laparoscopic approach.

References

1. Anderson CA, Kennedy FR, Potter M, Opie HL, Flowers S, Lewis S, Belmont M, Fowler DL (2002) Results of laparoscopically assisted colon resection for carcinoma. Surg Endosc 16:607–610
2. Anthuber M, Fuerst A, Elser F, Berger R, Jauch KW (2003) Outcome of laparoscopic surgery for rectal cancer in 101 patients. Dis Colon Rectum 46:1047–1053
3. Barlehner E, Decker T, Anders S, Heukrodt B (2001) [Laparoscopic surgery of rectal carcinoma. Radical oncology and late results]. Zentralbl Chir 126:302–306
4. Bennett CL, Stryker SJ, Ferreira MR, Adams J, Beart RW, Jr. (1997) The learning curve for laparoscopic colorectal surgery. Preliminary results from a prospective analysis of 1194 laparoscopic-assisted colectomies [published erratum appears in Arch Surg 1997 Jul;132(7):781] [see comments]. Arch Surg 132:41–44; discussion 45
5. Bohm B, Schwenk W, Muller JM (1999) [Long-term results after laparoscopic resection of colorectal carcinoma]. Chirurg 70:453–455

6. Bohm B, Rotting N, Schwenk W, Grebe S, Mansmann U (2001) A prospective randomized trial on heart rate variability of the surgical team during laparoscopic and conventional sigmoid resection. Arch Surg 136:305–310
7. Boulez J, Blanchet MC, Espalieu P (1999) [Colonic diverticulosis and laparoscopy. Analysis of a series of 60 cases]. Ann Chir 53:1033–1038
8. Braga M, Vignali A, Zuliani W, Radaelli G, Gianotti L, Martani C, Toussoun G, Di Carlo V (2002) Metabolic and functional results after laparoscopic colorectal surgery: a randomized, controlled trial. Dis Colon Rectum 45:1070–1077
9. Bruch HP, Schwandner O (2001) Current status of laparoscopic surgery in colorectal cancer. Onkologie 24:29–32
10. Bruch HP, Schiedeck TH, Schwandner O (1999) Laparoscopic colorectal surgery: a five-year experience. Dig Surg 16:45–54
11. Chen HH, Wexner SD, Weiss EG, Nogueras JJ, Alabaz O, Iroatulam AJ, Nessim A, Joo JS (1998) Laparoscopic colectomy for benign colorectal disease is associated with a significant reduction in disability as compared with laparotomy. Surg Endosc 12:1397–1400
12. Chung CC, Ha JP, Tsang WW, Li MK (2001) Laparoscopic-assisted total mesorectal excision and colonic J pouch reconstruction in the treatment of rectal cancer. Surg Endosc 15:1098–1101
13. Curet MJ, Putrakul K, Pitcher DE, Josloff RK, Zucker KA (2000) Laparoscopically assisted colon resection for colon carcinoma: perioperative results and long-term outcome. Surg Endosc 14:1062–1066
14. Decanini C, Milsom JW, Bohm B, Fazio VW (1994) Laparoscopic oncologic abdominoperineal resection. Dis Colon Rectum 37:552–558
15. Duepree HJ, Senagore AJ, Delaney CP, Brady KM, Fazio VW (2002) Advantages of laparoscopic resection for ileocecal Crohn's disease. Dis Colon Rectum 45:605–610
16. Dunker MS, Bemelman WA, Slors JF, van Duijvendijk P, Gouma DJ (2001) Functional outcome, quality of life, body image, and cosmesis in patients after laparoscopic-assisted and conventional restorative proctocolectomy: a comparative study. Dis Colon Rectum 44:1800–1807
17. Fleshman JW, Wexner SD, Anvari M, LaTulippe JF, Birnbaum EH, Kodner IJ, Read TE, Nogueras JJ, Weiss EG (1999) Laparoscopic vs. open abdominoperineal resection for cancer. Dis Colon Rectum 42:930–939
18. Franklin ME, Kazantsev GB, Abrego D, Diaz EJ, Balli J, Glass JL (2000) Laparoscopic surgery for stage III colon cancer: long-term follow-up. Surg Endosc 14:612–616
19. Hartley JE, Mehigan BJ, Qureshi AE, Duthie GS, Lee PW, Monson JR (2001) Total mesorectal excision: assessment of the laparoscopic approach. Dis Colon Rectum 44:315–321
20. Havenga K, Enker WE, McDermott K, Cohen AM, Minsky BD, Guillem J (1996) Male and female sexual and urinary function after total mesorectal excision with autonomic nerve preservation for carcinoma of the rectum. J Am Coll Surg 182:495–502
21. Heald RJ, Husband EM, Ryall RD (1982) The mesorectum in rectal cancer surgery—the clue to pelvic recurrence? Br J Surg 69:613–616
22. Heald RJ, Moran BJ, Ryall RD, Sexton R, MacFarlane JK (1998) Rectal cancer: the Basingstoke experience of total mesorectal excision, 1978–1997. Arch Surg 133:894–899
23. Hildebrandt U, Kessler K, Pistorius G, Lindemann W, Ecker KW, Feifel G, Menger MD (1999) Granulocyte elastase and systemic cytokine response after laparoscopic- assisted and open resections in Crohn's disease. Dis Colon Rectum 42:1480–1486
24. Hong D, Lewis M, Tabet J, Anvari M (2002) Prospective comparison of laparoscopic versus open resection for benign colorectal disease. Surg Laparosc Endosc Percutan Tech 12:238–242
25. Jacobi CA, Bonjer HJ, Puttick MI, O'Sullivan R, Lee SW, Schwalbach P, Tomita H, Kim ZG, Hewett P, Wittich P, Fleshman JW, Paraskeva P, Gessman T, Neuhaus SJ, Wildbrett P, Reymond MA, Gutt C, Whelan RI (2002) Oncologic implications of laparoscopic and open surgery. Surg Endosc 16:441–445
26. Jacobs M, Verdeja JC and Goldstein HS (1991) Minimally invasive colon resection (laparoscopic colectomy). Surg Laparosc Endosc 1:144–150
27. Kakisako K, Sato K, Adachi Y, Shiraishi N, Miyahara M, Kitano S (2000) Laparoscopic colectomy for Dukes A colon cancer. Surg Laparosc Endosc Percutan Tech 10:66–70
28. Kehlet H, Nielsen HJ (1998) Impact of laparoscopic surgery on stress responses, immunofunction, and risk of infectious complications. New Horiz 6: S80–88

29. Kockerling F, Scheidbach H (2000) Current status of laparoscopic colorectal surgery. Surg Endosc 14:777–778
30. Kockerling F, Scheuerlein H, Schneider C, Scheidbach H, Hohenberger W (2000) Colorectal surgery for cancer: conventional or laparoscopic? Semin Oncol 27:34–44
31. Lezoche E, Feliciotti F, Paganini AM, Guerrieri M, Campagnacci R, De Sanctis A (2000) Laparoscopic colonic resections versus open surgery: a prospective non- randomized study on 310 unselected cases. Hepatogastroenterology 47:697–708
32. Lezoche E, Feliciotti F, Paganini AM, Guerrieri M, De Sanctis A, Campagnacci R, D'Ambrosio G (2002) Results of laparoscopic versus open resections for non-early rectal cancer in patients with a minimum follow-up of four years. Hepatogastroenterology 49:1185–1190
33. Milsom JW, Bohm B, Decanini C, Fazio VW (1994) Laparoscopic oncologic proctosigmoidectomy with low colorectal anastomosis in a cadaver model. Surg Endosc 8:1117–1123
34. Milsom JW, Bohm B, Hammerhofer KA, Fazio V, Steiger E, Elson P (1998) A prospective, randomized trial comparing laparoscopic versus conventional techniques in colorectal cancer surgery: a preliminary report [see comments]. J Am Coll Surg 187:46–54; discussion 54–55
35. Morino M, Parini U, Giraudo G, Salval M, Brachet Contul R, Garrone C (2003) Laparoscopic total mesorectal excision: a consecutive series of 100 patients. Ann Surg 237:335–342
36. Patankar SK, Larach SW, Ferrara A, Williamson PR, Gallagher JT, DeJesus S, Narayanan S (2003) Prospective comparison of laparoscopic vs. open resections for colorectal adenocarcinoma over a ten-year period. Dis Colon Rectum 46:601–611
37. Pikarsky AJ, Rosenthal R, Weiss EG, Wexner SD (2002) Laparoscopic total mesorectal excision. Surg Endosc 16:558–562
38. Poulin EC, Schlachta CM, Gregoire R, Seshadri P, Cadeddu MO, Mamazza J (2002) Local recurrence and survival after laparoscopic mesorectal resection forrectal adenocarcinoma. Surg Endosc 16:989–995
39. Quah HM, Jayne DG, Eu KW, Seow-Choen F (2002) Bladder and sexual dysfunction following laparoscopically assisted and conventional open mesorectal resection for cancer. Br J Surg 89:1551–1556
40. Roblick UJ, Massmann A, Schwandner O, Sterk P, Krug F, Bruch HP, Schiedeck TH (2002) [Quality of life assessment after surgery for diverticulitis—a follow-up study]. Zentralbl Chir 127:31–35
41. Rullier E, Sa Cunha A, Couderc P, Rullier A, Gontier R, Saric J (2003) Laparoscopic intersphincteric resection with coloplasty and coloanal anastomosis for mid and low rectal cancer. Br J Surg 90:445–451
42. Scheidbach H, Schneider C, Konradt J, Barlehner E, Kohler L, Wittekind C, Kockerling F (2002) Laparoscopic abdominoperineal resection and anterior resection with curative intent for carcinoma of the rectum. Surg Endosc 16:7–13
43. Schiedeck TH, Schwandner O, Bruch HP (1999) [Laparoscopic therapy of chronic constipation]. Zentralbl Chir 124:818–824
44. Schiedeck TH, Schwandner O, Baca I, Baehrlehner E, Konradt J, Kockerling F, Kuthe A, Buerk C, Herold A, Bruch HP (2000) Laparoscopic surgery for the cure of colorectal cancer: results of a German five-center study. Dis Colon Rectum 43:1–8
45. Schlachta CM, Mamazza J, Poulin EC (1999) Laparoscopic sigmoid resection for acute and chronic diverticulitis. An outcomes comparison with laparoscopic resection for nondiverticular disease. Surg Endosc 13:649–653
46. Schwandner O, Schiedeck T, Bruch H (1999) Advanced age-indication or contraindication for laparoscopic colorectal surgery. Dis Colon Rectum 42:356–362
47. Schwandner O, Schiedeck TH, Killaitis C, Bruch HP (1999) A case-control-study comparing laparoscopic versus open surgery for rectosigmoidal and rectal cancer. Int J Colorectal Dis 14:158–163
48. Schwenk W, Bohm B, Haase O, Junghans T, Muller JM (1998) Laparoscopic versus conventional colorectal resection: a prospective randomised study of postoperative ileus and early postoperative feeding. Langenbecks Arch Surg 383:49–55
49. Schwenk W, Jacobi C, Mansmann U, Bohm B, Muller JM (2000) Inflammatory response after laparoscopic and conventional colorectal resections—results of a prospective randomized trial. Langenbecks Arch Surg 385:2–9
50. Senagore AJ, Duepree HJ, Delaney CP, Dissanaike S, Brady KM, Fazio VW (2002) Cost structure of laparoscopic and open sigmoid colectomy for diverticular disease: similarities and differences. Dis Colon Rectum 45:485–490

51. Seow-Choen F, Eu KW, Ho YH, Leong AF (1997) A preliminary comparison of a consecutive series of open versus laparoscopic abdomino-perineal resection for rectal adenocarcinoma. Int J Colorectal Dis 12:88–90
52. Sim R, Milsom JW (2000) Laparoscopic colectomy for malignancy. Semin Laparosc Surg 7:101–117
53. Stage JG, Schulze S, Moller P, Overgaard H, Andersen M, Rebsdorf-Pedersen VB, Nielsen HJ (1997) Prospective randomized study of laparoscopic versus open colonic resection for adenocarcinoma [see comments]. Br J Surg 84:391–396
54. Stelzner F (1962) [The current status of rectal resection with sphincter retention and rectal amputation in cancer of the rectum]. Bruns Beitr Klinischen Chir 204:41–63
55. Sterk P, Kasperk R, Opitz T, Schubert F, Klein P (2000) Vascular organization in the mesorectum: angiography of rectal resection specimens. Int J Colorectal Dis 15:225–228
56. Sterk P, Nagel T, Gunter S, Schubert F, Klein P (2000) [Methods for postoperative evaluation of complete excision of the mesorectum]. Zentralbl Chir 125:370–374
57. Stocchi L, Nelson H (2000) Wound recurrences following laparoscopic-assisted colectomy for cancer. Arch Surg 135:948–958
58. Watanabe M, Teramoto T, Hasegawa H, Kitajima M (2000) Laparoscopic ultralow anterior resection combined with per anum intersphincteric rectal dissection for lower rectal cancer. Dis Colon Rectum 43: S94–97
59. Watanabe M, Ohgami M, Teramoto T, Hibi T, Kitajima M (1999) Laparoscopic ileocecal resection for Crohn's disease associated with intestinal stenosis and ileorectal fistula. Surg Today 29:446–448
60. Weiser MR, Milsom JW (2000) Laparoscopic total mesorectal excision with autonomic nerve preservation. Semin Surg Oncol 19:396–403
61. Westhues H (1954) [Abdominosacral rectal resection]. Zentralbl Chir 79:257–362
62. Wu FP, Cuesta MA, Sietses C (2002) Randomized clinical trial of the effect of open versus laparoscopically assisted colectomy on systemic immunity in patients with colorectal cancer. Br J Surg 89:497
63. Yamamoto S, Watanabe M, Hasegawa H, Kitajima M (2001) Oncologic outcome of laparoscopic versus open surgery for advanced colorectal cancer. Hepatogastroenterology 48:1248–1251
64. Yamamoto S, Watanabe M, Hasegawa H, Kitajima M (2002) Prospective evaluation of laparoscopic surgery for rectosigmoidal and rectal carcinoma. Dis Colon Rectum 45:1648–1654
65. Young-Fadok TM, HallLong K, McConnell EJ, Gomez Rey G, Cabanela RL (2001) Advantages of laparoscopic resection for ileocolic Crohn's disease. Improved outcomes and reduced costs. Surg Endosc 15:450–454

Laparoscopic TME — The Surgeon's or the Patient's Preference

J. Göhl, S. Merkel, W. Hohenberger

J. Göhl (✉)
Department of Surgery, University of Erlangen, Erlangen, Germany
e-mail: jonas.goehl@chir.imed.uni-erlangen.de

Abstract

Since laparoscopic surgery in rectal cancer was introduced ten years ago large patient collectives have been published by several authors in the meantime. The literature was carefully reviewed to analyse data on postoperative complications, long term prognosis and quality of life after laparoscopic surgery for rectal cancer to answer the question whether laparoscopic surgery is still just feasible or maybe has even reached the golden standard.

The review showed that there is not a single prospectively randomized trial published comparing laparoscopic vs. open surgery for rectal cancer. It is clearly evident that until now the most laparoscopic series are published with patients selected according to criteria that vary significantly especially regarding the kind of procedures performed (anterior, low anterior, intersphincteric resections and abdomino-perineal excision), other demographic items like gender, body mass index, eventual prior laparotomies, emergencies and tumor related characteristics like tumor stage or T-categories.

At the moment any data concerning outcome from prospectively randomized trials comparing laparoscopic versus open surgery for rectal cancer are missing. Therefore, there is more speculation and belief concerning the true quality of laparoscopic surgery. The review in the literature only indicates, that laparoscopic surgery for rectal cancer is feasible. To prove the potential advantage of laparoscopic surgery in rectal cancer randomized trials are essential. If a surgeon discusses laparoscopic surgery outside a randomized trial, he should go through a questionnaire, presented in the paper which reflects the present situation without any proven advantage and not available long term results and should leave a final decision to the patient.

Recent Results in Cancer Research, Vol. 165

Introduction

The first laparoscopic operations for colorectal cancer were performed more than 10 years ago. Thus one could assume that there are enough data available in the literature to evaluate the outcome, quality of life and cost-effectiveness of this procedure and to judge whether a laparoscopic surgery is still simply feasible or whether it has become the golden standard. Focusing on rectal cancer including total mesorectal excision (TME), the literature was carefully reviewed to collect data on postoperative complications, long-term prognosis and quality of life figures after laparoscopic surgery for rectal cancer.

Facts

The first result of this review was that there is no single prospectively randomized trial published comparing laparoscopic versus open surgery for rectal cancer. It was clearly evident that till now only series are published with patients selected according to criteria that are never fully transparent and may vary significantly. This is true for the following:

1. The kind of procedures performed (anterior, low anterior, intersphincteric resections and abdominoperineal excision)
2. Other demographic items such as gender, body mass index, eventual prior laparotomies, emergencies
3. Tumor-related items such as UICC stage, T categories and others

In this context it should be noted that an equal distribution of stages in correlation to a conventional series does not exclude patient selection.

Any stage-III patient may have a very small pT1 carcinoma with a single lymph node metastasis which may cause no technical problem or adverse effect during preparation. However, a T4 lesion without any lymph node metastases is still stage II, which may even be impossible to be touched by laparoscopic instruments without laceration: the T category may be much more important when judging the extent of selection in a given report. For that reason, one needs reference figures from unselected series with open surgery including the procedures performed and all the demographic data needed.

Procedures Performed and Distribution of the pN Category at the Erlangen Registry of Colorectal Carcinoma

In our own department, over the last years, the rate of perineal excisions was 20.9% (n=80). In another one, the rate (n=307) of anterior or low anterior resection was 74.5%, including 49 cases with abdominoperineal intersphincteric resection and perineal anastomosis. In addition, a small number of local excisions were performed by a perineal approach (Table 1).

Table 1. Operative procedures in conventional rectal cancer surgery, Surgical Department, University of Erlangen 1995–2000 (UICC I—III, n=412)

Operative procedure	*n*	%
Anterior resection	307	74.5
(including intersphincteric resection)	49	11.9
Perineal excision	80	19.4
Local excision perineal	25	6.1

Table 2. Distribution of pT, pN and stage, Surgical Department, University of Erlangen 1995–2000 (UICC I—III, R0 resections, n=373, mean number of regional lymph nodes examined: 26)

	n	%
pT1	46	12.3
pT2	124	33.7
pT3	188	50.7
pT4	14	3.8
pN0	227	60.9
pN1	95	25.5
pN2	51	13.6
Stage I	132	35.4
Stage II	95	25.5
Stage III	146	39.2

In the same period, the majority of curatively resected patients (R0) without distant metastases presented with stage III (39.2%; n=146) disease. The rate of stage I disease was 35.4% (n=132).

pT4 tumors were found in 3.8% of the cases (n=14). The majority of the cases were pT3 tumors (n=188). In total, 60.9% had no lymph node involvement (n=227). The mean number of lymph nodes examined was 26 (Table 2). Of all patients, 3.6% presented as an emergency.

Locoregional Recurrence

The most important impact of rectal cancer surgery is the prevention of locoregional recurrence because it reduces survival significantly.

Potentially curative approaches include extended, mainly multidisciplinary therapeutic modalities that may affect the patient significantly. If, however, failure of locoregional control is inevitable, this will lead to intractable problems for the patient.

In the literature, including our own results, local recurrence rates are seen in between 2.6% and 17.1% of the cases, depending on the length of follow-up and eventual subgroup analysis including high-risk patients.

Table 3. Local recurrence rates (LR rate) after conventional surgery with TME

		LR rate	Median follow-up (months)
Simunovic et al. [13] (2003)	*n*=115: no RCT	2.6%	29
	n=35: with RCT	17.1%	
Kneist et al. [5] (2003)	*n*=87	4.9%	24
Bülow et al. [2] (2003)	*n*=311	11%	36
Erlangen 1995–2000	*n*=373	8,8%	52

Table 4. Local recurrence rates (LR rate) after laparoscopic TME (treatment series by individual surgeons or centers)

	n	LR rate	Median follow-up (months)
Fleshman [3] (1999)	31	19.0	19
Bärlehner [1] (2001)	138	3.8	40
Hartley [4] (2001)	21	5.0	38
Lezoche [6] (2002)	29 T2,T3	24.1	49
Quah [9] (2002)	40	–	–
Reis Neto [10] (2002)	32	3.1	–
Scheidbach [12] (2002)	380	6.6	25
Yamamoto [14] (2002)	70 Tis, T1, T2	3.0	23
Morino [7] (2003)	87 Evaluable malignancies	4.2	46
Patankar [8] (2003)	66	3.5	52
Rullier [11] (2003)	32	–	–

In our own department, without any patient selection, the locoregional recurrence rate is 8.8% after a follow-up period of 52 months (Table 3).

In the literature for laparoscopic total mesorectal excision for rectal cancer over the last 4 years, recurrence rates at various follow-up intervals ranged from 0% to 24.1%, or were not mentioned. The majority of reports do not specify T categories. In some series, even benign lesions are included. In not a single publication all the demographic data needed for adequate analysis were given (Table 4).

The largest series was published by Scheidbach et al. [12], including 380 patients. This paper presents the data of 23 institutions as a kind of patient care study. Stage distribution does not indicate a selection bias. However, as mentioned above, the T categories would be much more important to allow deeper analysis. In this series, the abdominal perineal excision rate was 39.2%, which nevertheless indicates a relevant selection (Table 5).

Clinical reality is probably best reflected by a study published by Hartley et al. [4], in which 42 patients entered an intention-to-treat study. Of these patients,

Table 5. Multicenter study, 23 institutions, 380 patients, 5-year period laparoscopic surgery

Scheidbach et al. [12]		
Ant. resection	*n*=231	60.8%
Abd. perineal excision	*n*=149	39.2%
Operating time (mean)	218 min	
Converting rate		6.1%
Morbidity rate postoperative		37.6%
Number of lymph nodes examined (mean)		13.0
Local recurrence rate		6.6%
Overall survival		86.6%
Stage distribution		
UICC I	*n*=129	34.0%
UICC II	*n*=112	29.5%
UICC III	*n*=139	36.5%

14 needed early conversion; 6 of the 28 remaining patients finally needed partial open dissection. Thus, only 21 curative total mesorectal excisions were completed laparoscopically (Fig. 1). Comparing early postoperative outcome figures within the three groups, it could be demonstrated that bowel movement started 1 day earlier in the laparoscopic group and hospital stay was 1.5 days shorter compared to the open group (10%). Operation time was 55 min longer (44%). The need of analgesic drugs was the same. However, in the conversion group, all parameters were worse, due to postoperative paralysis, which was the same compared to the open group. Astonishingly enough, the clinical leakage rate in the laparoscopic group was fourfold higher, for various reasons (Table 6).

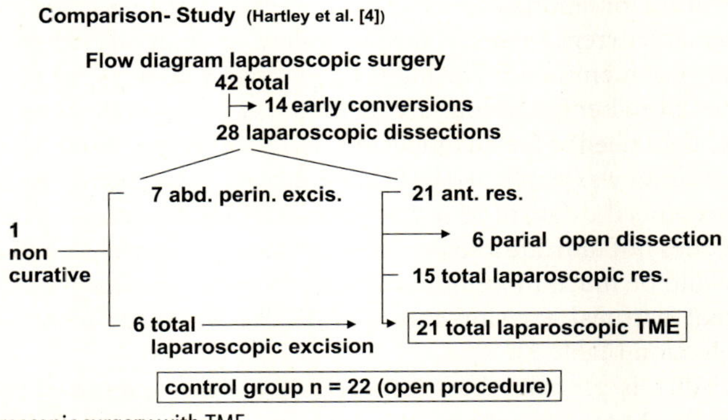

Figure 1. Laparoscopic surgery with TME

Table 6. Laparoscopic surgery with TME: comparison study, Hartley et al. [4], clinical data

Group	Operating time (min)	Postoperative paralyses (days)	Analgesia required (days)	Hospital stay (days)
Laparoscopic (*n*=21)	180 (168–218)	3 (3–4)	4 3–6	13.5 (10–27)
Converted (*n*=21)	146 (136–180)	4 (4–7)	5 (4–7)	16 (12–33)
Open (*n*=22)	125 (104–144)	4 (3–5)	4 (3–5)	15 12–29)

Survival

Again, the interpretation of survival figures from laparoscopic surgery for rectal cancer needs reference figures from open series for the reasons mentioned above.

In this context, it is important to postulate that optimal figures should be used for comparisons. Otherwise some results may be misinterpreted, for example those published by Patankar et al [8]. These authors demonstrated a nonsignificant better survival for laparoscopically operated patients with an advantage for all patients after 5 years and for stage I patients after 7 years. However, if one compares these figures with the survival rates from our department, including all patients prospectively documented without any selection with a cancer related 5-year survival of 83.6% (*n*=373) and for stage I patients 94.7%, these figures are much higher than the reference figures from open surgery in this study (Table 7). Thus the comparison

Table 7. Cancer-related 5-year survival rate, Surgical Department, University of Erlangen 1995–2000 (UICC I–III, R0 resections, *n*=373)

	n	5-Year survival rate (%)
All	373	83.6
pT1	46	100.0
pT2	124	90.2
pT3	188	78.9
pT4	14	39.1
pN0	227	93.9
pN1	95	72.3
pN2	51	59.9
Stage I	192	94.7
Stage II	95	93.0
Stage III	146	67.7

of absolute figures indicates that many results obtained in some studies comparing open versus laparoscopic approach do not represent optimally obtainable results.

Quality of Life

There is one prospectively documented trial comparing quality of life. In this study, postoperative male sexual dysfunction is found significantly more frequently in the laparoscopically operated group (Table 8).

Table 8. Quality of life: postoperative male sexual dysfunction, Quah et al. [8]

	Laparoscopic approach (*n*=15)	Open operation (*n*=22)	*p*
Erectile function			0.03*
No difference	9	19	
Reduced	1	2	
Impotent	5	1	
Able to ejaculate			0.01*
Yes	9	21	
No	6	1	
Overall sexual dysfunction[a]	7	1	0.004*
Median (i.q.r.) change in sexual satisfaction	-1 (-3.0)	1 (-0.25)	0.06**

* Fisher's exact test; ** Mann-Whitney *U* test.
[a] Some patients were both impotent and unable to ejaculate.
I.q.r., Interquartile range.

Summary

At present, data concerning outcome from prospectively randomized trials comparing laparoscopic versus open surgery for rectal cancer are missing. Therefore, there is more speculation and belief concerning the true quality of laparoscopic surgery. Surgeons are obliged to make their decisions on the basis of evidence. However, at the moment, the literature only indicates that laparoscopic surgery for rectal cancer is feasible. However, even the safety and quality of outcome figures cannot be substantiated adequately. Therefore, there is no argument at the moment to support why some surgeons prefer laparoscopic approach.

If one explained this situation to a patient, laparoscopic surgery would not even be discussed if the patient was asked to make the final decision on the approach to be used.

In some aspects, a patient is a customer who deserves our service. From that point of view, there is no big difference to a customer who wants to buy a car. If one translates our actual "testing result" into the language of a client who wants to buy a car, one must ask: Do you want to buy a car that:

1. Is certainly running (feasibility proven)?
2. Can drive you a short distance safely (small series, from selected institutions, no national wide registers including every laparoscopic case)?
3. May eventually run on selected roads only (the majority of papers published is based on patient selection of various degrees)?
4. May have a breakdown more frequently (conversions at different rates, the only unselected series published indicates a conversion rate of 50% if no preoperative selection was performed)?
5. Whose long-term function has not yet been proven (no single prospectively randomized trial or other well-designed study published, no adequate long-term figures allowing adequate interpretation)?
6. May cause you imminent significant health problems (more postoperative sexual dysfunction in males reported, increased adverse effects from conversion)?

If a surgeon discusses laparoscopic surgery for a patient with rectal cancer outside a randomized trial, he should go through this list with his patient, and should leave the final decision to the patient.

Even within randomized trials, it should be guaranteed that the performing surgeons are highly trained and are well aware of the potential complications. A protocol should be able to identify the selection criteria needed and should make the results comparable to those that are obtained by optimal open surgery. That means, however, that these studies should be performed only by surgeons who can guarantee the highest quality of surgery, both laparoscopic and open arm.

References

1. Barlehner E, Anders S, Heukrodt B (2001) Technique of rectum resection and excision with special reference to TME. Kongressbd Dtsch Ges Chir Kongr 118:101–103
2. Bülow S, Christensen IJ, Harling H, Kronborg O, Fenger C (2003) Recurrence and survival after mesorectal excision for rectal cancer. BJS 90:974–980
3. Fleshman JW, Wexner SD, Anvari M, LaTulippe JF, Birnbaum EH, Kodner IJ, Read TE, Nogueras JJ, Weiss EG (1999) Laparoscopic vs. open abdominoperineal resection for cancer. Dis Colon Rectum 42:930–939
4. Hartley JE, Mehigan BJ, Qureshi AE, Duthie GS, Lee PW, Monson (2001) Total mesorectal excision: assessment of the laparoscopic approach. Dis Colon Rectum 44:315–321
5. Kneist W, Heintz A, Wolf HK, Junginger T (2003) Totale Mesorektumexzision bei Karzinom des mittleren und unteren Rektumdrittels. Chirurg 4:125–131
6. Morino M, Parini U, Giraudo G, Salval M, Brachet Contul R, Garro C (2003) Laparoscopic total mesorectal excision: a consecutive series of 100 patients. Ann Surg 237:335–342
7. Lezoche E, Feliciotti F, Paganini AM, Guerrieri M, De Sanctis A, Campagnacci R, D'Ambrosio G (2002) Results of laparoscopic versus open resections for non-early rectal cancer in patients with a minimum follow-up of four years. Hepatogastroenterology 49:1185–1190
8. Patankar SK, Larach, Ferrara SW, Williamson PR, Gallagher JT, DeJesus S, Narayanan S (2003) Prospective comparison of laparoscopic vs. open resections for colorectal adenocarcinoma over a ten-year period. Dis Colon Rectum46:601–611

9. Quah, HM, Jayne DG, Eu KW, Seow-Choen F (2002) Bladder and sexual dysfunction following laparoscopically assisted and conventional open mesorectal resection for cancer. BJS 89,1551–1556
10. Reis Neto JA, Quilici FA, Cordeiro F, Reis JA Jr, Kagohara O, Simo Neto J (2002) Laparoscopic total mesorectum excision. JSLS 6:163–167
11. Rullier E, Sa Cunha A, Coudere P, Rullier A, Gontier R, Saric J (2003) Laparoscopic intersphincteric resection with coloplasty and coloanal anastomosis for mid and low rectal cancer. BJS 90:445–451
12. Scheidbach H, Schneider C, Konradt J, Bärlehner E, Köhler I, Wittekind Ch, Köckerling F (2002) Laparoscopic abdominoperineal resection and anterior resection with curative intent for carcinoma of the rectum. Surg Endosc 16:7–13
13. Simunovic M, Sexton R, Rempel E, Moran BJ, Heald RJ (2003) Optimal preoperative assessment and surgery for rectal cancer may greatly limit the need for radiotherapy. BJS 90:999–1000
14. Yamamoto S, Watanabe M, Hasegawa H, Kitajima M (2002) Prospective evaluation of laparoscopic surgery for rectosigmoidal and rectal carcinoma. Dis Colon Rectum 45:1648–1654

Laparoscopic Total Mesorectal Excision—The Turin Experience

M. Morino, G. Giraudo

M. Morino (✉)
II Department of Surgery, University of Turin, 14 C. so A.M. Dogliotti,
10126 Turin, Italy
e-mail: mario.morino@unito.it

Abstract

Improved local control and survival rates in the treatment of rectal cancer have been reported after total mesorectal excision (TME). We performed an analysis of TME for rectal cancer by laparoscopic approach during a prospective nonrandomized trial. A prospective consecutive series of 98 laparoscopic total mesorectal excision (LTME) procedures for low and mid-rectal tumors. All patients had a sphincter-saving procedure. Case selection, surgical technique, and clinical and oncological results were reviewed. The distal limit of rectal neoplasm was on average 5.4 cm (range 3–12) from the anal verge. The mean operative time was 192.5 min (range 125–360). The conversion rate was 18.4%. The mean postoperative stay was 11.6 days (range 4–61). The 30-day mortality rate was 1% (1/98) and the overall postoperative morbidity was 18.4% including 10 anastomotic leakages. Concerning long-term oncological results, we evaluated 93 (94.8%) patients with a median follow-up of 46.3 months (range 12–132). During this period, 15.1% (14/93) died of cancer and 7.5% (7/93) are alive with metastatic disease. The port-site metastases rate was 2.1% (2/93). The locoregional pelvic recurrence rate was 2.1% (2/93): 1 stage II at 12 months and 1 stage III at 18 postoperative months, respectively. LTME is a feasible but technically demanding procedure (18.4% conversion rate). Our series confirms the safety of the procedure, while oncological results are at present comparable to the open published series with the limitation of a short follow-up period. Further studies and possibly randomized series will be necessary to evaluate long-term clinical outcome in cancer patients.

Introduction

Improved local control and survival rates in the treatment of rectal cancer have been reported after total mesorectal excision (TME) [1]. At the same time, laparoscopy has become the gold standard for the surgical management of many digestive diseases, including benign colorectal pathologies. However, the oncological safety

Recent Results in Cancer Research, Vol. 165

of this approach is still controversial and laparoscopic methods have been less widely applied to colorectal malignancy.

At our institution, we started laparoscopic colorectal surgery at the beginning of 1992. Having obtained good experience with laparoscopic colon resections with satisfactory clinical results and having successfully performed a few laparoscopic abdominoperineal resections with an excellent view during the perineal dissection, in 1994 we decided to extend the routine use of laparoscopic approach to tumors of the middle and low rectum reproducing laparoscopically the so-called TME [1].

The present study reports an analysis of TME for low and mid-rectal cancer via a laparoscopic approach during a prospective nonrandomized trial.

Material and Methods

At our institution, between June 1994 and March 2003, 531 malignant neoplasms located in the colon and rectum underwent laparoscopic surgical treatment. Laparoscopic total mesorectal excision (LTME) for neoplasms sited in low and mid-rectum was performed in 98 patients. The site of rectal neoplasm was defined according to the International Guidelines for Cancer registrars [2]: 7 cm or less from the anal verge, low rectum; 7–12 cm, middle rectum. All patients treated in this period were included in a prospective study. The protocol was approved by the Ethical Committee of our institution and patients gave informed consent. In absence of specific contraindications to laparoscopy (i.e., severe cardiopulmonary diseases, glaucoma, etc.), patients with tumors located in the low and mid-rectum were selected for LTME according to the following criteria: elective surgery, absence of occlusion, American Society of Anaesthesiologist (ASA) status I to III. Neither morbid obesity nor prior pelvic surgery were considered as contraindication to LTME. When the neoplasm at digital examination reached the anatomical anal canal or was fixed to the pelvic floor, it was excluded from the study and a laparoscopic abdominoperineal resection was performed. Therefore, all patients included in this study had a sphincter-saving procedure. Preoperative work-up consisted of clinical evaluation, total colonoscopy, computed tomographic scan, upper abdominal ultrasound, and endoscopic ultrasound. Patients preoperatively staged T3 or T4 [3] without distant metastases were treated by preoperative radiochemotherapy (45 Gy for 4 weeks together with systemic 5-fluouracil intravenous infusion) and were re-evaluated with clinical examination and computed tomographic scan 20 days after completion of the treatment. Definitive inclusion in this study was decided at this moment, excluding locally advanced tumor, i.e., T4 in the TNM classification [3].

Clinical parameters analyzed included patient characteristics, operative variables, pathological examination, and short-term and long-term outcome. Analysis of patient characteristics included age and gender. Operative variables examined included length of operative procedure (from skin incision to the application of dressings), and conversion rate. Conversion to laparotomy was defined as unplanned incision or an incision made longer or earlier than planned. Pathological examination included type (adenoma or adenocarcinoma) and stage of diseases

(TNM). Parameters recorded included number of lymph nodes harvested and longitudinal and radial margins of excision. Short-term outcomes included intra-postoperative morbidity, 30-day mortality, and quality of life assessment evaluated by analgesic requirement. Long-term outcomes included tumor recurrence, disease-free survival, and overall survival for rectal cancer. Results were compared with literature data. Patients were followed up with physician examination, digital examination, serum carcinoembryonic antigen (CEA) assay, ultrasound of the liver, computed tomographic scan, chest X-ray, and colonoscopy. Every case of suspected local recurrence was histologically confirmed. Data were collected prospectively from the time of diagnosis using a custom-written computerized database. All analyses were performed using BMDP Statistical Software (University of California, Berkeley, LA, Oxford, Copyright 1992 by BMDP Statistical Software, Inc.). Chi-square tests were used to compare proportions. Actuarial survival was estimated with the Kaplan–Meier method, and the evaluation of differences between the groups was performed with the log-rank test. We considered a p value less than 0.05 as significant. The survival data are expressed as probability (percentage), with 95% confidence interval.

Surgical Technique

All patients were under general anesthesia when being operated. Intravenous antibiotics, such as second-generation cephalosporin and metronidazole, were administered prior to incision. The patient was placed on the operating table in a supine position; the legs were positioned in a 20–25-degree abducted position only minimally elevated above the abdomen (a higher elevation may cause the surgeon's hands to collide with the thigh when mobilizing the splenic flexure). Surgical devices used for the procedure were: a 3CCD TV camera (Karl Storz Endoscopy, Tuttlingen, Germany), a 30^{circ} angled scope, a high-flow insufflator (30 l/min) with a heating element and an adequate system of irrigation and aspiration, ultrasound scalpel, and an operating table permitting forced placement in the Trendelenburg and anti-Trendelenburg positions. Five trocars were positioned after carbon dioxide (CO_2) pneumoperitoneum at 12–14 mmHg was induced using a Veress needle or the open technique (Fig. 1).

The first phase of the procedure consisted of a careful exploration of the peritoneal cavity, the liver, and the pelvis; the small bowel with the epiploon were placed in the right upper quadrant, out of the area of dissection. Using 5-mm bowel graspers through the left-sided port, the assistant held the sigmoid ventrally under traction and to the left. The peritoneal serosa was incised starting at the sacral promontory. A window was made between the mesocolon containing the arch of the inferior mesenteric artery (IMA) and the posterior plane covered by Toldt's fascia, after which the left ureter and gonadal vessels were identified. Dissection then proceeded to the origin of the IMA, care being taken not to injure the sympathetic roots of dorsolumbar origin, which give rise to the superior hypogastric plexus located at the level of the sacral promontory. This phase of

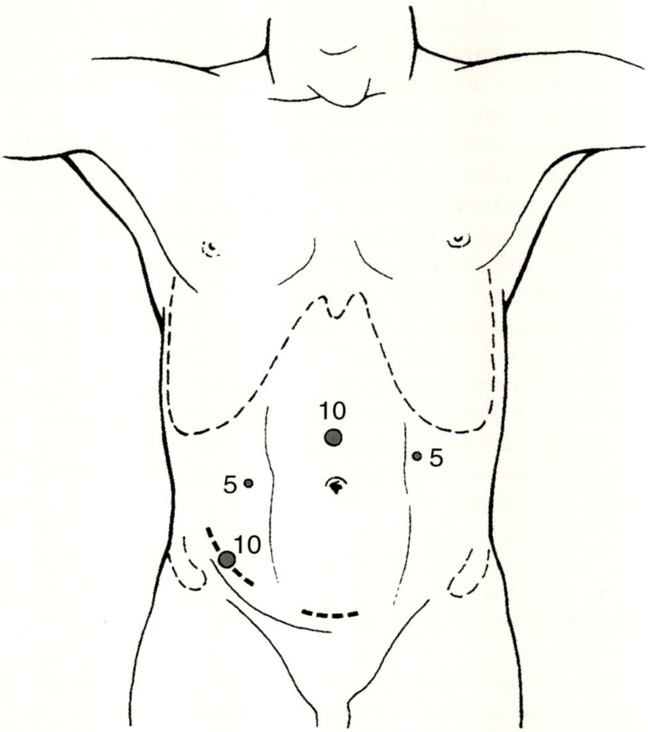

Figure 1. Trocar positions for laparoscopic total mesorectal excision; *dotted lines* represent possible sites of mini-laparotomy. The *numbers* represent the size of trocars (5 or 10 mm). (Licensed by UTET, Italy)

the procedure can be carried out using ultrasound scalpel or scissors. The IMA is divided 1 cm from the aorta after ligation with clips.

Next was the identification, dissection, and cutting of the inferior mesenteric vein under the duodenojejunal flexure. Following the avascular plane in front of Toldt's fascia and posterior to the mesocolon, the splenic flexure was routinely completely mobilized to obtain a proximal colonic segment long enough for a tension-free colorectal anastomosis at the level of the pelvic floor. Before starting pelvic dissection it is important to locate, at the level of the sacral promontory, the cleavage between the parietal layer (presacral fascia) of the pelvic fascia and the visceral layer that underlines the mesorectum. This space is practically avascular. By preserving the parietal layer, one avoids the risk of injuring the superior hypogastric plexus and the left and right hypogastric nerves (sympathetic). A deliberate attempt was made to identify and preserve the components of the pelvic autonomic nervous system, namely, the superior hypogastric nerves and the autonomic branches of S2, S3 and S4. Posterior dissection is carried out using ultrasound forceps, facilitated by pneumodissection. The peritoneum was then incised along the right side of the rectum down to the anterior reflection (retrovesical in males, retrovaginal in females). The incision was completed on the left side of the pelvis where the hypogastric nerve is found as well as the ureter, which must be identified and followed along its course. Next was the anterior dissection between the rectum and Denonvillier's fascia in males, and between the rectum and the posterior vaginal wall in females. In males, if the tumor was located on the anterior wall of the rectum, Denonvillier's fascia was removed for purposes of oncologic radicality, even at the risk of damaging the urogenital nerves. Laterally, descending towards the pelvic floor, the middle rectal artery was found. This vessel was sectioned between clips or coagulated with an ultrasound scalpel, not at its origin, but in its intermediate portion in order to preserve the pelvic plexus. Posteriorly, the rectosacral ligament was incised at the level of the fourth sacral vertebra. This incision gives access to the muscular plane of the pelvic floor (Fig. 2). Dissection proceeded posteriorly and laterally until circumferential mobilization of the bowel was accomplished. To verify the location of the tumor and the distance between its inferior margin and the line of resection, simple rectal exploration may suffice. Otherwise, rectoscopy was performed. A rectal washout was not performed routinely before transection, but a thorough irrigation of the pelvis was carried out after transection of the rectum. Division of the rectum was carried out with a linear endoscopic stapler inserted through the right iliac fossa or the suprapubic trocar. During the first part of our experience we used a 30-mm linear stapler; more recently we used a 45-mm roticulator stapler. During this step the assistant pushed from below on the perineum to elevate the pelvic floor to avoid an oblique transection of the rectum (Fig. 3). Recently, the availability of roticulator linear staplers has improved this maneuver. Proximal section of the vascular arcade was performed laparoscopically before specimen extraction to identify the level of proximal section of the colon,

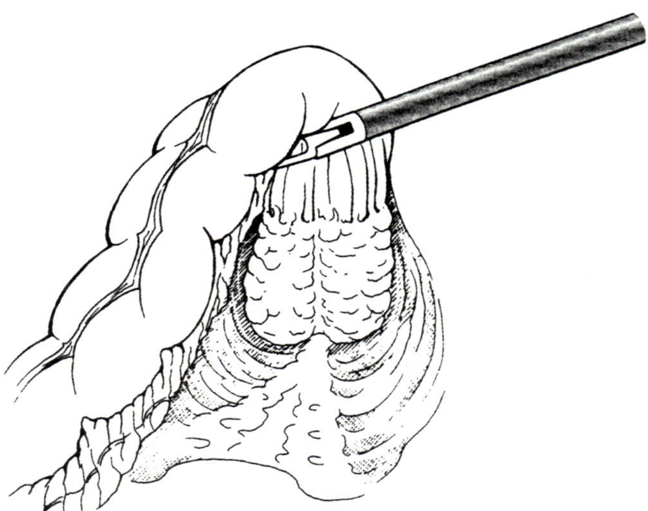

Figure 2. Laparoscopic view at the end of total mesorectal excision. (Licensed by UTET, Italy)

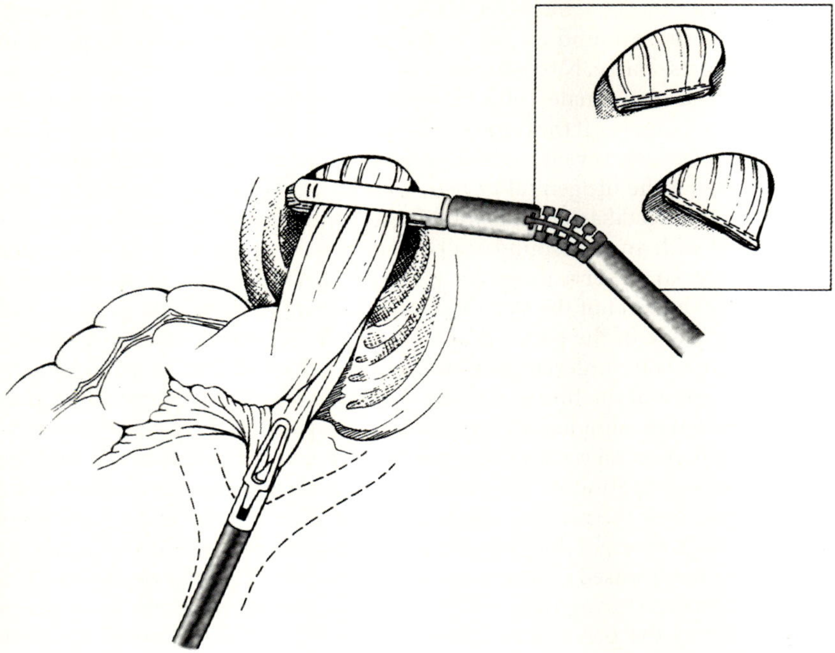

Figure 3. Distal transection of the rectum elevating the pelvic floor in order to avoid an oblique transection. (Licensed by UTET, Italy)

thus avoiding subsequent problems of tension or blood supply. The anastomosis is fashioned with a mechanical circular stapler PCEEA (Tyco Healthcare; Autosuture Co., US Surgical Corp., Norwalk, CT), usually 31 mm and occasionally 28 mm in diameter, according to the double-stapled technique, extracting the specimen and the descending colon through either a right lower quadrant or a transverse mini-laparotomy in the suprapubic area. The length of the mini-laparotomy depends on the size of the tumor and the mesorectum: mean incision length was 5.4 cm (range 4–7). The descending colon was transected, the specimen removed, and the anvil of the circular stapler placed into the lumen of the proximal colon. A wound protector was always utilized at this time. In performing LTME, the surgeon's hand is never inserted into the abdomen. After reestablishing the pneumoperitoneum, the circular stapler was inserted transanally under laparoscopic guidance and subsequently an end-to-end colorectal anastomosis was fashioned with a double-stapled technique (Fig. 4). When the distal clearance of the inferior margin of the tumor was at the level of the surgical anal canal, or in a narrow pelvis where a transverse stapled section was sometimes impossible, the technique of choice was to perform a coloanal anastomosis, executed manually from below, removing the specimen by the anal verge. This technique was used in 16 cases (16.1%).

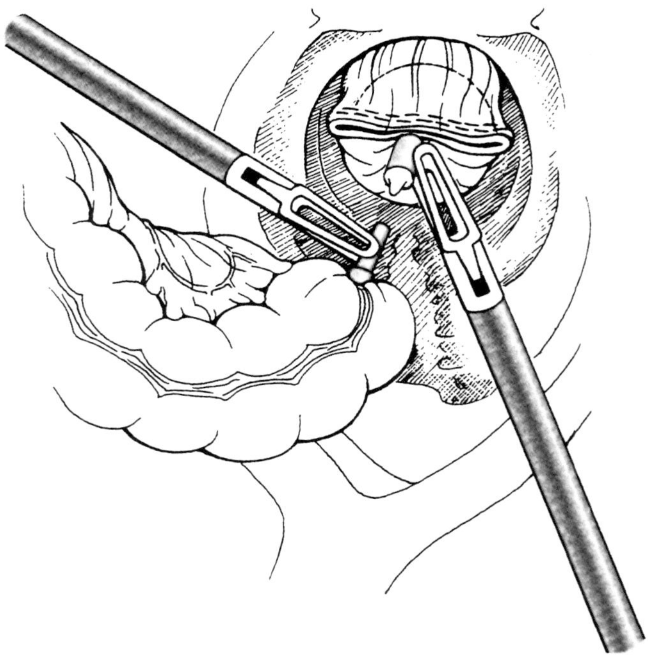

Figure 4. Laparoscopic-assisted end-to-end colorectal anastomosis with a double-stapled technique. (Licensed by UTET, Italy)

A protective ileostomy is performed at the end of the procedure, depending on the surgeon's technical evaluation of the quality of the anastomosis in the first part of our experience, routinely in the last 50 cases.

Results

LTME for neoplasms sited in the low or mid-rectum was performed on 98 patients between June 1994 and March 2003. The distal limit of the rectal neoplasm was on average 5.4 cm (range 3–12) from the anal verge. There were 59 male and 39 female subjects with a mean age of 64.9 years (range 28–89). The ASA status of the patients was: 38 ASA I, 45 ASA II, and 15 ASA III. Mean operative time was 192.5 min (range 125–360). Eighteen (18.4%) patients were converted to laparotomy: locally advanced tumors in 10 cases, technical difficulties in 7 cases, and severe obesity (body mass index 36) in 1 case.

Concerning short-term outcome, the mean time for complete patient mobilization was 1.7 days (range 1–4), for passing stools 3.8 days (range 2–9). The mean postoperative stay was 11.6 days (range 4–61).

The 30-day mortality rate was 1% (1/98): one case of intestinal infarction in an elderly patient at postoperative day 4. The overall postoperative morbidity rate was

18.4% (18/98). Complications related to anastomotic leakage clinically diagnosed occurred in ten patients (10%), treated in two cases with diverting stomas, in five cases with surgical or radiological drainages, and in three cases with prolonged total parenteral nutrition. There were three cases of prolonged postoperative ileus, treated surgically in two cases and by prolonged total parenteral nutrition in one case. Globally, six patients underwent an emergency postoperative reoperation (4 anastomotic leakages and 2 ileus).Two patients had transitory urinary and bladder dysfunction, two patients required postoperative blood transfusion, one patient had a wound infection. No general complications, pulmonary or cardiac, were observed.

Concerning quality of life assessment, no patient required narcotics for postoperative pain control, and parenteral nonsteroid analgesics (Ketorolac, Roche, Milan, Italy) were required in 35% of cases only up to postoperative day 2.

There was no case of tumor involvement of the distal or radial margin; in three cases the distal margin was inferior to 2 cm: 0.7, 1.3, and 1.6 cm respectively. Average distal clearance was 3.2pm 1.1 cm (range 0.7–8) on the fixed specimen. Median number of lymph nodes harvested was 11.6 (6–29). The stage of rectal cancer according to TNM classification [3] was: stage I in 27 patients, stage II in 23, stage III in 35, and stage IV in 13. Conversion rate was significantly higher in oncologically advanced cases: stage I 0%, stage II 13% (3/23), stage III 28.6% (10/35), stage IV 38.5% (5/13).

Concerning long-term oncological results, we evaluated 93 (94.8%) patients with a median follow-up of 46.3 months (range 12–132). Five (5%) patients were lost to follow-up. During this period, 15.1% (14/93) died of cancer and 7.5% (7/93) are alive with metastatic disease. The port-site metastases rate was 2.1% (2/93): a stage IV 17 months after surgery and a stage III 28 months after surgery, respectively. The locoregional pelvic recurrence rate was 2.1% (2/93): one stage II at 12 months and one stage III at 18 postoperative months. Concerning distant metastases, there were two (2.1%) isolated lung metastases, five (5.4%) isolated liver metastases, one (1%) isolated kidney metastases and seven (7.5%) multiple metastases. No patient presented simultaneous local and distant metastases.

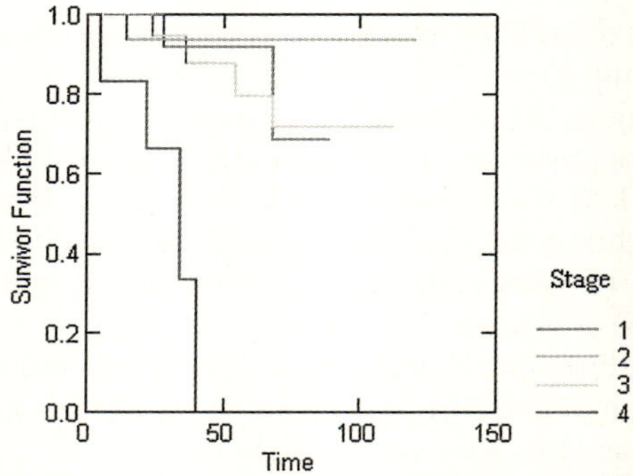

Figure 5. Survival rate by stage evaluated using Kaplan–Meier statistical analysis. Time represented in postoperative months

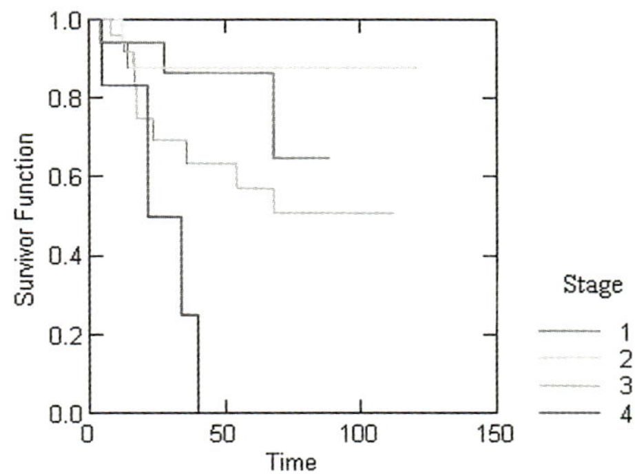

Figure 6. Disease-free rate by stage evaluated using Kaplan–Meier statistical analysis. Time represented in postoperative months

The survival rate and disease-free rate were evaluated using Kaplan–Meier statistical analysis as reported in Figs. 5 and 6. The 5-year survival rate for stage I was 94.1%, stage II 95%, and stage III 79.9%; no patient with stage IV disease was alive after 40 postoperative months, with a significance *p* value of less than 0.001 using the Log-rank test. The disease-free rate for stage I was 83.4%, stage II 90.2%, and stage III 59.2%; no stage-IV patient was disease free after 40 postoperative months, with a significance *p* value of less than 0.001 using Log-rank test.

Discussion

The technique of TME for the treatment of cancer of the mid and distal rectum is increasingly recognized as a new benchmark of quality. Developed and popularized by Heald [1], this technique presently represents the gold standard with a reported local recurrence rate at 5 and 10 years of 4% in curative cases and a 5-year tumor-free survival rate of 78% [4].

TME is a difficult and time-consuming procedure associated with a clinical leak rate in the range of 7%–20% [1, 2, 24] and a postoperative complication rate up to 50%; however, the optimal oncological results make TME an acceptable risk for rectal cancer.

One of the most controversial areas of laparoscopic surgery has been laparoscopic resection for cancer, more specifically for colon and rectal cancer [5–7]. The appearance of several reports of early wound recurrence after laparoscopic resection for malignancy [8, 9] has led to the suggestion that pattern of disease recurrence may be altered by the laparoscopic approach. Recently, a few clinical series presented results from the long-term follow-up of colon cancer patients operated laparoscopically; the majority of this series present a small number of uncontrolled patients, but some have control groups [7, 25] and some are randomized [10, 11]. Controlled studies concluded that oncological outcome at a minimum of 2 years is not compromised by the laparoscopic approach and there are no significant differences in terms of wound recurrence, survival and tumor-free survival between

Table 1. Clinical results from prospective series of LTME for rectal cancer

	Pts	Conv.	Mort.	Morbid.	An. leak	Loc. rec.
Morino–Parini [26]	100	12%	2%	36%	17%	4.7%
Leroy [27]	98	3%	2%	27%	17%	6%
Bretagnol [28]	50	12%	2%	28%	–	0%
Present series	98	18.4%	1%	18.4%	10%	2.1%

Pts, number of patients; Conv., conversion rate;Mort., 30-day mortality; Morbid., overall morbidity; An. leak, anastomotic leakages; Loc. rec., locoregional pelvic recurrence rate.

open and laparoscopic colorectal resections. The same conclusions were reached for the prospective randomized trials [10, 11].

The first consistent prospective series of LTME for rectal cancer were published in 2003 by Morino-Parini [26], Leroy [27] and Bretagnol [28], presenting clinical results similar to the present series (Table 1). LTME is feasible in the vast majority of patients with low and mid-rectal cancer with a conversion rate of 18.4% in the present series and varying from 3% to 17% in the literature [26–28]. The high conversion rate in the majority of series reflects the technical difficulty of the procedure and is related mainly to the oncological stage varying in our experience from 0% in stage I to 38.5% in stage IV.

Concerning morbidity and mortality, LTME is characterized by results at least as good as open surgery. We report a 1% mortality rate and an overall morbidity rate of 18.4% that compare favorably with mortality ranging from 3% to 7% [1, 2] and a morbidity as high as 53% [2] in open series. In particular, general morbidity is low after LTME [26–28], while the rate of anastomotic leakage in the present series compares favorably with open series: 10.2% versus 12% in Heald's series [1] and 16% in Carlsen's [2]. The 10.2% leakage rate of the present series compares favorably also with the 17% rate published in Leroy's series [27] and in our own earlier experience [26] showing a significant reduction in morbidity as a consequence of more experience and improved technique. There is a consensus in considering preoperative radio-chemotherapy and the absence of a diverting stoma as a relative risk factor for anastomotic leakage as shown by our results [26]; since 4 years ago, we routinely protect our LTME with ileostomy.

The postoperative course of LTME was characterized by early mobilization, early restoration of bowel function and low requirements of postoperative analgesics. These advantages of laparoscopic colorectal surgery have already been highlighted by many clinical series, both controlled and randomized [7, 10, 11, 15].

Other reports have shown that laparoscopic surgery for colorectal cancer is more expensive and time consuming [29]. The mean operative time for LTME in our series was 192.5 min. This figure compares favorably with data from Heald, who found a mean operative time of 4 h for open TME [1]. Although the laparoscopic approach has traditionally been associated with longer operating time than its open counterpart, we think that the enhanced magnification and improved visualization in the narrow pelvis offered by the laparoscope, coupled with the technical expertise in laparoscopic surgery of our surgical team, may have contributed to offsetting this difference.

Concerning oncological results, in the present series there were no cases of tumor involvement of the distal or radial margins. Three patients presented a distal margin inferior to 2 cm; nevertheless, these patients are disease-free at 33, 56 and 77 postoperative months, respectively. The true assessment of the safety of LTME in neoplasia must come from long-term follow-up studies of patients operated on using this technique. At present, such results are not available in the literature. Nevertheless, if we consider the present series with a median follow-up of 46.3 months, results are encouraging. There were two cases of port-site metastases (2/93, 2.1%) in one stage IV and one stage III patient. A recent review of 20 laparoscopic colectomy studies performed between 1994 and 1998 found 30 port-site recurrences in 2,365 operations, for an overall rate of port-site metastases of 1.1% after a mean follow-up of 10–33 months [6]. Our data add to the growing body of evidence attesting to the fact that port-site recurrences in laparoscopic surgery do not represent a frequent clinical problem. The locoregional pelvic recurrence rate was 2.1% (2/93), well within the range of 2%–13% local recurrence rate reported in studies of laparotomic TME for rectal cancer [1, 16–22]. Considering together port-site metastases and local recurrences, overall surgical recurrence rate was 4.3%, still an excellent oncological result even when compared with the best open series [1, 2, 24].

Concerning overall survival and disease-free survival, the mean follow-up of LTME is too short to draw any conclusion. Nevertheless, the projected Kaplan–Meier 5-year overall survival and disease-free survival rate of LTME are well within the range of published open TME series [16–22], but fail to equal the exceptional results reported by Heald [23].

In accordance with Leroy [27], in our opinion one of the major advantages of laparoscopy lies in the magnification that is offered by the endoscopic camera, which enables greater surgical precision and better identification of critical structures such as the nerve plexus, significantly aiding in their preservation. This may be particularly important in the deep narrow pelvis. Furthermore, the ability to perform deep pelvic dissection in full view of the whole operating team will undoubtedly accelerate the teaching of rectal cancer surgery and may also lead to greater standardization of the surgical procedure.

Large-scale randomized studies comparing laparoscopic and open resection for colon cancer currently ongoing on both sides of the Atlantic will hopefully provide evidence-based data on cancer-free survival in the coming future. Unfortunately, all these studies exclude extraperitoneal rectal cancer. LTME is a feasible but technically demanding procedure. Specific results of laparoscopic treatment of mid and low rectal cancer published recently [26–28] do not present any adverse oncological effect but follow-up is still limited. Our series confirms the safety of the procedure while oncological results are at present comparable to the open published series with the limitation of a short follow-up period. Further studies and possibly randomized series will be necessary to evaluate quality of life benefits and long-term clinical outcome in rectal cancer patients.

References

1. Heald RJ, Moran BJ, Ryall RDH et al (1998) The Basingstoke experience of total mesorectal excision, 1978–1997. Arch Surg 133:894–899
2. Carlsen E, Schlichting E, Gudvog I et al (1998) Effect of the introduction of total mesorectal excision for the treatment of rectal cancer. Br J Surg 85:526–529
3. Sobin LH, Wittekind C (1997) TNM classification of malignant tumours, 5th edn. Wiley
4. MacFarlane JK, Ryall RDH, Heald RJ (1993) Mesorectal excision for rectal cancer. Lancet 341:457–460
5. Fleshman JW, Wexner SD, Anvari M et al (1999) Laparoscopic vs open abdominoperineal resection for cancer. Dis Colon Rectum 42:930–939
6. Tomita H, Marcello PW, Milsom JW (1999) Laparoscopic surgery of the colon and rectum. Word J Surg 23:397–405
7. Hartley JE, Mehigan BJ, MacDonald AW et al (2000) Patterns of recurrence and survival after laparoscopic and conventional resection for colorectal carcinoma. Ann Surg 232: 181–186
8. Nduka CC, Monson JRT, Menzies-Gow N et al (1994) Abdominal wall metastases following laparoscopy. Br J Surg 81:648–652
9. Wexner SD, Cohen SM (1995) Port site metastases after laparoscopic colorectal surgery for cure of malignancy. Br J Surg 82:295–298
10. Lacy AM, Garcia-Valdecasas JC, Delgado S, Castells A, Taura P, Piqué JM et al (2002) Laparoscopic-assisted colectomy versus open colectomy for treatment of non-metastatic colon cancer: a randomised trial. Lancet 359:2224–2229
11. Milsom JW, Bohm B, Hammerhofer KA et al (1998) A prospective, randomized trial comparing laparoscopic versus conventional techniques in colorectal cancer surgery: preliminary report. J Am Coll Surg 187:46–57
12. Lord SA, Larach SW, Ferrara A et al (1996) Laparoscopic resections for colorectal carcinoma. A three-year experience. Dis Colon Rectum 39:148–154
13. Bokey EL, Moore JW, Chapuis PH et al (1996) Morbidity and mortality following laparoscopic-assisted right hemicolectomy for cancer. Dis Colon Rectum 39: S24-S28
14. Gellman L, Salky B, Edye M (1996) Laparoscopic assisted colectomy. Surg Endosc 10:1041–1044
15. Weeks JC, Nelson H, Gelber S et al (2002) Short-term quality-of-life outcomes following laparoscopic-assisted colectomy vs open colectomy for colon cancer: a randomized trial. JAMA 287:321–328
16. Arbam G, Nilsson E, Hallbook O et al (1996) Local recurrence following total mesorectal excision for rectal cancer. Br J Surg 63:375–379
17. Arenas RB, Fischera H, Mhoon D et al (1998) Total mesenteric excision in the surgical treatment of rectal cancer. Arch Surg 133:608–612
18. Enker WE, Thaler H, Cranor M et al (1995) Total mesorectal excision in the operative treatment of carcinoma of the rectum. J Am Coll Surg 181:335–346
19. Aitken RJ (1996) Mesorectal excision for rectal cancer. Br J Surg 83:214–226
20. Dixon AR, Maxwell WA, Thornton Holmes J (1991) Carcinoma of the rectum: a 10-years experience. Br J Surg 78:308–311
21. Jatzko G, Lisborg P, Welte V (1992) Improving survival rates for patients with colorectal cancer. Br J Surg 79:588–591
22. Cawthorn SJ, Parums DV, Gibbs NM et al (1990) Extent of mesorectal spread and involvement of lateral resection margin as prognostic factors after surgery for rectal cancer. Lancet 335:1055–1059
23. Heald RJ, Ryall RDH (1986) Recurrence and survival after total mesorectal excision for rectal cancer. Lancet 1:1479–1482
24. Zaheer S, Pemberton JH, Farouk R et al (1998) Surgical treatment of adenocarcinoma of the rectum. Ann Surg 227:800–811
25. Lezoche E, Feliciotti F, Paganini AM et al (2002) Laparoscopic vs open hemicolectomy for colon cancer. Surg Endosc 16:596–602
26. Morino M, Parini U, Giraudo G et al (2003) Laparoscopic total mesorectal excision: a consecutive series of 100 patients. Ann Surg 237:335–342
27. Leroy J, Jamali F, Forbes L et al (2004) Laparoscopic total mesorectal excision (TME) for rectal cancer surgery: long-term outcomes. Surg Endosc18:281–289

28. Bretagnol F, Rullier E, Couderc P, Roullier A, Saric J (2003) Technical and oncological feasibility of laparoscopic total mesorectal excision with pouch coloanal anastomosis for rectal cancer. Colorectal Dis 5:451–453
29. Philipson BM, Bokey EL, Moore JW, Chapuis PH, Bagge E (1997) Cost of open versus laparoscopically assisted right hemicolectomy for cancer. World J Surg 21:214–217

Evacuation of Neorectal Reservoirs after TME

J. S. Köninger, M. Butters, J. D. Redecke, K. Z'graggen

J.S. Köninger (✉)
Department of General Surgery, University of Heidelberg,
Im Neuenheimer Feld 110, 69120 Heidelberg, Germany
e-mail: joerg_koeninger@med.uni-heidelberg.de

Abstract

Colon pouch reconstruction after deep rectal resection is functionally superior to straight colorectal/anal anastomosis. However, stool evacuation difficulties could jeopardize the functional benefit of neorectal reservoirs. Beside the well proven colon J-pouch, the transverse coloplasty pouch may represent a viable alternative. We examined evacuation and functional outcome after total mesorectal excision and transverse coloplasty pouch reconstruction. Thirty consecutive patients with cancer of the middle and distal third of rectum underwent a total mesorectal excision. In all patients, reconstruction was performed with a transverse coloplasty pouch. Pouch and anastomosis were checked by Gastrografin enema postoperatively. Eight months after surgery, video defecography, anal manometry and pouch volumetry were performed and the patients were interviewed according to a standardized continence questionnaire. Rectal resection and reconstruction with transverse coloplasty pouch anastomosis could be performed in all patients. No insufficiency of the pouch occurred. In the follow-up, no patient had difficulties to evacuate the pouch, none of these patients needed enemas or suppositories to facilitate defecation. All patients were continent for solid stools. Twenty-five of 27 patients had up to three bowel movements per day. Patients with reduced pelvic floor movement in the defecography proved more likely to suffer from urgency, fragmented evacuation and incontinence. Transverse coloplasty pouch reconstruction after total mesorectal excision is not associated with stool evacuation problems. Urgency and incontinence, which are rarely seen after this type of reconstruction, correlate with impaired pelvic floor movement rather than with pouch size or anal sphincter tonus.

Introduction

The surgical strategy of rectal cancer has seen significant modification over the last 15 years. The concept of total mesorectal excision (TME) [1–5] in combination

Recent Results in Cancer Research, Vol. 165

with a smaller tumor-free distal margin [6–9] leads to a higher rate of continence-preserving surgeries. Nevertheless, anal dysfunction following low colorectal or coloanal anastomosis may impair quality of life in as many as 40% of patients. As a consequence of the complete removal of the rectum, patients may suffer from complex disturbances of defecation concerning both continence and stool evacuation. This is especially true over the 1st year after rectal resection [10–15].

It has already been well documented that a short colon J-pouch (CJP) is functionally superior to straight coloanal anastomosis (CAA) [16–22]. Lower stool frequencies, less urgency and an almost normal social life can be predicted for the majority of patients. Nevertheless, incomplete evacuation and constipation may be a problem after CJP [20, 23, 24]. Up to 35% of the elderly patients will need laxatives or enemas to avoid constipation and fecal impaction [20, 25, 26]. At present, it is widely accepted that construction of a short CJP reduces these problems. Whether routine resection of the sigmoid colon will improve functional outcome is still uncertain [14, 15, 17, 22, 27].

In 1997, Z'graggen and Büchler from Bern, Switzerland, described a novel technique of constructing a small-volume colonic reservoir designed in analogy to a stricturoplasty [28, 29]. This technique was originally described as the transverse coloplasty pouch (TCP), but is variably termed as colonic coloplasty or coloplasty pouch in the literature [30]. The comparison with a short colonic J-pouch (CJP) and straight coloanal anastomosis (CAA) in pigs demonstrated superior functional outcome and morphometric data [29]. Pigs with TCP showed a moderately reduced velocity of colonic transit compared to those with CAA and there were no signs of marker accumulation above the pouch or fecal impaction. The stool frequency after TCP lies between the results of the CAA and those of the CJP. In contrast, the colonic transit time after CJP was significantly delayed. In the colon passage with opaque radio markers, a relative J-pouch obstruction led to substantial fecal impaction and marker accumulation above rather than in the J-pouch [29] and this was in accordance with the known evacuation problems in humans with CJPs.

Clinical series demonstrated that patients with TCP did not develop evacuation difficulties in the follow-up [31, 32]. Defecography is the currently used standard examination to investigate impaired defecation. Defecography results after TME and TCP reconstruction have not yet been reported and the aim of the current study was to prospectively investigate functional outcome after TCP and correlate the results with defecography.

Patients and Methods

Thirty consecutive patients with cancer of the middle and lower third of the rectum underwent a TME. All interventions were done by three experienced surgeons who had each performed more than 50 TMCs. The trial was approved by the local ethical committee and informed consent was given by all patients. Table 1 shows patient data. R0 resection was confirmed in all patients by the pathologist. The important steps during reconstruction included: mobilization of the splenic flexure up to the middle colic artery and resection of the sigmoid colon. After

Table 1. Characteristics of 30 consecutive patients with rectal cancer who underwent TME and reconstruction with the transverse coloplasty pouch

Gender (F/M)		*n*=9/21
Median age in years (range)		65 (52–80)
Median body mass index (range)		25.3 (16.2–35.3)
Dukes' stage	A	11
	B	7
	C	12
Mean operating time in minutes (range)		168 (130–220)
Median follow up in weeks (range)		34 (24–72)

insertion of the anvil of a circular stapler (all anastomoses were performed by means of a circular stapling device, Proximate ILS, Ethicon Endosurgery, Johnson-Johnson, Cincinnati, OH), the descending colon was opened longitudinally at the antimesocolic border, starting 2 cm proximal to the rim of the anvil, over a distance of 10 cm. In analogy to a stricturoplasty (Heineke-Mikulicz), the incision was then closed transversally, by a two-layered running suture (4.0 PDS). Twenty-five patients had a protective loop ileostomy. Continuity was restored in median 6 weeks (2–18 weeks) after surgery. All the anastomoses were checked on the 10th postoperative day by radiografin enema. All patients with Dukes' B and C stage of the disease underwent adjuvant radiochemotherapy.

Patients were reexamined within 8 months after ileostomy-closure by interview and defecography. The standardized questionnaire according to Kirwan and Parks contained questions about incontinence, stool frequency, urgency and fragmented evacuation. A fragmented bowel movement was defined as an evacuation in a multiple consecutive manner within 1 h after defecation. Urgency was defined as the inability to defer defecation for more than 15 min.

Defecography was performed according to a standard procedure as an enema with semi-solid water-soluble contrast medium, with the patient in a squatting position. The following sequence was standardized:

1. The patient was asked to squeeze the levator ani muscles, especially the puborectalis sling contracts maximally, causing an impression at the posterior border of the anorectal junction and an acute anorectal angulation.
2. The patient was asked to relax the levator ani muscles. At this stage the puborectalis remains in a state of contraction, but not as accentuated as while squeezing. This can be observed by the partial obliteration of the impression, a slight decrease of the anorectal angle and a slight descent of the anorectal junction.
3. The patient was requested to defecate: a further obliteration of the impression, a decrease of the anorectal angle, a descent of the anorectal junction and a widening of the anal canal could be seen.
4. At the end of defecation, the ampulla recti should be empty (<10 ml), and there should be no further urge to defecate.

The change of the anorectal angle was noted during the squeezing, relaxing and defecation as an expression of the motility of the pelvic floor as well as the completeness of evacuation.

Anal manometry was performed with a water-perfused four-channel manometric catheter (MUI Scientific, Mississagua, ON, Canada). Normal values are 37–114 cm H_2O for maximum resting pressure and 37–213 cm H_2O for maximum squeeze increment pressure.

Volumetry was performed by means of a balloon inserted into the pouch, which was then filled with water at 37°C in portions of 10 ml. The first sensation was taken as threshold volume. The balloon was filled in further 10-ml steps up to the point when the patient had any discomfort or pain (maximum tolerable volume).

Results

The transverse coloplasty pouch was constructed in all 30 patients. One 78-year-old patient with severe cardiac risks died of myocardial infarction on the 3rd postoperative day (3% mortality). One patient without ileostomy underwent another operation on the 4th day because of anastomotic dehiscence and pelvic sepsis. A lavage of the abdominal cavity and a protective ileostomy were performed. In four patients, asymptomatic anastomotic leakage was detected radiologically (4/30; 13%). No insufficiency of the pouch, e.g., leakage from the transverse suture, occurred. One patient died of toxic agranulocytosis following adjuvant chemotherapy 7 weeks after surgery. One 81-year-old patient could not be examined because of rapid deterioration of his general condition (Table 2). Twenty-seven patients entered the follow-up.

Table 2. Postoperative complications

Surgical complications	Number of patients
Anastomotic leakage	
Clinically detected	2
Radiologically detected	4
Pelvic sepsis	1
Anastomotic stricture	0
Urinary dysfunction	0
Other complications	
Acute heart failure	1
Toxic agranulocytosis	1

Defecography

The TCP was constructed according to a stricturoplasty. The shortening of the anterior wall led to angulation and gave the pouch a shape similar to that of the original rectum as seen in a lateral radiograph control. Measurement of the anorectal angle could therefore be performed in analogy to that in patients who did not undergo colorectal surgery.

There was a wide variety of anorectal angles under defecation (normal values, 25–40°). The median value was 20° (range, 0–40°). Eighteen patients (67%) showed a normal mobility of the pelvic floor with a change of the ano-neorectal angle of 20–40° during defecation. All but one patient (96%) could evacuate the pouch spontaneously during defecography. One patient with Parkinson's disease was not able to evacuate the pouch during defecography (4%). All other patients emptied the neorectum according to the above-mentioned criteria, with seven patients

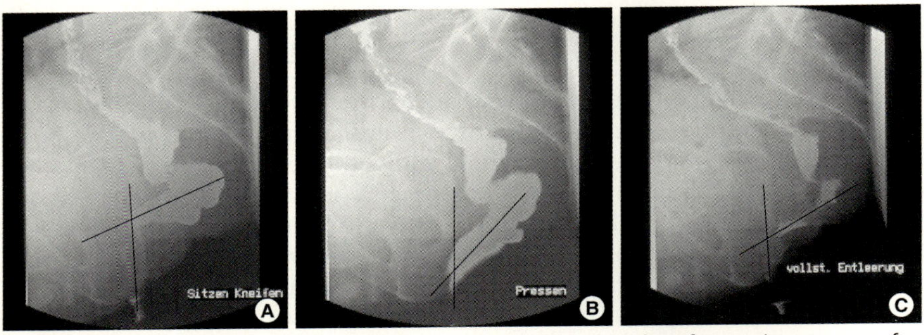

Figure 1A–C. Defecography after TME and TCP reconstruction. Patient with perfect continence status after rectal resection. Preserved continence due to acute anorectal angulation of approximately 25°, which is the result of the contraction state of the puborectalis and levator ani muscle at rest. As a result of the forward pull exerted by the puborectalis on the dorsal border of the anorectal junction, the posterior and anterior wall of this region are forced together and act as a mechanical flutter valve occluding the anal canal. During defecation, the puborectalis and levator ani muscle relaxes, resulting in obliteration of the impression of the posterior wall of the anorectal junction, abasement of the pelvic floor and the anus, with a consequent widening of the anorectal angulation. The anorectum is converted into a tunnel-like shape, enabling passage of the rectal content. The evacuation of the rectum is a result of an interaction of propulsive forces of the rectal wall and reflectory relaxation of the sphincter muscles. During defecography, the interaction between the levator ani musculature and the sphincter ani muscles with the dorsal part of the anorectum can be observed

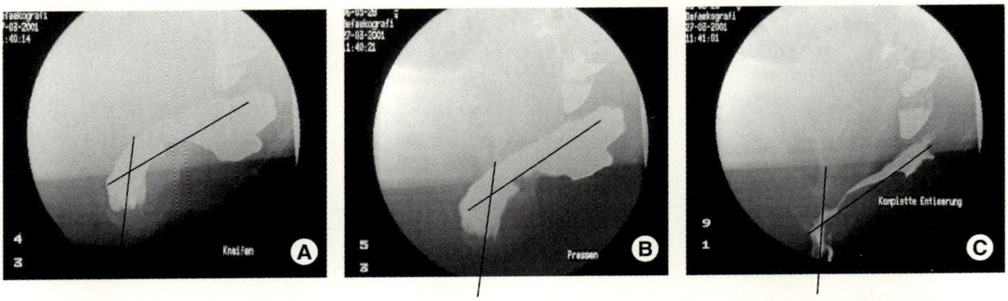

Figure 2A–C. Defecography after TME and TCP reconstruction. Patient suffering from urgency and fecal incontinence after TME and TCP reconstruction. The patient has fragmented evacuation but no evacuation difficulties with need for medical treatment or enemas. In the defecography, nearly complete evacuation of the pouch despite of minimal pelvic movement retaining less than 10 ml of the semiliquid contrast medium after defecation. Two patients showed no pelvic floor movement, but spontaneous defecation was possible. There were no signs of neorectal intussusception or mucosal prolapse in any of the patients (Figs. 1, 2).

Manometry

Maximum resting sphincter pressure was moderately reduced in a majority of the patients (Table 3), but all exceeded the lower limit of normal values (35 cm H_2O). Seven patients had a reduced maximum increment squeeze pressure and did not reach normal values (38 cm H_2O). Patients with reduced pelvic floor movement (0–25°) tended to have reduced maximum sphincter pressure, although this observation failed to reach statistical significance.

Table 3. Postoperative anorectal physiology (*n*=27)

Maximum resting pressure in cm H_2O	70 (40–140)[a]
Maximum squeeze pressure in cm H_2O	40 (30–80)
Threshold volume in ml	110 (60–130)
Maximum tolerated volume in ml	220 (180–270)
Change of anorectal angle under defecation in degrees	25 (0–40)

[a] All values are median (range).

Pouch Volumetry

The median threshold volume was 110 ml (range, 60–130 ml), the median maximum tolerated volume (MTV) 220 ml (range, 180–270 ml). The sensation described by the patients was heterogenous and only few described it similar to urgency. We discontinued the filling of the neorectal reservoir as soon as the patients reported discomfort or pain, but most (17) of the patients could not define an exact limit.

Functional Outcome

Seven months after TME and TCP anastomosis, 25 of 27 patients had one to three bowel movements per day, with a median of 2.7 patients reported occasionally uncontrolled flatus and five were occasionally incontinent for liquid stools. Two patients had difficulties to defer defecation for more than 15 min. Fourteen of 27 patients reported stool fragmentation, but all could evacuate the pouch without the help of enemas or suppositories. None of the patients used laxatives or enemas to facilitate defecation. Twenty-five of 27 patients had no limitations in social life or daily activities (see Table 4). Patients with reduced pelvic floor movement tended to have worse functional results; however, this was not statistically significant. There

Table 4. Functional results 7 months after TME and TCP anastomosis

		Number of patients
Stool frequency/day	<1	5
	1–3	20
	>3	2
Uncontrolled flatus	Always	–
	Sporadic	7
	No	20
Incontinence for liquid stool	Always	0
	Sporadic	5
	No	22
Incontinence for solid stool	Always	0
	Sporadic	2
	No	25
Ability to defer defecation always for more than 15 min	Yes	25
	No	2
Fragmented stools	Yes	14
	No	13
Inability to evacuate pouch		0

was no correlation between anal sphincter tonus and pouch volume and functional results. In addition, statistical analysis did not reveal a correlation between anastomotic leakage, postoperative radiation therapy and anal continence.

Discussion

Functional outcome after TME for rectal cancer depends on the quality of the primary surgery, the technique of reconstruction and the functional state of the pelvic floor and sphincter apparatus. A distinct "anterior resection syndrome" consists of increased stool frequency, urgency to defecate and minor degrees of incontinence/fecal leakage. Anal continence is widely reported to improve over time postoperatively. Most patients achieve relatively normal bowel function by the end of the 1st year after the operation. However, in about one-third of patients after CAA, these symptoms persist and have significant impact on the quality of life [15, 22, 24, 25, 33, 34]. The ideal rectal surgery therefore combines an optimal TME involving the preservation of nerves, bladder and genital functions and preservation of continence with a reconstruction that minimizes early and late functional problems.

Compared with CAA, functional results after CJP are superior, mainly in the 1st year after surgery, but in the long term, evacuation difficulties can jeopardize the functional benefit that results from the formation of a colonic pouch [31].

Even in the case of smaller J-pouches with a limb length of 5–7 cm, up to 20% of patients [25, 34, 35], and more frequently elderly patients [26], need suppositories and small enemas to avoid fecal impaction as early as 6 months after surgery.

A possible explanation for this phenomenon is the design of the J-pouch with its anisoperistaltic limb resulting in a neutralization of the properistaltic vector (the counter-current principle) [14, 23, 28, 36, 37]. It is also documented that size of the reservoir may play a role in the malfunctioning CJP. Larger pouches tend to dilate and favor constipation and fecal impaction [14, 36].

Seow-Choen and colleagues, however, could not show a significant difference in neorectal volume, compliance or rectal sensation after J-pouch-anal and straight descendoanal anastomosis, but nevertheless the functional results have proven to be better after pouch-anal anastomosis [14]. This implies that the brake on the propulsive wave may be more important than the volume of the neorectal reservoir [31].

The TCP may represent an ideal compromise between CAA and short CJP. A relatively small volume pouch is formed without a complete anisoperistaltic segment. This design leads to a certain degree of counter-current action, which seems to result in a moderate braking of the propulsive wave and perhaps retaining enough propulsion to allow complete evacuation.

In our series of defecographies, evacuation of the pouch was possible in all but one patient suffering from advanced Parkinson's disease who was not able to follow the instructions. All other patients evacuated the pouch spontaneously and completely—less than 10 ml of contrast medium retention—during defecography.

Preservation of anal continence depends mainly on proper function of the levator ani and the sphincter ani muscles. During defecography, the interaction between these functional units can be appreciated. A decisive factor seems to be the acute anorectal angulation. It is the result of the contraction and positioning of the puborectalis sling and the levator ani muscle at rest. As a result of the forward pull exerted by the puborectalis sling on the anorectal junction, the posterior and anterior wall are forced together and act as a mechanical flutter valve occluding the anal canal. During defecation, the puborectalis and levator ani muscle relax, which leads to an abasement of the pelvic floor and the anus with a widening of the anorectal angulation. The anorectum is converted into a tunnel-like shape, enabling passage of the rectal content. The evacuation of the rectum is then a result of an interaction of propulsive forces of the rectal wall and reflectory relaxation of the sphincter muscles.

The neorectal reservoir does not functionally replace the normal rectum. We have observed that evacuation after TME and pouch reconstruction depends on proper function of the pelvic floor and straining. There was a wide variety of pelvic floor movement in our patients. Change in anorectal angle under defecation was between 0 and 40° and correlated with functional results. In the subgroup of ten patients with physiologic floor movement (change in anorectal angle between 25–40°), none suffered from urgency and only a single patient was sporadically incontinent for flatus. Urgency and incontinence were more frequent in patients with limited pelvic floor motility. A lack of pelvic floor movement seemed to be associated with fragmented evacuation.

Besides evacuation, functional outcome significantly depends on the preservation of anal continence. Reduced anal sphincter tonus can be expected after low anterior rectal resection [15, 36]. In our study, patients with physiologic pelvic floor movement tended to have higher sphincter tonus, but in accordance with other investigators [23, 33, 35] there was no correlation between anal sphincter tonus and continence.

During pouch volumetry, we found an average threshold volume of 70 ml and average maximum tolerated volume of 220 ml after TCP, which is comparable to other reports on short J-pouches [18, 23, 36]. No correlation was found between threshold/maximum tolerated volume and either urgency, fragmented evacuation or continence status. These findings again underline that it is not so much the volume of the reservoir, but rather its antipropulsive effect that is fundamental for the functional outcome after TME.

Conclusion

Transverse coloplasty pouch reconstruction after total mesorectal excision leads to good functional results and is not associated with stool evacuation problems. Urgency and incontinence correlate more with impaired pelvic floor movement than with pouch size or anal sphincter tonus. It may be interesting to investigate whether preoperative defecography can predict functional outcome after total mesorectal excision.

References

1. Heald RJ (1988) The 'Holy Plane' of rectal surgery. J R Soc Med 81:503–508
2. MacFarlane JK, Ryall RD, Heald RJ (1993) Mesorectal excision for rectal cancer. Lancet 41:457–460
3. Nymann T, Jess P, Christiansen J (1995) Rate and treatment of pelvic recurrence after abdominoperineal resection and low anterior resection for rectal cancer. Dis Colon Rectum 38:799–802
4. Quirke P, Durdey P, Dixon MF, Williams NS (1986) Local recurrence of rectal adenocarcinoma due to inadequate surgical resection. Histopathological study of lateral tumour spread and surgical excision. Lancet 2:996–999
5. Schumpelick V, Braun J (1996) [Intersphincteric rectum resection with radical mesorectum excision and colo-anal anastomosis]. Chirurg 67:110–120
6. Amato A, Pescatori M, Butti A (1991) Local recurrence following abdominoperineal excision and anterior resection for rectal carcinoma. Dis Colon Rectum 34:317–322
7. Curti G, Maurer CA, Büchler MW (1998) Colorectal carcinoma: is lymphadenectomy useful? Dig Surg 15:193–208
8. Pollett WG, Nicholls RJ (1983) The relationship between the extent of distal clearance and survival and local recurrence rates after curative anterior resection for carcinoma of the rectum. Ann Surg 198:159–163
9. Shirouzu K, Isomoto H, Kakegawa T (1995) Distal spread of rectal cancer and optimal distal margin of resection for sphincter-preserving surgery. Cancer 76:388–392
10. Lewis WG, Martin IG, Williamson ME et al (1995) Why do some patients experience poor functional results after anterior resection of the rectum for carcinoma? Dis Colon Rectum 38:259–263

11. Braun J, Treutner KH, Winkeltau G, Heidenreich U, Lerch MM, Schumpelick V (1992) Results of intersphincteric resection of the rectum with direct coloanal anastomosis for rectal carcinoma. Am J Surg 163:407–412
12. Joo JS, Latulippe JF, Alabaz O, Weiss EG, Nogueras JJ, Wexner SD (1998) Long-term functional evaluation of straight coloanal anastomosis and colonic J-pouch: is the functional superiority of colonic J-pouch sustained? Dis Colon Rectum 1:740–746
13. Pedersen IK, Christiansen J, Hint K, Jensen P, Olsen J, Mortensen PE (1986) Anorectal function after low anterior resection for carcinoma. Ann Surg 204:133–135
14. Seow-Choen F (1996) Colonic pouches in the treatment of low rectal cancer. Br J Surg 83:881–882
15. Williamson ME, Lewis WG, Finan PJ, Miller AS, Holdsworth PJ, Johnston D (1995) Recovery of physiologic and clinical function after low anterior resection of the rectum for carcinoma: myth or reality? Dis Colon Rectum 38:411–418
16. Harris GJ, Lavery IC, Fazio VW (2001) Function of a colonic J pouch continues to improve with time. Br J Surg 88:1623–1627
17. Berger A, Tiret E, Parc R, Frileux P et al (1992) Excision of the rectum with colonic J pouch-anal anastomosis for adenocarcinoma of the low and mid rectum. World J Surg 16:470–477
18. Kusunoki M, Yanagi H, Shoji Y, Yamamura T, Utsunomiya J (1997) Anoabdominal rectal resection and colonic J pouch-anal anastomosis: 10 years' experience. Br J Surg 84:1277–1280
19. Lazorthes F, Fages P, Chiotasso P, Lemozy J, Bloom E (1986) Resection of the rectum with construction of a colonic reservoir and colo-anal anastomosis for carcinoma of the rectum. Br J Surg 73:136–138
20. Lazorthes F, Gamagami R, Chiotasso P, Istvan G, Muhammad S (1997) Prospective, randomized study comparing clinical results between small and large colonic J-pouch following coloanal anastomosis. Dis Colon Rectum 40:1409–1413
21. Mortensen NJ, Ramirez JM, Takeuchi N, Humphreys MM (1995) Colonic J pouch-anal anastomosis after rectal excision for carcinoma: functional outcome. Br J Surg 82:611–613
22. Seow-Choen F, Goh HS (1995) Prospective randomized trial comparing J colonic pouch-anal anastomosis and straight coloanal reconstruction. Br J Surg 82:608–610
23. Ho YH, Tan M, Seow-Choen F (1996) Prospective randomized controlled study of clinical function and anorectal physiology after low anterior resection: comparison of straight and colonic J pouch anastomoses. Br J Surg 83:978–980
24. Lazorthes F, Chiotasso P, Gamagami RA, Istvan G, Chevreau P (1997) Late clinical outcome in a randomized prospective comparison of colonic J pouch and straight coloanal anastomosis. Br J Surg 84:1449–1451
25. Dehni N, Tiret E, Singland JD et al (1998) Long-term functional outcome after low anterior resection: comparison of low colorectal anastomosis and colonic J-pouch-anal anastomosis. Dis Colon Rectum 41:817–822
26. Dehni N, Schlegel D, Tiret E, Singland JD, Guiguet M, Parc R (1998) Effects of aging on the functional outcome of coloanal anastomosis with colonic J-pouch. Am J Surg 175:209–212
27. Heah SM, Seow-Choen F, Eu KW, Ho YH, Tang CL (2002) Prospective, randomized trial comparing sigmoid vs descending colonic J-pouch after total rectal excision. Dis Colon Rectum 45:322–328
28. Maurer CA, Z'graggen K, Zimmermann W, Hani HJ, Mettler D, Büchler MW (1999) Experimental study of neorectal physiology after formation of a transverse coloplasty pouch. Br J Surg 86:1451–1458
29. Z'graggen K, Maurer CA, Mettler D, Stoupis C, Wildi S, Büchler MW (1999) A novel colon pouch and its comparison with a straight coloanal and colon J-pouch–anal anastomosis: preliminary results in pigs. Surgery 125:105–112
30. Fazio VW, Mantyh CR, Hull TL (2000) Colonic "coloplasty": novel technique to enhance low colorectal or coloanal anastomosis. Dis Colon Rectum 43:1448–1450
31. Mantyh CR, Hull TL, Fazio VW (2001) Coloplasty in low colorectal anastomosis: manometric and functional comparison with straight and colonic J-pouch anastomosis. Dis Colon Rectum 44:37–42
32. Z'graggen K, Maurer CA, Birrer S, Giachino D, Kern B, Büchler MW (2001) A new surgical concept for rectal replacement after low anterior resection: the transverse coloplasty pouch. Ann Surg 234:780–785
33. Hallbook O, Sjodahl R (1997) Comparison between the colonic J pouch-anal anastomosis and healthy rectum: clinical and physiological function. Br J Surg 84:1437–1441

34. Miller AS, Lewis WG, Williamson ME, Holdsworth PJ, Johnston D, Finan PJ (1995) Factors that influence functional outcome after coloanal anastomosis for carcinoma of the rectum. Br J Surg 82:1327–1330
35. Hallbook O, Pahlman L, Krog M, Wexner SD, Sjodahl R (1996) Randomized comparison of straight and colonic J pouch anastomosis after low anterior resection. Ann Surg 224:58–65
36. Huber FT, Herter B, Siewert JR (1999) Colonic pouch vs side-to-end anastomosis in low anterior resection. Dis Colon Rectum 42:896–902
37. Schumpelick V, Willis S (1999) [Colonic pouch]. Chirurg 70:543–551

Long-Term Functional Results After Straight or Colonic J-Pouch Coloanal Anastomosis

Guillaume Portier, Ivan Platonoff, Frank Lazorthes

G. Portier (✉)
Service de Chirurgie Digestive, CHU Purpan, Place du Dr. Baylac,
31059 Toulouse, France
e-mail: portier.g@chu-toulouse.fr

Abstract

Proctectomy followed by straight coloanal anastomosis (CAA) often results in poor functional outcome known as the anterior resection syndrome. It is now based on evidence that a colonic J-pouch CAA improves outcome in the first 2 years. We assessed the very late functional outcome of CAA patients with or without a pouch. These results show that the functional benefit of the J-pouch anastomoses is sustained over the very long term.

Introduction

Proctectomy and coloanal anastomosis makes it possible to cure a majority of patients with cancer of the mid and low rectum. However, functional results are often disappointing and patients' quality of life can be altered seriously. Attempts to ameliorate the function have been made. The colonic J-pouch, first described in 1986, is now being challenged by other techniques, still under evaluation. The aim of this work was to assess the very long-term functional results of coloanal anastomoses (CAA) with or without a colonic J-pouch (CJP).

Patients and Methods

Among all consecutive patients treated for rectal cancer between 1980 and 1996, we specifically analyzed CAA for mid and lower rectal tumors, after at least 5 years of follow-up.

In June 2001, a functional questionnaire was sent to patients who were still alive, without recurrence.

Items recorded were increased stool frequency, stool fragmentation, evacuating difficulties, and continence. Quality of life related to incontinence was also assessed

Recent Results in Cancer Research, Vol. 165

by the FIQL (Fecal Incontinence Quality of Life) questionnaire [1]. Patients who had had postoperative radiotherapy were excluded.

Statistical analysis was comparative between straight and J-pouch anastomoses. A multivariate analysis was made including factors such as preoperative radiotherapy, age, gender, and partial internal sphincter resection.

Results

A total of 190 consecutive patients were treated in the study period. In 2001, 95 were alive without recurrence. Six postoperatively irradiated patients were excluded, and seven were lost to follow-up. Mean follow-up was 156 months (SE, 54). There were 52 males and 30 females. Mean age was 71.5 years (SE, 9.1). Patient characteristics are detailed in Table 1.

There were no significant differences between the two groups for age, sex ratio, neoadjuvant radiotherapy, partial internal sphincter excision.

Functional results are detailed in Table 2.

Table 1. Characteristics of 82 patients after proctectomy and coloanal anastomosis

		n	%
Dukes'	A	41	50
	B	25	30.5
	C	15	18.3
	M+	1	1.2
Radiotherapy	None	43	52.4
	Preoperative	33	40.2
	postoperative	6	7.3

Table 2. Long-term functional results after proctectomy between straight coloanal anastomosis (CAA) and colonic J-pouch coloanal anastomosis (CJP)

		CAA (%)	CJP (%)	*p*
Continence	Fazio I+II	53	72	0.04
	III+IV	47	28	
	Cleveland score	6.44	4.56	NS
	Nocturnal soiling	56.3	32	0.03
	Gas/stool discrimination	84.5	92	NS
Evacuation disorders	Yes	59	48	
	Urgencies	47	21	0.014
	>2 movements /24h	68.8	50	0.03
	Need to stay near toilets	22	6	0.038
	Incomplete evacuation	50	27	0.028

Table 3. Long-term Fecal Incontinence Quality of Life scores after proctectomy between straight coloanal anastomosis (CAA) and colonic J-pouch coloanal anastomosis (CJP); *n*=45. Scales are from 0 (worse) to 4 (excellent)

	CAA	CJP	*p*
Lifestyle	3.07	3.35	NS
Coping/behavior	2.95	3.25	NS
Depression/self-perception	3.71	3.81	NS
Embarrassment	3.1	3.29	NS

No patients had a diverting stoma attributable to functional reasons.

More patients were continent to stools in the CJP group than in the straight CAA group (72% vs. 53%; p=0.04). They also had less nocturnal soiling (32% vs. 56%), fewer urgencies (21% vs. 47%), lower frequency, and less incomplete evacuation.

FIQL scores are detailed in Table 3.

FIQL scores were available for 45 patients. The four domains studied were higher in the CJP group, but did not reach statistical significance.

Discussion

Proctectomy results in a well-described functional outcome : the anterior resection syndrome [2]. This syndrome associates several troubles such as increased stool frequency, stool fragmentation, incomplete exoneration, incapacity to defer exoneration, soiling or incontinence.

This is due to the loss of rectal capacity and compliance, and by sphincter alterations due to partial internal resection (for ultralow CAA) and adjuvant treatments [3, 4].Its severity is increased by the extent of rectal resection, and thus is mostly observed after straight coloanal anastomosis [5]. In addition, pelvic septic complications due to anastomotic leakages occur in about 15% of cases after straight CAA in published series [6–9].

The colonic J-pouch, described in 1986 [10, 11], offered several theoretical advantages: it creates a neorectal reservoir, with the aim of increasing rectal capacity [12]. In a scintigraphic randomized study, retention of colonic liquids was improved in the pouch group [13]. It also brings more healthy tissue to the pelvis. The tension-free anastomosis is lateroterminal, with, in theory, better vascularization, and less anastomotic leakages.

Since 1986, a large number of comparative prospective, and even randomized trials between CJP and straight CAA have been published. In all studies, CJP resulted in a better functional outcome in the first 2 years [5, 8, 9, 14–17].

Fragmentation, urgency, nocturnal defecation and continence were all improved in these series. They also confirmed a decreased anastomotic leakage rate with J-pouches, compared to straight anastomosis [6–9].

A new problem appeared in the first experience, represented by evacuation difficulties, probably due to a J-pouch that was too long (10 cm) [18]. A randomized trial assessed this problem specifically, and showed that a 5-cm J-pouch can avoid this poor outcome [19].

More recent studies assessed quality of life, and were concordant with previous results.

Evidence-based studies have now led to the conclusion that a pouch offers a functional benefit, at least in the first 2 years.

Since straight anastomosis patients usually experience a functional improvement with time [16], it is not known whether the functional superiority of pouch anastomoses is sustained in the long term.

Very few data about long-term functional outcome are available since only one series had more than 5 years of follow-up [20].

Our work compared functional results between CJP and straight CAA after more than 10 years.

It suggests that the functional benefit of a colonic pouch persists, and moreover, that no outlet obstruction appears, as has been previously described with 10-cm pouches [18].

Still, about 30% of our patients experience occasional soiling or stool fragmentation. The satisfactory quality-of-life scores in our study reflect that in the long term, most of them are adapted to this situation and prefer not to have a definitive stoma. FIQL scores were all higher in the CJP group but not significantly different, probably because of a lack of statistical power, since only 45 patients returned the questionnaire.

Our data do not predict the individual functional outcome. This is why experimental studies must carry on with new techniques of rectal reconstruction after proctectomy, such as transverse coloplasty pouch, or lateroterminal anastomosis [21]. Influence of adjuvant treatments, especially preoperative chemoradiotherapy, and of partial sphincter excision, must be taken into consideration for the subgroup analysis.

Conclusion

The functional benefit of a colonic J-pouch is now based on evidence, at least for the first 2 years. Our study suggests that this superiority is maintained over the very long term, and that CJP function does not deteriorate with time. Nevertheless, these results are not perfect, and efforts should be made to ameliorate patients' anorectal function and quality of life after curative proctectomy for cancer.

References

1. Rockwood TH, Church JM, Fleshman JW, Kane RL, Mavrantonis C, Thorson AG, Wexner SD, Bliss D, Lowry AC (2000) Fecal Incontinence Quality of Life Scale: quality of life instrument for patients with fecal incontinence. Dis Colon Rectum 43:9–16; discussion 16–17
2. Lewis WG, Martin IG, Williamson ME, Stephenson BM, Holdsworth PJ, Finan PJ, Johnston D (1995) Why do some patients experience poor functional results after anterior resection of the rectum for carcinoma? Dis Colon Rectum 8:259–263

3. Dahlberg M, Glimelius B, Graf W, Pahlman L (1998) Preoperative irradiation affects functional results after surgery for rectal cancer: results from a randomized study. Dis Colon Rectum 41:543–549; discussion 549–551
4. Gervaz P, Rotholtz N, Wexner SD, You SY, Saigusa N, Kaplan E, Secic M, Weiss EG, Nogueras JJ, Belin B (2001) Colonic J-pouch function in rectal cancer patients: impact of adjuvant chemoradiotherapy. Dis Colon Rectum 44:1667–1675
5. Hida J, Yasutomi M, Maruyama T, Fujimoto K, Nakajima A, Uchida T, Wakano T, Tokoro T, Kubo R, Shindo K (1998) Indications for colonic J-pouch reconstruction after anterior resection for rectal cancer: determining the optimum level of anastomosis. Dis Colon Rectum 41:558–563
6. Hallbook O, Sjodahl R (1996) Anastomotic leakage and functional outcome after anterior resection of the rectum. Br J Surg 83:60–62
7. Ho YH, Tan M, Seow-Choen F (1996) Prospective randomized controlled study of clinical function and anorectal physiology after low anterior resection: comparison of straight and colonic J pouch anastomoses. Br J Surg 83:978–980
8. Hallbook O, Pahlman L, Krog M, Wexner SD, Sjodahl R (1996) Randomized comparison of straight and colonic J pouch anastomosis after low anterior resection. Ann Surg 224:58–65
9. Joo JS, Latulippe JF, Alabaz O, Weiss EG, Nogueras JJ, Wexner SD (1998) Long-term functional evaluation of straight coloanal anastomosis and colonic J-pouch: is the functional superiority of colonic J-pouch sustained? Dis Colon Rectum 41:740–746
10. Lazorthes F, Fages P, Chiotasso P, Lemozy J, Bloom E (1986) Resection of the rectum with construction of a colonic reservoir and colo-anal anastomosis for carcinoma of the rectum. Br J Surg 73:136–138
11. Parc R, Tiret E, Frileux P, Moszkowski E, Loygue J (1986) Resection and colo-anal anastomosis with colonic reservoir for rectal carcinoma. Br J Surg 73:139–141
12. Hallbook O, Sjodahl R (1997) Comparison between the colonic J pouch-anal anastomosis and healthy rectum: clinical and physiological function. Br J Surg 84:1437–1441
13. Ho YH, Yu S, Ang ES, Seow-Choen F, Sundram F (2002) Small colonic J-pouch improves colonic retention of liquids—randomized, controlled trial with scintigraphy. Dis Colon Rectum 45:76–82
14. Ortiz H, De Miguel M, Armendariz P, Rodriguez J, Chocarro C (1995) Coloanal anastomosis: are functional results better with a pouch? Dis Colon Rectum 38:375–377
15. Kusunoki M, Shoji Y, Yanagi H, Hatada T, Fujita S, Sakanoue Y, Yamamura T, Utsunomiya J (1991) Function after anoabdominal rectal resection and colonic J pouch - anal anastomosis. Br J Surg 78:1434–1438
16. Lazorthes F, Chiotasso P, Gamagami RA, Istvan G, Chevreau P (1997) Late clinical outcome in a randomized prospective comparison of colonic J pouch and straight coloanal anastomosis. Br J Surg 84:1449–1451
17. Seow-Choen F, Goh HS (1995) Prospective randomized trial comparing J colonic pouch-anal anastomosis and straight coloanal reconstruction. Br J Surg 82:608–610
18. Hida J, Yasutomi M, Maruyama T, Tokoro T, Wakano T, Uchida T (1999) Enlargement of colonic pouch after proctectomy and coloanal anastomosis: potential cause for evacuation difficulty. Dis Colon Rectum 42:1181–1188
19. Lazorthes F, Gamagami R, Chiotasso P, Istvan G, Muhammad S (1997) Prospective, randomized study comparing clinical results between small and large colonic J-pouch following coloanal anastomosis. Dis Colon Rectum 40:1409–1413
20. Harris GJ, Lavery IC, Fazio VW (2001) Function of a colonic J pouch continues to improve with time. Br J Surg 88:1623–1627
21. Mantyh CR, Hull TL, Fazio VW (2001) Coloplasty in low colorectal anastomosis: manometric and functional comparison with straight and colonic J-pouch anastomosis. Dis Colon Rectum 44:37–42

Urinary and Sexual Function After Total Mesorectal Excision

Christoph A. Maurer

C.A. Maurer (✉)
Surgical Department, Kantonsspital, Rheinstrasse 26, 4410 Liestal, Switzerland
e-mail: christoph.maurer@ksli.ch

Abstract

The autonomous pelvic nerves are in close contact to the visceral pelvic fascia that surrounds the mesorectum. The concept of total mesorectal excsion (TME) in rectal cancer treatment has led to a substantial improvement of autonomous pelvic nerve preservation. Consecutively, this highly precise and sharp dissection technique under direct vision reduces the problem of accidental bladder denervation from 50–60% with conventional rectal cancer surgery to less than 20% with TME and the problem of postoperative impotence from 70–100% to less than 30%. The learning curve in this technically demanding procedure plays a major role with regard to a satisfying nerve preservation. The laparoscopic approach for TME allows to obtain similarly favorable results with regard to postoperative urogenital function, at least for tumors situated in the middle and upper third of the rectum, compared with open surgery. The present paper describes and depictures in detail the anatomy and the pathophysiology of autonomic pelvic nerves, the surgical technique for nerve preservation and gives a short overview of the results in the literature including own data.

Introduction

Rectal cancer is the number one cancer with regard to the incidence of abdominal malignancies [26, 32]. The two main problems of rectal cancer surgery are local recurrence and pelvic autonomic nerve damage. Whereas enormous efforts have been made recently to improve local recurrence rates, only few studies have investigated postoperative urinary and sexual function, which has a large impact on the patients' postoperative quality of life. This chapter focuses on the issue of pelvic autonomic nerve function, particularly in the context of total mesorectal excision (TME) [2, 9, 20]. As described in detail elsewhere in this book, the TME technique is characterized by a sharp dissection between the parietal and visceral planes of the pelvic fascia, resulting in a complete removal of the rectum together

Recent Results in Cancer Research, Vol. 165

with the mesorectum. Compared to conventional rectal resection, TME is more extensive and radical, and therefore has a potentially adverse effect on pelvic nerve preservation. On the other hand, TME is a more precise technique, respecting the anatomical planes and preserving the autonomic pelvic nerves that are adjacent to the resection plane.

new

Anatomy and Pathophysiology of Autonomic Pelvic Nerves

A plexus of sympathetic nerves lies in extraperitoneal connective tissue on the anterior aspect of the aorta and surrounds the origin of the inferior mesenteric artery. This inferior mesenteric plexus (upper part) and the superior hypogastric plexus (lower part) of the preaortic plexus is preserved by ligating and dividing the inferior mesenteric artery not flush to the aorta but 1–2 cm from its aortic origin. Hence, a "preaortic strip" is avoided, except when indicated by lymph node involvement at this site. Resection of the superior hypogastric plexus and/or resection of the hypogastric nerve on both sides will cause retrograde ejaculation since the reflectory activation of urinary bladder sphincter during ejaculation is lost. The superior hypogastric plexus divides in the manner of an inverted Y into

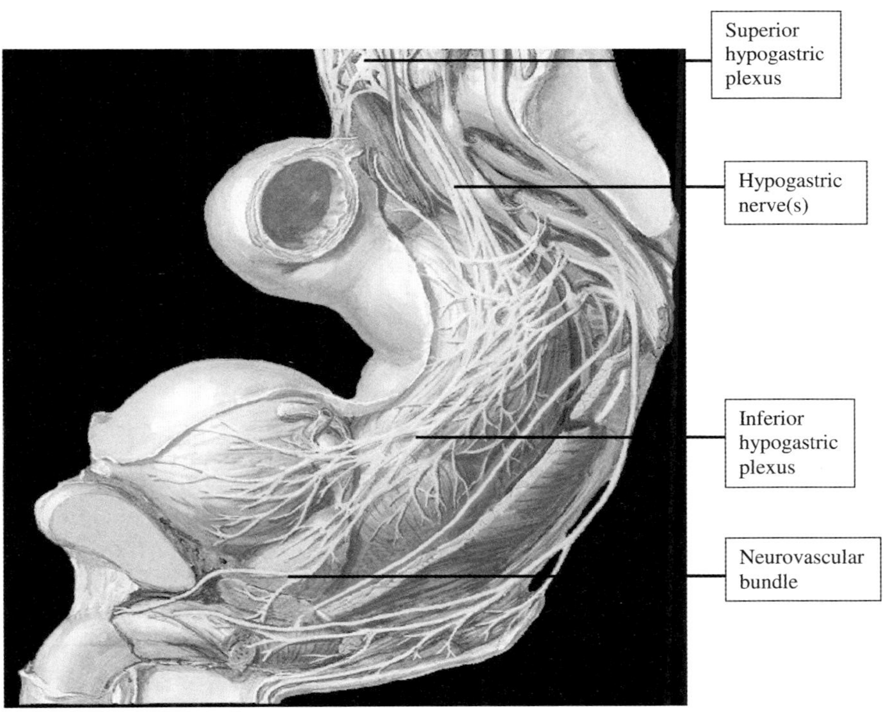

Figure 1. Anatomy of autonomous pelvic nerves

Table 1. Autonomic pelvic nerve structures and consequences of lost function corresponding to site of nerve damage

Site of nerve damage	Nerve failure	Bladder disorder	Male genital disorder	Female genital disorder	Anal sphincter disorder
Superior hypogastric plexus	S partially both sides	Incontinence (partial)	Retrograde ejaculation	Diminished orgasm	None
N. hypogastricus one side	S partially one side	None	Ev. retrograde ejaculation	None	None
Nn. hypogastrici both sides	S partially both sides	Incontinence (partial)	Retrograde ejaculation	Diminished orgasm	None
Inferior hypogastric plexus one side	S+PS completely one side	Voiding disorder	Incomplete erection+ejaculation	Incomplete erection/lubrication	None
Inferior hypogastric plexus both sides	S+PS completely both sides	Atonia, severe voiding disorder	Lack of erection+ejaculation	Lack of erection/lubrication	Incontinence I–II
Neurovascular bundle one side	S+PS completely one side	None	Incomplete erection+ejaculation	Incomplete erection/lubrication	None
Neurovascular bundle both sides	S+PS completely both sides	None	Lack of erection+ejaculation	Lack of erection/lubrication	None

S, pelvic sympathetic nerve; PS, pelvic parasympathetic nerve.

a pair of hypogastric nerves, each of which may be a single nerve or an elongated network of anastomosing fibers, which run to the side walls of the pelvis, where they merge with parasympathetic fibers (Nn. erigentes, "the erigent pillar" according to Heald) from the second to fourth sacral nerve roots and fibers from the sacral sympathetic ganglia to form the inferior hypogastric plexus on each side (Fig. 1). This almost rectangular plaque of nervous tissue is firmly attached to the anterolateral aspect of the mesorectum on both sides, i.e. between 10 and 2 o'clock, due to nerve branches directly entering the mesorectum for autonomic innervation of the rectum. These nerve fibers together with an inconsistently (less than 20%) found small artery (the middle rectal artery) must be carefully dissected; meanwhile the inferior hypogastric plexus itself must be preserved. Damage to the latter on one side will cause (temporary) voiding difficulties of the urinary bladder and at least diminished erection and ejaculation or diminished vaginal lubrication and arousal; damage on both sides will lead to denervated bladder requiring catheterism, and impotence/dyspareunia. Communicating predominantly parasympathetic nerves between bilateral splanchnic nerves may take over an important function in patients with hemilateral nerve damage [31]. Neurovascular bundles from the inferior hypogastric plexus and internal iliac vessel branches pass forwards from their posterolateral relationship to seminal vesicles, prostate and bladder, as the lateral edges of Denonvilliers' fascia, and they need to be preserved as the fascia is resected with the rectum [1, 6, 11, 18]. Autonomic pelvic nerve structures and loss of their function corresponding to the site of nerve damage are summarized in Table 1.

Urinary and Sexual Function After Conventional Rectal Cancer Surgery

For many years severe urogenital dysfunction has been accepted as normal faith following rectal cancer surgery. Reasons for the high rates of denervated bladder and impotence (Table 2) were the anatomy and pathophysiology of autonomic pelvic nerves that were only poorly understood by surgeons, and the commonly used blunt dissection technique. There was even a period where some surgeons recommended stripping the aorta and the iliac vessels for an increase in radicality. Nowadays, we know that this is not only of no benefit with regard to survival, but it deteriorates quality of life substantially.

Table 2. Urinary and male sexual function after conventional rectal cancer surgery

Author	Year	No. of patients	Bladder dysfunction	Loss of erection	Lack of ejaculation
Kinn and Ohman [14]	1986	22	50%	80%	n.a.
Cunsolo et al. [3]	1990	46	57%	59%	59%
Hojo et L; [10]	1991	134	58%	69%	81%
Koukouras et al. [15]	1991	40	n.a.	53%	30%

Nerve Preservation Using the Total Mesorectal Excision Technique

Recent studies reported improved urinary and sexual function (Table 3) in comparison to older data (Table 2). We hypothesized that this improvement is the result of the introduction and growing acceptance of the TME technique [8, 9, 20, 22]. Therefore, we analyzed our own series of 133 patients with resected rectal cancer between November 1993 and September 1998 at the university of Bern [21]. The TME technique was introduced in 1995. A questionnaire regarding preoperative and current urogenital function was sent to all 87 patients who were alive in December 1998. Sixty patients answered reliably to the questionnaire: 29 patients in group 1 underwent conventional rectal cancer surgery from 1993 to 1995, and 31 patients in group 2 underwent mesorectal excision from 1996 to 1998. Three out of 31 patients in group 2 had only partial mesorectal excision. There was no significant difference between group 1 and group 2 regarding gender, tumor location, tumor stage, radiation therapy, or surgical complications. However, group 2 patients had a significantly higher median age at operation (71.2 vs. 63.9 years) and smaller distance of anastomosis from anal verge (4.7 vs. 6.4 cm) than group 1 patients. Regarding urinary function both groups were similar. Regarding male sexual function, however, the ability to achieve orgasm and to ejaculate was significantly better preserved in the TME patients (group 2) than in the conventionally operated patients (group 1). Overall, the postoperative deterioration in male sexual function was significantly more common in group 1 (Fig. 2). The high rate of preexisting sexual disorders in both groups needs to be mentioned.

Table 3. Urinary and male sexual function after introduction of TME

Author	Year	No. of patients	Bladder dysfunction	Loss reduction of erection	Lack of ejaculation
Enker [4]	1992	42	5%	13%	24%
Leveckis et al. [17]	1995	20	15%	19%	NA
Havenga et al. [7]	1996	136	32%	17%	42%
Maas et al. [19]	1998	47	28%	11%	42%
Saito et al. [30]	1998	91	26%	24%	45%
Nesbakken et al. [25]	2000	27	13%[a]	28%	43%
Nagawa et al. [24]	2001	22	27%	45%	45%
Maurer et al. [21]	2001	19	21%[a]	55%	30%
Quah et al. [28]	2002	37	3%	24%	19%
Pocard et al. [27]	2002	9	0%	44%	11%
Kim et al. [13]	2002	68	26%	25%	38%

[a]Women additionally included.

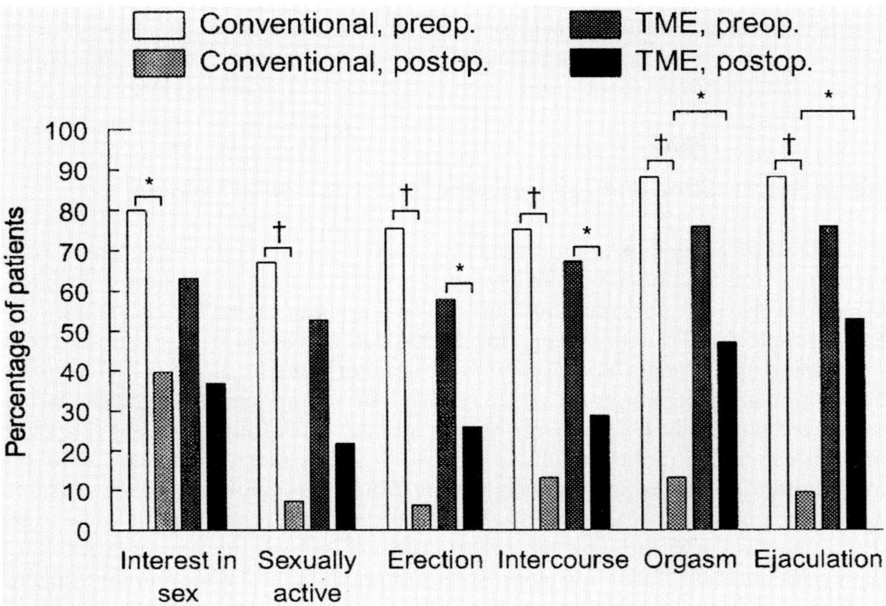

Figure 2. Frequency of six different features of male genital function in group 1 (conventional rectal surgery) and group 2 (total mesorectal excision; TME) before and after operation. *Preop.*, before operation; *postop.*, after operation. *$p<0.05$, † $p<0.001$ (χ^2 test). (From [21], with permission of Blackwell Science)

Impact of Learning Curve on Pelvic Autonomic Nerve Preservation

In a recent personal series (unpublished data) of 45 low anterior resections (30 of them with coloanal reconstruction) and eight abdominoperineal resections for rectal cancer from July 2002 to December 2004, none of these patients had to be sent home with a urinary catheter and only one male patient complained of diminished erection and ejaculation. Rectal dissection in this patient was more difficult because of previous rectal surgery. A second male patient with hemilateral pelvic nerve resection resulting from direct tumor infiltration was no longer sexually active before operation and did not complain of sexual dysfunction postoperatively. All other patients did not experience any alteration in urinary or sexual function. These data strongly suggest further improvement of the author's precision of the nerve-sparing TME technique when compared to our recently published results [21]. Similarly good results were reported by Quah et al. for open rectal cancer surgery [28]: 0/40 required long-term intermittent self-catheterization, 3/22 men had erectile dysfunction and 1/22 were unable to ejaculate.

After introduction of TME, Junginger et al. were able to identify and preserve the pelvic autonomic nerves in 60%, 94% and 92% within the first 50 patients, the second 50 patients and the third 50 patients, respectively [12]. Correspondingly, the frequency of bladder voiding disturbance requiring catheterization decreased from 26% to 2% and 4%, respectively.

Intraoperative parasympathetic nerve stimulation with penile tumescence monitoring may be an aid to less experienced pelvic surgeons and may help in learning to identify and preserve autonomic nerves during total mesorectal excision [5].

Nerve Preservation and Laparoscopic Total Mesorectal Excision

Evidence is growing that laparoscopically resected patients with rectal cancer do at least not worse than open resected patients in terms of long-term survival [16, 23]. Therefore, the next question must address urinary and sexual function following laparoscopic rectal cancer surgery. In a retrospective analysis of a randomized trial comparing open versus laparoscopic rectal cancer resection, 7/15 (47%) sexually active men in the laparoscopic group reported impotence or impaired ejaculation compared with only 1/22 patients having an open operation ($p<0.01$) [28]. The authors concluded that especially in patients with low rectal cancers or bulky tumors, autonomic nerve preservation is more difficult to achieve by the laparoscopic approach, probably because of insufficient tension on the planes that have to be dissected. Similarly, Rullier et al. reported loss of sexual function in 8 out of 18 male patients (44%) following laparoscopic intersphincteric resection for mid and low rectal cancers [29]. Further studies will have to show whether laparoscopy will be able to overcome this problem in future.

Conclusion

The autonomous pelvic nerves are in close contact with the visceral pelvic fascia, the "holy plane" that surrounds the mesorectum. The growing acceptance of the concept of total mesorectal excision in rectal cancer treatment has led to a substantial improvement in autonomous pelvic nerve preservation. Consecutively, postoperative genital function—and to a lesser extent the urinary function, too—is significantly better preserved after TME than after conventional rectal cancer surgery. The learning curve in this highly precise and technically demanding procedure plays a major role with regard to satisfactory nerve preservation. The laparoscopic approach for TME makes it possible to obtain similarly favorable results in terms of postoperative urogenital function, at least for tumors situated in the middle and upper third of the rectum.

References

1. Baader B, Herrmann M (2003) Topography of the pelvic autonomic nervous system and its potential impact on surgical intervention in the pelvis. Clin Anat 16:119–130
2. Büchler MW, Heald RJ, Maurer CA, Ulrich B (eds) (1998) Rektumkarzinom: das Konzept der totalen mesorektalen Exzision, S. Karger, Basel
3. Cunsolo A, Bragaglia RB, Manara G, Poggioli G, Gozzetti G (1990) Urogenital dysfunction after abdominoperineal resection for carcinoma of the rectum. Dis Colon Rectum 33:918–922

4. Enker WE (1992) Potency, cure, and local control in the operative treatment of rectal cancer. Arch Surg 127:1396–1401; discussion 1402
5. Hanna NN, Guillem J, Dosoretz A, Steckelman E, Minsky BD, Cohen AM (2002) Intraoperative parasympathetic nerve stimulation with tumescence monitoring during total mesorectal excision for rectal cancer. J Am Coll Surg 195:506–512
6. Havenga K, DeRuiter MC, Enker WE, Welvaart K (1996) Anatomical basis of autonomic nerve-preserving total mesorectal excision for rectal cancer. Br J Surg 83:384–388
7. Havenga K, Enker WE, McDermott K, Cohen AM, Minsky BD, Guillem J (1996) Male and female sexual and urinary function after total mesorectal excision with autonomic nerve preservation for carcinoma of the rectum. J Am Coll Surg 182:495–502
8. Heald RJ (1995) Total mesorectal excision is optimal surgery for rectal cancer: a Scandinavian consensus. Br J Surg 82:1297–1299
9. Heald RJ, Husband EM, Ryall RD (1982) The mesorectum in rectal cancer surgery—the clue to pelvic recurrence? Br J Surg 69:613–616
10. Hojo K, Vernava AM 3rd, Sugihara K, Katumata K (1991) Preservation of urine voiding and sexual function after rectal cancer surgery. Dis Colon Rectum 34:532–539
11. Hollabaugh RS, Steiner MS, Dmochowski RR (2001) Neuroanatomy of the female continence complex: clinical implications. Urology 57:382–388
12. Junginger T, Kneist W, Heintz A (2003) Influence of identification and preservation of pelvic autonomic nerves in rectal cancer surgery on bladder dysfunction after total mesorectal excision. Dis Colon Rectum 46:621–628
13. Kim NK, Aahn TW, Park JK, Lee KY, Lee WH, Sohn SK, Min JS (2002) Assessment of sexual and voiding function after total mesorectal excision with pelvic autonomic nerve preservation in males with rectal cancer. Dis Colon Rectum 45:1178–1185
14. Kinn AC, Ohman U (1986) Bladder and sexual function after surgery for rectal cancer. Dis Colon Rectum 29:43–48
15. Koukouras D, Spiliotis J, Scopa CD, Dragotis K, Kalfarentzos F, Tzoracoleftherakis E, Androulakis J (1991) Radical consequence in the sexuality of male patients operated for colorectal carcinoma. Eur J Surg Oncol 17:285–288
16. Lacy AM, Garcia-Valdecasas JC, Delgado S, Castells A, Taura P, Pique JM, Visa J (2002) Laparoscopy-assisted colectomy versus open colectomy for treatment of non-metastatic colon cancer: a randomised trial. Lancet 359:2224–2229
17. Leveckis J, Boucher NR, Parys BT, Reed MW, Shorthouse AJ, Anderson JB (1995) Bladder and erectile dysfunction before and after rectal surgery for cancer. Br J Urol 76:752–756
18. Lindsey I, Guy RJ, Warren BF, Mortensen NJ (2000) Anatomy of Denonvilliers' fascia and pelvic nerves, impotence, and implications for the colorectal surgeon. Br J Surg 87:1288–1299
19. Maas CP, Moriya Y, Steup WH, Kiebert GM, Kranenbarg WM, van de Velde CJ (1998) Radical and nerve-preserving surgery for rectal cancer in The Netherlands: a prospective study on morbidity and functional outcome. Br J Surg 85:92–97
20. Maurer CA, Renzulli P, Meyer JD, Buchler MW (1999) Rectal carcinoma. Optimizing therapy by partial or total mesorectum removal. Zentralbl Chir 124:428–435
21. Maurer CA, Z'Graggen K, Renzulli P, Schilling MK, Netzer P, Buchler MW (2001) Total mesorectal excision preserves male genital function compared with conventional rectal cancer surgery. Br J Surg 88:1501–1505
22. McCall JL (1997) Total mesorectal excision: evaluating the evidence. Aust N Z J Surg 67:599–602
23. Morino M, Parini U, Giraudo G, Salval M, Brachet Contul R, Garrone C (2003) Laparoscopic total mesorectal excision: a consecutive series of 100 patients. Ann Surg 237:335–342
24. Nagawa H, Muto T, Sunouchi K, Higuchi Y, Tsurita G, Watanabe T, Sawada T (2001) Randomized, controlled trial of lateral node dissection vs. nerve-preserving resection in patients with rectal cancer after preoperative radiotherapy. Dis Colon Rectum 44:1274–1280
25. Nesbakken A, Nygaard K, Bull-Njaa T, Carlsen E, Eri LM (2000) Bladder and sexual dysfunction after mesorectal excision for rectal cancer. Br J Surg 87:206–210
26. Parker SL, Tong T, Bolden S, Wingo PA (1997) Cancer statistics. CA Cancer J Clin. 47:5–27
27. Pocard M, Zinzindohoue F, Haab F, Caplin S, Parc R, Tiret E (2002) A prospective study of sexual and urinary function before and after total mesorectal excision with autonomic nerve preservation for rectal cancer. Surgery 131:368–372

28. Quah HM, Jayne DG, Eu KW, Seow-Choen F (2002) Bladder and sexual dysfunction following laparoscopically assisted and conventional open mesorectal resection for cancer. Br J Surg 89:1551–1556
29. Rullier E, Sa Cunha A, Couderc P, Rullier A, Gontier R, Saric J (2003) Laparoscopic intersphincteric resection with coloplasty and coloanal anastomosis for mid and low rectal cancer. Br J Surg 90:445–451
30. Saito N, Sarashina H, Nunomura M, Koda K, Takiguchi N, Nakajima N (1998) Clinical evaluation of nerve-sparing surgery combined with preoperative radiotherapy in advanced rectal cancer patients. Am J Surg 175:277–282
31. Taguchi K, Tsukamoto T, Murakami G (1999) Anatomical studies of the autonomic nervous system in the human pelvis by the whole-mount staining method: left-right communicating nerves between bilateral pelvic plexuses. J Urol 161:320–325
32. Winawer SJ, Fletcher RH, Miller L, Godlee F, Stolar MH, Mulrow CD, Woolf SH, Glick SN, Ganiats TG, Bond JH, Rosen L, Zapka JG, Olsen SJ, Giardiello FM, Sisk JE, Van Antwerp R, Brown-Davis C, Marciniak DA, Mayer RJ (1997) Colorectal cancer screening: clinical guidelines and rationale. Gastroenterology 112:594–642

Functional Results of the Colon J-Pouch Versus Transverse Coloplasty Pouch in Heidelberg

Alexis Ulrich, Kaspar Z'graggen, Jürgen Weitz, Markus W. Büchler

A. Ulrich (✉)
Department of General, Visceral and Trauma Surgery,
Ruprecht-Karls-University Heidelberg, Im Neuenheimer Feld 110,
69120 Heidelberg, Germany
e-mail: alexis.ulrich@med.uni-heidelberg.de

Abstract

Within the last 20 years various achievements have been made in the treatment of rectal cancer, improving survival and quality of life of rectal cancer patients. Especially the introduction of the total mesorectal excision (TME) and the use of modern staplers, making anastomoses possible in the deep pelvis, have increased our ability to cure more and more low rectal cancers by sphincter-preserving low anterior resections. Consequently, the interest in functional results after rectal reservoir reconstruction has increased significantly. Various randomized controlled trials have shown that the colon J-pouch (CJP) as a rectal reservoir reconstruction leads to better early functional results compared to the straight coloanal anastomosis (CAA). However, 30% of the patients with CJP faced late evacuation problems, requiring the chronic use of enemas or laxatives. This rate could be decreased to 10% by shortening the limb of the CJP from 8–10 cm to 5–6 cm. The transverse coloplasty pouch (TCP) was developed to provide early functional results comparable to the CJP, while avoiding these late evacuation problems. We report the early postoperative and functional results of 106 patients undergoing low anterior resections with TCP due to rectal cancer between October 2001 and the end of September 2003. Furthermore, we report on a single-center randomized controlled trial to compare the new TCP technique with the gold standard technique of CJP, which we started in October 2002. The objectives were to compare the two pouch reconstruction techniques in terms of morbidity, mortality and functional results.

Introduction

The significance of improving treatment modalities for patients with rectal cancer is highlighted by the high incidence of the disease (10–20/100,000 inhabitants), making it the fourth leading cancer in men and third leading cancer in women in Western countries. Approximately 300,000 new cases and 200,000 deaths occur in Europe and the USA combined, each year [1].

Recent Results in Cancer Research, Vol. 165

Within the last 20 years various achievements have been made in the treatment of rectal cancer, improving survival and quality of life of rectal cancer patients. The introduction of total mesorectal excision (TME) by Heald and its acceptance as the gold standard in rectal cancer surgery has to be recognized as the most significant contribution. Just by adopting the rules of TME, local recurrence rates can be reduced from 20%–50% down to 4%–10% [2, 3, 6].

The use of modern circular staplers, making anastomoses possible in the deep pelvis, as well as the widespread belief that 1–2 cm of safety distance to the distal border of the tumor are sufficient enough from an oncological point of view [2, 13, 22], have increased our ability to cure more and more low rectal cancers by sphincter-preserving low anterior resections [2]. Consequently, the interest in functional results after rectal reservoir reconstruction has increased significantly.

Colon J-Pouch

The straight coloanal anastomosis (CAA) had been the most commonly used technique until Lazorthes and Parcs described the colon J-pouch independently of each other in 1986 [15, 20]. Various randomized controlled trials have shown the superiority of the colon-J-pouch as a rectal reservoir reconstruction leading to better early functional results compared to the straight CAA [5, 10, 14, 23]. However, 30% of the patients with CJP faced late evacuation problems requiring the chronic use of enemas or laxatives [11, 18, 19]. This rate could be decreased by shortening the limb of the CJP from 8–10 cm to 5–6 cm, but the late evacuation problems remained in approximately 10% of the patients [7, 16]. Two years after the operation, no differences could be observed between CAA and CJP in terms of frequency, urge and incontinence [9].

Transverse Coloplasty Pouch

In 1999 a new technique for rectal reservoir reconstruction, the transverse coloplasty pouch (TCP), was introduced by Z'graggen and Büchler.

It was developed to provide early functional results comparable to the CJP, but avoiding the problems of late evacuation [25–29].

The technique is very simple, as an anti-mesenteric longitudinal colotomy is performed at the cut end of the descending colon. The incision should be 8 cm long, starting about 2 cm proximal to the rim of the anvil of the stapler. Stay sutures are placed 6 cm above the rim of the anvil lateral of both teniae, the pouch is then created by lateral traction of these sutures. Afterwards the colotomy is closed by transverse running sutures, starting from the pouch corners.

The importance and impact of this new technique in the surgical community is highlighted by the fact that, according to a Medline search, already 16 papers, including one randomized controlled trial, were published between 1999 and October 2003, with more to come.

CJP Versus TCP

The results of the first randomized controlled trial comparing the CJP with the TCP in terms of complications and functional results were published by Ho et al. in 2002 [10]. Forty-four patients received a CJP or TCP, respectively, after low anterior resection stemming from rectal cancer. Only minimal differences in the bowel function were observed 1 year after the operation between the two groups; however, significantly more anastomotic leaks were seen in the TCP group (15.9% vs. 0%, p=0,0121). Four of the seven patients with an anastomotic leak in the study from Singapore were asymptomatic, resulting in an symptomatic leakage rate of 6.7% [10]. The authors concluded that the CJP remains the benchmark of pouch reconstruction after low anterior resection.

Is this statement according to the currently available literature really undisputable?

TCP and Anastomotic Leakage

Z'graggen and Büchler reported in the first prospective phase I/II study, which included 41 patients with TCP after low anterior resection, an anastomotic leakage rate of 7.3% (3/41 patients) [27]. In a recently published study from Heidelberg, looking at the early postoperative results after 82 TCPs between October 2001 and May 2003, anastomotic leakages were seen in seven patients (8.5%). Two of the seven patients had only radiological leaks without clinical signs, as all patients received a protective loop ileostomy for at least 3 months [24]. Four months later (October 2003), the anastomotic leakage rate dropped to 7.5% (see Sect. 2.2).

In comparison, anastomotic leakage rates in a range of 0%–10% have been reported for the CJP. The leakage rates of the TCP in our own two series and of others fall within these limits [4, 5, 7, 9, 12, 17, 21]. Fürst et al. and Pimentel et al. came to the same conclusion when they published their preliminary results of a randomized controlled trial comparing CJP and TCP. No significant difference was observed between the two groups in terms of anastomotic leakages [4, 5, 21].

Early Postoperative Results After TCP

Between October 2001 and the end of September 2003, we performed 180 low anterior resections due to rectal cancer: 106 patients received a TCP. The patient data is shown in Table 1.

The median operation time was 260 min, the median blood loss was 600 ml with in median no transfusions (range, 0–12), the median hospital stay 12 days (range, 7–48). The postoperative results are shown in Table 2. Three patients died within the first 60 days (3%), one patient due to pulmonary embolism, the other two patients due to aspiration pneumonia.

Twenty-four patients (23%) developed surgical complications such as anastomotic leakage, bleeding, wound infection and voiding problems, five patients

Table 1. Patient data (01.10.2001–30.09.2003)

	TCP (n=106)	Range
Age (median, years)	60	39–89
Male:female	76:30	
Tumor above anal verge (cm)	7	3–12
Preoperative radiotherapy (5×5 Gy)[a]	30 (28%)	
Preoperative radiochemotherapy	22 (21%)	

[a]Since February 2002.

Table 2. Postoperative results

TCP (n=106)	n	%
Mortality (within 60 days)	3	3
Morbidity	29	27
Anastomotic leakage	8	7.5
Bleeding	2	2
Wound infection	8	7.5
Voiding problems	10	9
Cardiopulmonary complications	5	5
Reoperation	9	8

cardiopulmonary complications. Reoperations had to be performed in nine cases (8%) due to anastomotic leakages or bleeding (Table 2).

Functional Results after TCP

All studies published so far showed comparable early functional results for stool frequency, soiling, passing flatus, the ability to discriminate flatus from feces, need of antidiarrheal drugs, tenesmus and incomplete evacuation between the TCP and CJP reconstruction [10, 17, 21, 27].

To assess the bowel function after TCP, we sent a questionnaire to 106 patients. Seventy patients (66%) with a median follow-up of 11 months (range, 2–22) returned the completed questionnaire and stated a mean of three bowel movements per day (range, 1–10); 14% of these patients complained about incontinence for liquid stool, 28% about stool fragmentation, 41% could discriminate between flatus and feces. Overall, 76% of the patients were satisfied with their bowel function. The interpretation of these data is still difficult, as the follow-up of each patient was different and very often rather short. Bowel function 1 year after closure of the ileostomy will give more valid data.

CJP Versus TCP

To compare the new TCP technique with the gold standard technique of CJP, we started a single-center randomized controlled trial in October 2002. The objectives were to compare the two pouch reconstruction techniques in terms of morbidity, mortality and functional results. The sample size was calculated with 65 patients in each group.

As of October 2003, 59 patients were screened and 46 patients enrolled in the study. Twenty-two patients were randomized to the CJP, the other 24 patients to the TCP. The baseline characteristics of the patients are shown in Tables 3 and 4.

No significant differences were seen in terms of median age, gender ratio, preoperative treatment modalities, tumor stage and height of the tumor above the anal verge.

This data shows that the randomization worked. However, the small number of patients included so far and the short follow-up are not adequate for preliminary results at the moment.

Table 3. Baseline characteristics of the randomized controlled trial CJP vs. TCP

	CJP (*n*=22)	TCP (*n*=24)
Age (mean, range)	60 (46–76)	59 (39–78)
Male:female	15:7	16:8
Preop RT (5×5 Gy)	14	10
Preop RCT	4	2

RT, radiotherapy; RCT, radiochemotherapy.

Table 4. Baseline characteristics of the randomized controlled trial CJP vs. TCP

	CJP (*n*=22)	TCP (*n*=24)
UICC I	7	9
UICC II	8	6
UICC III	5	6
UICC IV	1	1
Adenoma	1	2
Tumor above anal verge (cm)	7	7

Conclusion

In conclusion, the TCP proved to be a safe method with low complication rates and anastomotic leakage rates within the limits of rates published for the CJP. The favorable early and late functional results, the technically easy and time-saving surgical procedure and the low morbidity and mortality rates make the TCP a good candidate for wide clinical application. Further randomized controlled trials are necessary to determine the indications for various pouch procedures in the future.

References

1. Boyle P (1998) Some recent developments in the epidemiology of colorectal cancer. In: Bleiberg H, Rougier P, Wilke HJ (eds) Management of colorectal cancer. Martin Dunitz London, pp 19–34
2. Bruch HP, Schwandner O, Farke S, Nolde J (2003) Pouch reconstruction in the pelvis. Langenbecks Arch Surg 388:60–75
3. Buchler MW, Heald RJ, Maurer CA, Ulrich B (1998) Rektumkarzinom: das Konzept der Totalen Mesorektalen Exzision. Karger, Basel
4. Furst A, Suttner S, Agha A, Beham A, Jauch KW (2003) Colonic J-pouch vs. coloplasty following resection of distal rectal cancer: early results of a prospective, randomized, pilot study. Dis Colon Rectum 46:1161–1166
5. Hallbook O, Pahlman L, Krog M, Wexner SD, Sjodahl R (1996) Randomized comparison of straight and colonic J pouch anastomosis after low anterior resection. Ann Surg 224:58–65
6. Heald RJ, Ryall RD (1986) Recurrence and survival after total mesorectal excision for rectal cancer. Lancet 1:1479–1482
7. Hida J, Yasutomi M, Fujimoto K, Okuno K, Ieda S, Machidera N, Kubo R, Shindo K, Koh K (1996) Functional outcome after low anterior resection with low anastomosis for rectal cancer using the colonic J-pouch. Prospective randomized study for determination of optimum pouch size. Dis Colon Rectum 39:986–991
8. Ho YH, Tan M, Seow-Choen F (1996) Prospective randomized controlled study of clinical function and anorectal physiology after low anterior resection: comparison of straight and colonic J pouch anastomoses. Br J Surg 83:978–980
9. Ho YH, Seow-Choen F, Tan M (2001) Colonic J-pouch function at six months versus straight coloanal anastomosis at two years: randomized controlled trial. World J Surg 25:876–881
10. Ho YH, Brown S, Heah SM, Tsang C, Seow-Choen F, Eu KW, Tang CL (2002) Comparison of J-pouch and coloplasty pouch for low rectal cancers: a randomized, controlled trial investigating functional results and comparative anastomotic leak rates. Ann Surg 236:49–55
11. Joo JS, Latulippe JF, Alabaz O, Weiss EG, Nogueras JJ, Wexner SD (1998) Long-term functional evaluation of straight coloanal anastomosis and colonic J-pouch: is the functional superiority of colonic J-pouch sustained? Dis Colon Rectum 41:740–746
12. Kanne V, Kim NH, Ulrich B (2002) [The transverse coloplasty pouch (TCP)—function and subjective judgement in comparison with the surgically more complicated J-Pouch]. Zentralbl Chir 127:781–785
13. Kapiteijn E, van de Velde CJ (2002) Developments and quality assurance in rectal cancer surgery. Eur J Cancer 38:919–936
14. Lazorthes F, Chiotasso P, Gamagami RA, Istvan G, Chevreau P (1997) Late clinical outcome in a randomized prospective comparison of colonic J pouch and straight coloanal anastomosis. Br J Surg 84:1449–1451
15. Lazorthes F, Fages P, Chiotasso P, Lemozy J, Bloom E (1986) Resection of the rectum with construction of a colonic reservoir and colo-anal anastomosis for carcinoma of the rectum. Br J Surg 73:136–138
16. Lazorthes F, Gamagami R, Chiotasso P, Istvan G, Muhammad S (1997) Prospective, randomized study comparing clinical results between small and large colonic J-pouch following coloanal anastomosis. Dis Colon Rectum 40:1409–1413
17. Mantyh CR, Hull TL, Fazio VW (2001) Coloplasty in low colorectal anastomosis: manometric and functional comparison with straight and colonic J-pouch anastomosis. Dis Colon Rectum 44:37–42
18. Mortensen NJ, Ramirez JM, Takeuchi N, Humphreys MM (1995) Colonic J pouch-anal anastomosis after rectal excision for carcinoma: functional outcome. Br J Surg 82:611–613
19. Nicholls RJ, Lubowski DZ, Donaldson DR (1988) Comparison of colonic reservoir and straight colo-anal reconstruction after rectal excision. Br J Surg 75:318–320

20. Parc R, Tiret E, Frileux P, Moszkowski E, Loygue J (1986) Resection and colo-anal anastomosis with colonic reservoir for rectal carcinoma. Br J Surg 73:139–141
21. Pimentel JM, Duarte A, Gregorio C, Souto P, Patricio J (2003) Transverse coloplasty pouch and colonic J-pouch for rectal cancer—a comparative study. Colorectal Dis 5:465–470
22. Ruo L, Guillem JG (1999) Major 20th-century advancements in the management of rectal cancer. Dis Colon Rectum 42:563–578
23. Seow-Choen F, Goh HS (1995) Prospective randomized trial comparing J colonic pouch-anal anastomosis and straight coloanal reconstruction. Br J Surg 82:608–610
24. Ulrich A, Z'graggen K, Schmied B, Weitz J, Buchler MW (2004) [The transverse coloplasty pouch after low anterior resection: early postoperative results]. Chirurg 75:430–435
25. Z'graggen K, Maurer CA, Buchler MW (1999) Transverse coloplasty pouch. A novel neorectal reservoir. Dig Surg 1999; 16:363–366
26. Z'graggen K, Maurer CA, Mettler D, Stoupis C, Wildi S, Buchler MW (1999) A novel colon pouch and its comparison with a straight coloanal and colon J-pouch—anal anastomosis: preliminary results in pigs. Surgery 125:105–112
27. Z'graggen K, Maurer CA, Birrer S, Giachino D, Kern B, Buchler MW (2001) A new surgical concept for rectal replacement after low anterior resection: the transverse coloplasty pouch. Ann Surg 234:780–785
28. Z'graggen K, Maurer CA, Buchler MW (2001) "Colonic coloplasty" equals "transverse coloplasty pouch made in Switzerland". Dis Colon Rectum 44:1222–1223
29. Z'graggen K, Maurer CA, Buchler MW (2001) [The transverse coloplasty pouch. Review of experimental data and clinical application]. Zentralbl Chir 126 [Suppl 1]:64–66

Indications for Neoadjuvant Long-Term Radiotherapy

Lars Påhlman

L. Påhlman (✉)
Department of Surgery, Colorectal Unit, University Hospital, 75185 Uppsala, Sweden
e-mail: lars.pahlman@surgsci.uu.se

Abstract

If radiotherapy is considered in the management of a rectal cancer, there is very strong evidence supporting preoperative settings. To avoid treatment to cases where surgery alone is enough, exact preoperative staging with MRI is crucial.

Introduction

The indication for radiotherapy in the treatment of rectal cancer can be divided into four main topics.

1. To lower local failure rates and improve survival in resectable rectal cancer
2. To allow surgery in non-resectable rectal cancer
3. To facilitate sphincter-preserving procedures in low lying rectal cancer
4. A totally curative procedure without major surgery

This short review will cover the first three options of using radiotherapy. The fourth one, curative treatment with radiotherapy alone, will not be covered at all.

Radiotherapy in Resectable Rectal Cancer

In the late 1970s it was obvious that a local recurrence in rectal cancer was a major problem for many patients. Most hospital-based series reported a recurrence rate around 30% and up to, in some centres, 50% [1]. This was thought to be a matter of tumour biology and aggressiveness of the tumour growth and therefore, in analogy with breast cancer, adjuvant radiotherapy was proposed. This treatment could be given either pre- or postoperatively. The drawbacks with preoperative radiotherapy was the lack of staging, and many patients had the treatment needlessly

Recent Results in Cancer Research, Vol. 165

due to an early stage of the disease or due to distant metastases. Therefore postoperative radiotherapy was considered in many countries. However, based upon tumour biology a better rational should be to use radiotherapy preoperatively given the way radiotherapy works. Radiotherapy needs well-oxygenated tissues, which are present in the preoperative setting [2]. Postoperatively the tissue is more fibrotic and therefore the effect might not be that good. Moreover, the time period from surgery to the start of radiotherapy will sometimes be long, giving a risk of repopulation of tumour cells [3].

During the last three decades 22 trials, including a total of 8,200 patients, have tried to evaluate the role of the use of radiotherapy by comparing surgery alone in one arm vs. radiotherapy given pre- or postoperatively in the experimental arm. Three well-written meta-analyses have been published within a 3-year period [4–6]. To summarise the data from all trials analysed in the three meta-analyses, radiotherapy decreases the local failure rates if standard surgery is performed and this reduction will improve survival. Moreover, there is a clear dose–response relationship with preoperative radiotherapy, indicating that a very low dose is ineffective [6]. The third very important message is the relative reduction in the local recurrence rate, which is numerically better if radiotherapy is given preoperatively compared to trials using postoperative radiotherapy. One trial, the Uppsala trial, actually compared pre- and postoperative radiotherapy and the result from this trial supports the view that preoperative radiotherapy reduces the local recurrence rate more effectively than postoperative radiotherapy and the survival figures are better after preoperative radiotherapy [7]. However, when radiotherapy is used postoperatively there are rather strong data supporting that radiotherapy should be combined with chemotherapy in order to improve not only the local recurrence rate but also survival [8–10]. However, there are very few trials and the data are not as solid from postoperative radiotherapy with chemotherapy as the data from preoperative radiotherapy, and only one trial testing preoperative radiotherapy, using radiotherapy alone, has shown a survival benefit [11].

An important question is the quality of surgery. Most trials involved in the three meta-analyses have used what could be considered standard surgery and this is probably not sufficient enough. Several reports from the mid 1980s came from centres claiming that the high local recurrence rate is not only a matter of tumour biology but also a problem of bad surgery [12–14]. Those centres advocated meticulous dissection in the lower pelvis taking into account the surrounding tissues. Mr. Heald from the UK has called this procedure total mesorectal excision (TME) and this has become the name for this more exact type of dissection called optimised surgery. These centres reporting very low local recurrence rates have even better results in terms of local recurrence rate than trials using standard surgery and radiotherapy. This has been claimed to be a matter of patient selection, but many modern studies do support the notion that surgery is important. With population-based studies from Norway and Sweden, it has been proven that radiotherapy might be superfluous in several patients [15–17].

In the midst of this discussion of good or suboptimal surgery in relation to adjuvant radiotherapy, a Dutch trial was conducted [18], in which a quality assurance programme was built in for surgeons trained to do a proper TME procedure.

Moreover, pathologists were trained to examine the specimen with special reference to the circumferential margin, and radiotherapy was delivered in a very strict and reproducible way. Several Swedish centres joined the Dutch group and the Dutch TME trial recruited 1,700 patients over a 3-year period. After a follow-up of a median of 3.5 years, data regarding the local recurrence rate have shown a 50% reduction from just above 10% down to 5%–6%. This reduction is of the same magnitude as has been seen in all other trials. No data on survival are available yet [18]. One could speculate if there ever will be a change in survival given the rather low frequency of local recurrences. In the trials where the old surgical technique was used, the local recurrence rate was so high (mean, >30%), the effect on outcome was more obvious, not only on local recurrences but also on survival because the reduction in local recurrences was quantitatively much larger [11].

In summary, we have learnt that in the management of resectable rectal cancer, the local recurrence rate after curative surgery with or without radiotherapy has more or less disappeared and should be below 3%. The overall local recurrence rate in any setting should not be above 10%. Based upon data from individual centres but also from nationwide register studies, it is possible to reach those figures [15,19]. We have also learnt that in standard surgery this reduction in local recurrences will slightly improve survival with approximately 10% [11]. However, there will be acute toxicity to radiotherapy with increased postoperative morbidity and mortality. Most of the morbidity can be explained with suboptimal radiotherapy [20]. An increased risk for a perineal wound infections after abdominal perineal excision is real, but there are no indication from randomised trials of an increase in anastomotic dehisces [20]. In the long-term follow-up, there is an increased risk of impaired bowel function. This has been seen for both preoperative [21] and postoperative radiotherapy [22].

There is still some concern about how to deliver radiotherapy and to whom we should give it. Radiotherapy has been given preoperatively with conventional fractionations, i.e. 45–50 Gy during a 4- to 5-week period followed by surgery after 1 month. Another technique is an accelerated fractionation system, which has been used in all Swedish trials, 5×5 Gy to a total dose of 25 Gy given over 1 week and with surgery immediately the week afterwards. It has been claimed not only short-term but also long-term toxicity is higher if the accelerated fractionation is used, the so-called short-course radiotherapy. However, the literature is rather biased because most data on late toxicity to radiotherapy in rectal cancer has been published from the Swedish trials where short-course radiotherapy has been used. Since it still is a concern whether this short-course treatment or the prolonged course is better in terms of toxicity, a three-armed prospective randomised trial is running in Sweden comparing 5×5 Gy over 1 week with immediate surgery vs. 5×5 Gy within a week and delayed surgery (6–7 weeks) vs. 25×2 Gy for 5 weeks and delayed surgery. This trial has not been finished and we are awaiting the results.

Another concern is whether or not chemotherapy should be included in the treatment schedule in patients with resectable rectal cancer. There are very few data on how to use this type of treatment, but in analogy with the experience with postoperative radiotherapy, it might be valuable [8–10]. There is only one randomised trial on preoperative radiotherapy where this specific question of the need for chemoradiotherapy in resectable rectal cancer is addressed. This is an EORTC trial, which has just been finished, where patients were randomised to have chemoradiotherapy vs. radiotherapy alone and after surgery there is a second randomisation, where patients are randomised to have chemotherapy or not. More than 1,000 patients have been included but no data are available from this trial.

Since all evidence-based data do support preoperative radiotherapy, it is crucial to know how to select patients for radiotherapy. We need a perfect preoperative local staging, which starts with an evaluation by the surgeons with a digital examination. If there is a very tiny superficial tumour endo-anal ultrasound is appropriate enough to distinguish whether or not the tumour is growing into the muscle layer (muscularis propria) [23]. If it turns out to be a T1 tumour one could consider local excision; if it is a T2 tumour, however, a more aggressive abdominal procedure is advocated. On the other hand, if the tumour is considered to be at least a T2 or even a tumour with a deeper penetration MRI is probably the staging method of choice [24–25]. This is because the rectal fascia can define on MRI and this is the area where the surgeon will dissect the tumour. Based upon MRI findings and the distance from the tumour to the rectal fascia, the circumferential resection margin can be evaluated, and a tumour could be classified according to the system proposed by the MERCURY group as good, bad or ugly (I. Daniels, personal communication). A good tumour indicates a tumour where there is a long distance to the circumferential resection margin (more than 1 cm) and many data support that there is no need for radiotherapy at all in this patient [26]. However, when the tumour is considered bad, indicating a tumour growing very close to the circumferential margin, there is strong evidence supporting that in this specific group of patients radiotherapy should be used [27]. Whether the treatment will be short- course (5×5 Gy) or long course (25×2 Gy) is probably optional. Although we have no firm data and conclusion require waiting for the results of the new Swedish trial, there are probably no differences in the local recurrence rate. There might be differences with toxicity. The major question is whether or not we need chemoradiotherapy in this specific group of patients, which be solved in trials. The third option is a tumour growing outside or into the perirectal fascia. Such a tumour, a very aggressive T3 or T4 tumour, indicates that the tumour has gone outside the normal resection area and by definition should be called a non-resectable rectal cancer. Although some of the T3 tumours could be resected in this setting, the surgeon's attitude should advocate preoperative radiotherapy and preferably chemoradiotherapy in these patients, according to a protocol of non-resectable rectal cancer (see below).

Non-resectable Rectal Cancer

A non-resectable rectal cancer is by definition a tumour that cannot be resected without a very high risk of a local recurrence, i.e. a tumour with involvement of the rectal fascia. Accordingly there is a high risk of having an involved circumferential resection margin. These are tumours which are tethered or fixed but it is difficult to know whether or not the fixity is due to cancer overgrowth or fibrosis. From the literature it is obvious that there is no uniform definition, but available data show that patients with such large tumours do benefit from preoperative radiotherapy with the aim to downsize the tumour. Approximately 10%–15% of all patients with a rectal cancer do have an advanced cancer, which could be considered non-resectable and half of those patients have no metastases, indicating that there is potential for a curative procedure [28]. Surgery alone is likely to cure very few and therefore these patients should be offered radiotherapy. The question is whether this should be combined with chemotherapy.

There is very little solid evidence for chemoradiotherapy based upon randomised trials. There is one old positive trial in gastrointestinal cancer published in 1969 [29]. There are two negative trials with increased toxicity published in the late 1980s [30–31]. One Swedish trial published in 2001 showed a benefit effect in terms of both the local recurrence rate and survival in patients having been randomised to chemoradiotherapy vs. radiotherapy alone followed by surgery [32]. This trial was very under-powered and new trials are necessary. However, several phase II trials have reported a good reduction in the local recurrence rate and these data are also very impressive in terms of survival [33–34]. However, the case-mix in those trials makes it difficult to interpret the results, and the definition of non-resectability differs enormously. Despite this, most radiotherapists and medical oncologists have more or less accepted the concept of using chemoradiotherapy in this specific group of non-resectable rectal cancer patients. However, the evidence-based data are very few and there is another Nordic trial, the LARCS trial, where patients were randomised to either 50 Gy preoperatively or 50 Gy and chemotherapy preoperatively. The trial has just been closed so no data are yet available. Despite a lack of good evidence-based data, the movement is strong and many patients will be offered chemoradiotherapy, and probably no more trials with a radiotherapy arm will be undertaken. One specific reason for this is the new drugs on the market [35].

Radiotherapy as a Tool to Increase Sphincter Preservation

It has been claimed from several series that preoperative radiotherapy and preferably chemoradiotherapy will downsize the tumour to the extent that it is possible to increase the number of patients where the sphincter can be preserved [36–37]. There are reports with complete response to chemoradiotherapy even in patients with T4 tumours; from this report some patients were not operated on and are alive and well [38]. However, in these phase II trials authors report the results and compare them with historical controls from their own unit. It is important to realise that the change in surgery and the philosophy for rectal cancer treatment has seen dramatic change during the last ten decades. We do accept a much more narrow margin distally and today a 5- to 10-mm margin is considered a curative procedure if a stapled anastomosis is done [39–40]. Therefore, randomised comparisons with patients treated with different options have to be conducted. There is a French trial from Lyon, the R9001 trial, where patients with T2 and T3 tumours had preoperative 39 Gy (13×3 Gy) and were randomised to immediate surgery or surgery 5 weeks after irradiation. In that trial the surgeons were asked before any treatment to evaluate the possibility of preserving the sphincter. There is a slight increase in numbers where the sphincter could be preserved if surgery was delayed [40]. However, in this trial the overall recurrence rate was 9%, which is considered a rather high figure today. But more important, among those patients where the surgeons had planned an abdominal perineal excision but changed it to a sphincter-preserving procedure as a result of the downsizing effect of radiotherapy, the local recurrence rate was 12% [40]. This is a rather small trial but the data indicate that there might be a downstaging effect and this downsizing might increase sphincter preservation.

The German trial (CAO/ARO/AIO-trial), where patients were randomised to pre- or postoperative chemoradiotherapy, has recently been closed. Preliminary data have shown a clear tendency to more favourable stage in patients having had preoperative treatment compared to postoperative chemoradiotherapy. In a subgroup analysis from this preliminary report there was an increase from 18% sphincter preservation in the postoperative chemoradiotherapy group compared to 35% in the preoperative irradiated group (Sauer and Rödel, personal communication). However, we do not have any data on survival and local recurrence rate from this trial.

Another very important trial is the Polish trial, where patients were randomised to short-course radiotherapy with immediate surgery vs. a long-course chemoradiotherapy and delayed surgery. The inclusion criteria in this trial was a tumour that could be reached by a digital examination but no sphincter infiltration. It had to be a T3 or a resectable T4 tumour and 1 cm microscopic distant margin was sufficient. The end-points in this trial included sphincter preservation and local recurrence rate. More than 300 patients were randomised and after closure of the trial the percentage of preserved sphincters were identical in both groups, 61% in the short-course radiotherapy with immediate surgery vs. 59% in the prolonged chemoradiotherapy course and delayed surgery [41]. This trial was conducted to see whether chemoradiotherapy and delayed surgery would have an impact on sphincter preservation. Accordingly this is not a subset analysis of the data from the trial, indicating the strength of the results. Therefore, there is still no good data supporting the notion that a prolonged course radiotherapy combined with chemotherapy with delayed surgery will have an impact on sphincter preservation. A very important drawback of having too many sphincters preserved is actually poor function. In some reports, up to 20% of all patients are incontinent for solid stools [36]. This cannot be a good quality of life! Moreover, there are data supporting that, as a group, patients with a stoma have a better quality of life compared to those with an anterior resection [42].

Conclusion

In summary, the main question is the choice of patients for preoperative radiotherapy. We know that radiotherapy has not only acute, but also late toxicity, with impaired bowel function among other side effects, and therefore we must select patients and avoid radiotherapy in as many as we can. Based upon proper preoperative staging using ultrasound and MRI, patients with a stage I disease could be revealed. This group should not have radiotherapy with, in my opinion, one exception, and that is a very low-stage cancer, where an abdominal perineal excision is the option. Given the difficulties of finding the correct planes in the perineal part of the procedure, it could be advisable to use radiotherapy. If there are indications in the preoperative imaging that is the cancer is a stage II or stage III tumour, i.e. at leased a T3 cancer, and MRI shows a very good margin to the circumferential resection area there is no real place for radiotherapy. However, in a T3 tumour with a compromised area, or those with T3 and N1 tumours, most data support radiotherapy, and if this is the case preoperative radiotherapy is best. For these patients either short-course treatment (5×5 Gy) or long-course radiotherapy up to 50 Gy is sufficient, but there are no good data supporting chemoradiotherapy. We know for sure that toxicity will increase if chemotherapy is added to radiotherapy. The third group of patients, those with a T4 tethered or fixed cancer, where the circumferential resection margin is compromised on the preoperative MRI examination, most data today support treating with preoperative chemoradiotherapy. The best chemotherapy technique has not yet not been defined, and trials should continue to explore this issue.

The only way to know whether or not one unit's treatment policy is correct is to have a perfect audit. In patients where a tumour has been resected with a curative resection, i.e. a local R0 resection, despite additional radiotherapy or not, the local recurrence rate should not exceed 3%. That is the guideline we should strive to reach. In T4 tumours where surgery is much more tricky and when there is more often R0–R2 resections, the local recurrence rate should still not exceed 10%.

References

1. Påhlman L, Glimelius B (1984) Local recurrences after surgical treatment for rectal carcinoma. Acta Chir Scand 150:331–335
2. Glimelius B, Isacsson U, Jung B, Påhlman L (1997) Radiotherapy in addition to radical surgery in rectal cancer—evidence for a dose-response effect favouring preoperative treatment. Int J Radiat Oncol Biol Phys 37:281–287
3. Withers HR, Taylor JMC, Maciejewski B (1988) The hazard of accelerated tumor clonogen repopulation during radiotherapy. Acta Oncol 27:131–146
4. Camma C, Giunta M, Fiorica F, Pagliaro L, Craxi A, Cottone M (2000) Preoperative radiotherapy for resectable rectal cancer: a meta-analysis. JAMA 284:1008–1015
5. Glimelius B, Grönberg H, Järhult J, Wallgren A, Cavallin-Ståhl E (2003) A systematic overview of radiation therapy in rectal cancer. Acta Oncologica 42; 476–492
6. Colorectal Cancer Collaborative Group (2001) Adjuvant radiotherapy for rectal cancer: a systematic overview of 8,507 patients from 22 randomised trials. Lancet 358:1291–1304
7. Påhlman L, Glimelius B (1990) Pre- or postoperative radiotherapy in rectal and rectosigmoid carcinoma—report from a randomized multicentre trial. Ann Surg 211:187–195
8. Krook JE, Moertel CG, Gunderson LL et al (1991) Effective surgical adjuvant therapy for high-risk rectal cancer. New Engl J Med 324:709–915
9. Gastrointestinal Tumor Study Group (1985) Prolongation of the disease-free interval in surgically treated rectal carcinoma. New Engl J Med 312:1464–1472
10. Tveit KM, Guldvog I, Hagen S et al (1997) Randomised controlled trial of postoperative radiotherapy and short-term time-scheduled 5-fluorouracil against surgery alone in the treatment of Dukes B and C rectal cancer. Br J Surg 84:1130–1135

11. Anonymous (1997) Improved survival with preoperative radiotherapy in resectable rectal cancer. Swedish Rectal Cancer Trial. New Eng J Med 336:980–987
12. Heald RJ, Karanjia ND. (1992) Results of radical surgery for rectal cancer. World J Surg 16:848–857
13. Enker WE (1992) Potency, cure, and local control in the operative treatment of rectal cancer. Arch Surg 127:1396–1401
14. Moriya Y, Hojo K, Sawada T, Koyama Y (1989) Significance of lateral node dissection for advanced rectal carcinoma at or below the peritoneal reflection. Dis Colon Rectum 32:307–315
15. Wibe A, Rendedal PR, Svensson E, Norstein J, Eide TJ, Myrvold HE, Soreide O (2002) Prognostic significance of the circumferential resection margin following total mesorectal excision for rectal cancer. Br J Surg 89:327–334
16. Dahlberg M, Glimelius B, Påhlman L (1999) Changing strategy for rectal cancer is associated with improved outcome. Br J Surg 86:379–384
17. Martling AL, Holm T et al (2000) Effect of a surgical training programme on the outcome of rectal cancer in the County of Stockholm. Lancet 356:93–96
18. Kapiteijn E, Marijnen CAM, Nagtegaal ID, Putter H, Steup WH, Wiggers T, Rutten HJT, Leer JWH, van Krieken JHJM, Påhlman L, Glimelius B, van de Velde CJH (2001) for the Dutch Colo Rectal Cancer Group and other cooperative investigators. Preoperative radiotherapy combined with total mesorectal excision for resectable rectal cancer. N Engl J Med 345:638–646
19. Swedish Rectal Cancer Register. http://www.SOS.se/mars/kvaflik.htm (Swe)
20. Påhlman L, Glimelius B (2002) Radiotherapy for rectal cancer: the European approach. In: Bleiberg H, Kemeny N, Rougier P, Wilke H-J (eds) Colorectal cancer: a clinical guide to therapy. Dunitz, London, pp 229–238
21. Dahlberg M, Glimelius B, Graf W, Påhlman L (1998) Preoperative irradiation for rectal cancer affects the functional results after colorectal anastomosis—results from the Swedish Rectal Cancer Trial. Dis Colon Rectum 41:543–551
22. Kollmorgen CF, Meagher AP, Pemberton JH et al (1994) The long-term effect of adjuvant postoperative chemoradiotherapy for rectal cancer on bowel function. Ann Surg 220:676–682
23. Akbari RP, Wong WD (2003) Endorectal ultrasound and the preoperative staging in rectal cancer. Scand J Surg 92:25–33
24. Brown G, Richards CJ, Newcombe RG et al (1999) Rectal carcinoma: thin-section MR imaging for staging in 28 patients. Radiology 211:215–222
25. Beets-Tan RGH, Beets GL, Vliegen RFA et al (2001) Accuracy of magnetic resonance imaging in prediction of tumour-free resection margin in rectal cancer surgery. Lancet 357:497–504
26. Adam IJ, Mohamdee MO, Martin IG et al (1994) Role of circumferential resection margin involvement in the local recurrence of rectal cancer. Lancet 344:707–711
27. Nagtegaal ID, van de Velde CJH, van der Worp E, Kapiteijn E, Phil Quirke J, van Krieken J, Han JM (2002) Macroscopic evaluation of rectal cancer resection specimen: clinical significance of the pathologist in quality control. J Clin Onc 20:1729–1734
28. Påhlman L, Enblad P, Glimelius B (1985) Clinical characteristics and their relation to surgical curability in adenocarcinoma of the rectum and recto-sigmoid: a population-based study in 279 consecutive patients. Acta Chir Scand 151:685–693
29. Moertel CG, Childs DS, Reitemeier RJ et al (1969) Combined 5-fluorouracil and supervoltage radiation therapy of locally unresectable gastrointestinal carcinoma. Lancet 2:865–867
30. Overgaard M, Berthelsen K, Dahlmark M, Gadeberg CG, van der Maase H, Overgaard J, Sell A (1989) A randomized trial of radiotherapy alone or combined with 5-FU in the treatment of locally advanced colorectal carcinoma (abstract). ECCO 5 meeting, 0-0626, Vienna
31. Wassif-Boulis S (1982) The role of preoperative adjuvant therapy in management of borderline operability of rectal cancer. Clin Radiol 33:353–358
32. Frykholm GJ, Pahlman L, Glimelius B (2001) Combined chemo and radiotherapy versus radiotherapy alone in the treatment of primary, non-resectable adenocarcinoma of the rectum. Int J Rad Onc Biol Phys 50:433–440
33. Janjan NA, Abbruzzese J, Pazdur R, Khoo VS, Cleary K, Dubrow R, Ajani J, Rich TA, Goswitz MS, Evetts PA, Allen PK, Lynch PM, Skibber JM (1999) Prognostic implications of response to preoperative infusional chemoradiation in locally advanced rectal cancer. Radiother Oncol 51:153–160

34. Bouzourene H, Bosman FT, Seelentag W, Matter M, Coucke P (2002) Importance of tumor regression assessment in predicting the outcome in patients with locally advanced rectal carcinoma who are treated with preoperative radiotherapy. Cancer 94:1121–1130
35. Glynne-Jones R, Sebag-Montefiore D (2002) Chemoradiation schedules—what radiotherapy? Eur J Cancer 38:258–569
36. Rouanet P, Saint-Aubert B, Lemanski C et. al (2002) Restorative and nonrestorative surgery for low rectal cancer after high-dose radiation. Dis Colon Rectum 45:305–315
37. Mohiuddin M, Regine WF, Marks GJ, Marks JW (1998) High dose preoperative radiation and the challenge of sphincter-preservation surgery for rectal cancer of the distal 2 cm of the rectum. Int J Radiat Oncol Biol Phys 40:569–574
38. Habr-Gama A, de Souza PM, Ribeiro U et al (1998) Low rectal cancer: impact of radiation and chemotherapy on surgical treatment. Dis Colon Rectum 41:1087–1096
39. Moore HG, Riedel E, Minsky BD et al (2003) Adequacy of 1 cm distal margin after restorative rectal cancer resection with sharp mesorectal excision and preoperative combined-modality therapy. Ann Surg Oncol 1:80–85
40. Karnjia ND, Schache DJ, Nort WR, Heald RJ (1990) 'Close shave' in anterior resection. Br J Surg 63:673–677
41. Francois Y, Nemoz CJ, Baulieux J et al (1999) Influence of the interval between preoperative radiation therapy and surgery on downstaging and on the rate of sphincter-sparing surgery for rectal cancer: the Lyon R90-01 randomized trial. J Clin Oncol 17:2396–2402
42. Bujko K, Nowacki MP, Bebenek M et al (2004) Sphincter preservation following preoperative radiotherapy for rectal cancer: report of a randomised trial comparing short-term radiotherapy versus conventionally fractionated radiochemotherapy. Radiation Oncol 72:15–24
43. Frigell A, Ottander M, Stenbeck H, Påhlman L (1990) Quality of life of patients treated with abdominoperineal resection or anterior resection for rectal carcinoma. Ann Chir Gynaecol 79:26–30

Neoadjuvant Radiotherapy and Radiochemotherapy for Rectal Cancer

Claus Rödel, Rolf Sauer

C. Rödel (✉)
Department of Radiation Therapy, University of Erlangen-Nürnberg,
Universitätsstr. 27, 91054 Erlangen, Germany
e-mail: claus.roedel@strahlen.med.uni-erlangen.de

Abstract

Combined radiochemotherapy is the recommended standard postoperative therapy for patients with stage II and III rectal cancer in the USA and in Germany. During the last decade, substantial progress has been made in treatment modalities: surgical management currently includes a broad spectrum of operative procedures ranging from radical operations such as abdominoperineal resections to innovative sphincter-preserving techniques. Specialized groups have reported excellent local control rates with total mesorectal excision (TME) alone without the addition of neoadjuvant or adjuvant treatment. New and improved radiation techniques using conformal radiotherapy as well as innovative chemotherapy schedules and combinations (capecitabine, oxaliplatin, irinotecan) of chemotherapy may have the potential to further increase the therapeutic benefit of (neo-)adjuvant treatment. Moreover, the basic issue of timing of radiotherapy—preoperative versus postoperative—within a multimodality regimen is currently being addressed in prospective trials. Evidently, the current monolithic approach established by studies conducted more than a decade ago, to either apply the same schedule of postoperative radiochemotherapy to all patients with UICC stage II and III rectal cancer or to give preoperative short-course radiation according to the Swedish concept for all patients with resectable rectal cancer irrespective of tumor stage and treatment goal (e.g., sphincter preservation), need to be questioned.

Introduction

Peri-operative radiotherapy with or without chemotherapy has been used widely in addition to surgery in an attempt to reduce local recurrence rates and to improve overall survival in rectal cancer. At least two conclusions can be drawn from randomized studies now available (Rödel and Sauer 2001). First, the combination of postoperative radiotherapy and 5-fluorouracil-based chemotherapy has

Recent Results in Cancer Research, Vol. 165

been shown to reduce local recurrence rates and to improve overall survival compared with (conventional) surgery alone or surgery plus postoperative radiotherapy alone. Second, irradiation seems to be more effective if given preoperatively compared with postoperatively.

The first conclusion prompted a National Cancer Institute Consensus Conference in the United States in 1990 and a German Cancer Society Consensus Conference in 1999 to recommend postoperative combined chemoradiation therapy for patients with UICC stage II and III rectal cancer as standard treatment (NIH 1990; Junginger et al. 1999). The second conclusion can be drawn from numerous studies conducted, especially in the northern countries of Europe: The Swedish Rectal Cancer Trial demonstrated reduced local recurrence rates and improved overall survival with a short-term preoperative 5×5 Gy regimen compared with conventional surgery alone (Swedish Rectal Cancer Trial 1997). The Dutch Colorectal Cancer Group has recently demonstrated that short-term preoperative radiotherapy significantly reduces the risk of local recurrences, even when surgery was optimized, and included total mesorectal excision (Kapiteijn et al. 2001). A recent meta-analysis also concluded that the combination of preoperative radiotherapy and surgery, as compared with surgery alone, significantly improved local control and overall survival (Camma et al. 2000). The only randomized trial by now that directly compared short-term preoperative to prolonged postoperative radiotherapy established the superiority of the preoperative approach for local control (Frykholm et al. 1993).

Adjuvant and Neoadjuvant Radiation Therapy: Pros and Cons

Among the potential advantages of the preoperative approach are downstaging and downsizing effects that possibly enhance curative (R0) surgery in locally advanced, e.g., T4-rectal cancer, and sphincter preservation in low-lying rectal cancer. Moreover, neoadjuvant therapy may be advantageous also in resectable rectal cancer as sterilization of the tumor cells prior to surgery may reduce the risk of tumor cell spillage during surgery. The small bowel in an unviolated abdomen will be mobile and less likely to be within a pelvic radiation portal; the irradiated volume does not require coverage of the perineum, as in the cases after abdominoperineal resection, and there is no irradiation of the anastomotic region. Thus, preoperative irradiation may cause less acute and late toxicity, and more patients will receive full-dose radiation therapy. In addition, a certain dose of irradiation seems to be more effective if given preoperatively compared with postoperatively, most probably because oxygen tension within the tumor may be higher prior to surgical compromise of the regional blood flow. This may improve the radiosensitivity of the tumor by decreasing the more radioresistent hypoxic fraction.

A major concern regarding preoperative radiation therapy is that patients with early-stage tumors or disseminated disease will often receive unnecessary treatment, necessitating improved imaging techniques that allow more accurate staging and selection of patients. Moreover, neoadjuvant combined modality treatment usually postpones definitive surgery considerably and may also be associated with increased postoperative morbidity.

Technically, there are two approaches to preoperative radiation therapy. The first one is an intensive short-course radiation with large fractions, e.g., 5×5 Gy, for 1 week followed by immediate surgery. The second includes 5–6 weeks of conventional fractionation (1.8–2.0 Gy), possibly combined with concurrent chemotherapy, and surgery 4–6 weeks later.

Preoperative Short-Course Radiation Therapy

In an attempt to improve results in "resectable" rectal cancer, a number of studies with various preoperative fractionation schedules, mainly intensive, short courses of radiation, were carried out in the 1970s and 1980s. In summary, while a significant decrease in local failure was shown at least in studies with higher doses, e.g., 25 Gy in five fractions, either no significant improvement in survival was observed or the benefit was restricted to subgroups.

The Swedish Rectal Cancer Trial, conducted between 1987 and 1990, was the first randomized trial to show a survival advantage for the total patient group according to an intention-to-treat analysis (Swedish Rectal Cancer Trial 1997). One thousand one hundred sixty-eight patients with resectable rectal cancer (T1–3) were randomized to one of the two treatment arms: surgery alone or 25 Gy in five fractions followed by surgery within 1 week. The addition of preoperative radiation significantly decreased the rate of local failure from 27% to 12% ($p<0.001$) and improved 5-year survival from 48% to 58% ($p=0.004$). This benefit was seen in all stages. Thus, the results of this large study with a clear and simple design once again supported the oncological paradigm that survival is improved by better local control. Because of short overall treatment time, early operation, low costs and patient convenience, the concept of a 1-week preoperative radiation therapy has been adopted in many institutions in resectable rectal cancer.

The most recent trial to report results of the preoperative short-course radiotherapy regimen was the Dutch CKVO 95–04 trial which randomized 1,805 patients with clinically resectable disease (T1–3) to optimized surgery with total mesorectal excision (TME) alone or to a regimen of 5×5 Gy applied immediately prior to TME surgery (Kapiteijn et al. 2001). Although overall local recurrence rates were low after 2 years of median follow-up in the TME-alone arm (8.2%), preoperative radiation therapy further significantly decreased local recurrences to 2.4% ($p<0.001$). With longer follow-up, 5-year local failure was higher with TME (12%) but was still significantly decreased to 6% with preoperative irradiation (Van de Velde 2002). Until now, this gain in local control did not translate to an overall survival benefit (82% in both arms after 2 years).

In subgroup analysis of this study, it became evident that preoperative radiotherapy mainly reduced the risk of local recurrence in patients who had tumors with an inferior margin less than or equal to 5 cm ($p=0.05$) or 5.1–10 cm ($p<0.001$) from the anal verge, whereas the addition of radiotherapy had no significant effect on tumors in the upper part of the rectum (10.1–15 cm, $p=0.17$). Likewise, the benefit of preoperative radiotherapy was restricted to TNM stage II and III tumors, an effect that was not observed for TNM stage I and IV tumors.

This trial also once again demonstrated that no significant downstaging occurs after short-term preoperative radiotherapy, with only a modest reduction in the mean diameter of irradiated tumors compared with nonirradiated tumors (4.0 cm for irradiated tumors to 4.5 cm for nonirradiated tumors; $p<0.001$) (Marijnen et al. 2001). Thus, in this trial no attempt was made to select patients with low-lying tumors for a sphincter-sparing procedure and the rate of APR was equal in both randomization arms (28% for RT+TME and 27% for TME alone) Moreover, radiotherapy did not influence the number of positive resection margins, both circumferential and distal. Positive circumferential resection margins (CRM+) were present in 16% of patients treated with radiotherapy, compared with 19% in the TME only group ($p=0.82$), suggesting that short-term preoperative irradiation is not able to downsize or sterilize tumors extending through the bowel wall and spreading very close to the mesorectal fascia in a way that leaves no positive margins after total mesorectal excision (Marijnen et al. 2003). With modern MRI technology, these patients at risk for CRM+ can be identified (Beets-Tan et al. 2001) and should, in our opinion, be selected for more intense preoperative radiochemotherapy schedules.

Preoperative Radiotherapy and Radiochemotherapy in T4 Rectal Cancer

Several institutions have applied preoperative radiation in conventional fractionation in the treatment of locally advanced or even fixed (T4) rectal lesions (Chan et al. 1993; Marsh et al. 1996; Videtic et al. 1998). The goal is to convert (downsize) a tumor, which is clinically not amenable to curative resection at presentation, to a resectable status. Minsky et al. (1992) compared preoperative radiotherapy (50.4 Gy) with or without 5-FU high-dose folinic acid and showed that 90% of the patients with initially unresectable tumors were converted to resectable lesions by preoperative combined therapy, as compared with only 64% of those who received radiation therapy alone. Moreover, a complete pathologic response was found in 20% of patients receiving combined modality therapy as compared to 6% receiving radiotherapy alone, indicating an enhancement of radiation-induced downstaging by concomitant 5-FU-based chemotherapy.

Several phase II trials of preoperative radiochemotherapy, including our own study at the University of Erlangen (Rödel et al. 2000), confirmed overall and complete resectability rates between 79% and 100% and 62% and 94%, respectively, and overall-survival rates in the range of 69% at 3 years and 51% at 5 years. In a recent randomized phase III study comparing combined radiochemotherapy with radiotherapy alone in primarily unresectable rectal cancer, Frykholm et al. (2001) demonstrated that the addition of chemotherapy to radiotherapy significantly improved local control rates, although no significant difference in survival was found between the groups. Thus, there is now compelling evidence that in locally advanced T4-rectal cancer, conventionally fractionated radiotherapy combined with chemotherapy should be applied, although there is still little evidence-based data

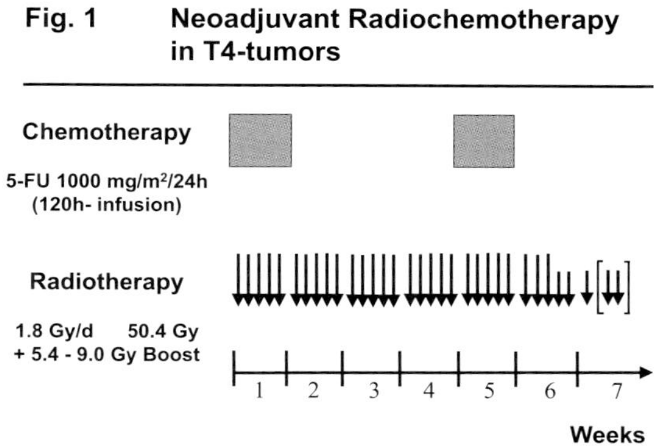

Figure 1. Erlangen radiochemotherapy regimen for locally advanced T4 rectal cancer not amenable to radical (R0) surgery at presentation

with regard to the optimal doses of radiation and chemotherapy as well as the type of 5-FU administration and combination with other cytotoxic agents. Figure 1 shows the Erlangen treatment regimen in T4-rectal cancer. Note that the interval between completion of radiotherapy and surgery should be at least 4 weeks to allow for tumor shrinkage.

In a subset of patients, even more aggressive attempts to achieve local tumor control, including preoperative radio-chemo-thermo-therapy (Rau et al. 1998) or intraoperative radiation boost techniques (Mannerts 2000) may be indicated. Moreover, as there is a substantial risk of systemic tumor cell dissemination in these locally advanced tumors, more effective chemotherapy schedules are urgently needed. A phase I II study at the University of Erlangen, using a combination of oxaliplatin and capecitabine together with preoperative radiotherapy in locally advanced rectal cancer (Fig. 2) has already proven the feasibility of such a regimen

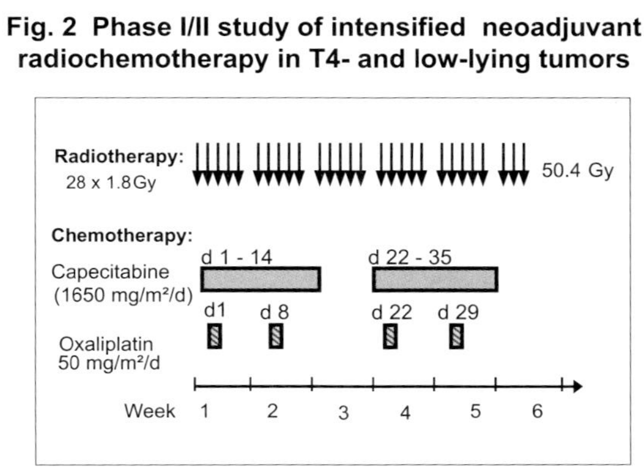

Figure 2. Preoperative conventionally fractionated radiotherapy with intensified chemotherapy using capecitabine and oxaliplatin. Schedule of a phase I II study at the University of Erlangen in locally advanced or low-lying rectal cancer patients. (Rödel et al. 2003)

(Rödel et al. 2003). Preliminary data suggest a high percentage of pathologically confirmed complete remissions (19%); however, longer follow-up is necessary to draw any firm conclusion with respect to the systemic efficacy of such an intensified chemotherapy schedule.

Preoperative Radiochemotherapy in Low-Lying Tumors with Intended Sphincter Preservation

Another major goal of neoadjuvant therapy is the conversion of a low-lying tumor, i.e., a tumor located in close proximity to the dentate line, that was declared by the surgeon to require an abdominoperineal resection (APR), into a lesion amenable to sphincter-preserving procedures. Technically, two surgical approaches have been used after preoperative therapy: local excision and a low anterior (intersphincteric) resection with coloanal anastomosis. While the first technique should be restricted to patients with clinical stage T1 lesions with favorable histopathologic features (G1–2, no evidence of lymph vascular invasion), the second approach has the advantage of allowing a more complete resection of the tumor and the perirectal soft tissue. It must be emphasized, however, that equivalent local control and survival rates compared to conventional APR as well as the quality of long-term rectal function is of the utmost importance in this setting.

Minsky reviewed seven series that have reported on patients with clinically resectable rectal cancer who underwent a prospective clinical assessment by their surgeons and were declared to need an APR (Minsky 2002). All have applied conventional doses of radiation therapy, four used concurrent chemotherapy (François et al. 1999; Grann et al. 1997; Hyams et al. 1997; Maghfoor et al. 1997; Rouanet et al. 1995; Valentini et al. 1998; Wagman et al. 1998). A sphincter-sparing approach, mostly low-anterior resection with coloanal anastomosis, was accomplished in 23%–85% of patients, local control ranged from 83% to 100% and sphincter function was declared to be "perfect" (71%) or "good to excellent" (85%) in two studies. However, these preliminary data need to be interpreted with caution. In a French trial of preoperative radiation in low-lying rectal cancer, the overall recurrence rate was 9%, but increased to 12% in those patients in whom sphincter preservation seemed impossible at presentation, but who had an anterior resection following preoperative downsizing of their tumor (François et al. 1999). Further studies are urgently needed to adequately select patients for the respective treatment alternatives.

Preoperative Radiochemotherapy in Resectable Rectal Cancer

The interest in preoperative radiochemotherapy for resectable tumors of the rectum is based not only on the success of the combined modality approach in the postoperative setting, but also on the many aforementioned advantages of delivering radiation treatment preoperatively. Until recently, the only randomized trial that directly compared preoperative to postoperative radiation therapy in rectal cancer has been the Uppsala trial, which was carried out between 1980 and 1985 in Sweden. In the preoperative arm, patients received intensive short-course radiation (five fractions of 5.1 Gy to a total dose of 25.5 Gy in 1 week); postoperatively conventional radiation therapy (2 Gy to a total of 60 Gy with a 2-week split after 40 Gy) was applied. Preoperative radiation significantly decreased the local failure rate (13% vs. 22%; p=0.02); however, there was no significant difference in 5-year survival rates (42% vs. 38%) (Frykholm et al. 1993).

Prospective randomized trials comparing the efficacy of preoperative radiochemotherapy to standard postoperative radiochemotherapy in UICC stage II and III rectal cancer were initiated both in the United States through the Radiation Therapy Oncology Group (RTOG 94–01) and the NSABP (R-03) as well as in Germany (Protocol CAO ARO AIO-94). Unfortunately, both US trials suffered from lack of accrual and have already been closed. A preliminary report of the NSABP R-03 trial (with a median follow-up of only 1 year) revealed that the percentage of patients who underwent sphincter-sparing surgery and were without evidence of disease was higher in the preoperative versus the postoperative arm (44% vs. 34%) (Roh et al. 2001)

The accrual of the German multicenter study has been going well with more than 820 patients included until September 2002. The design and treatment schedule is depicted in Fig. 3. As it has become increasingly clear in recent years that the surgeon himself is an important prognostic factor in controlling the local tumor, techniques of surgery were strictly standardized in this German trial and include total mesorectal excision for tumors of the lower and middle part of the rectum. In addition, stratification according to the individual surgeon has been provided for in order to help remove surgical bias. Moreover, prerandomization assessment of the intended surgical procedure (sphincter preservation possible or not) was included to evaluate the efficacy of preoperative radiochemotherapy to enable

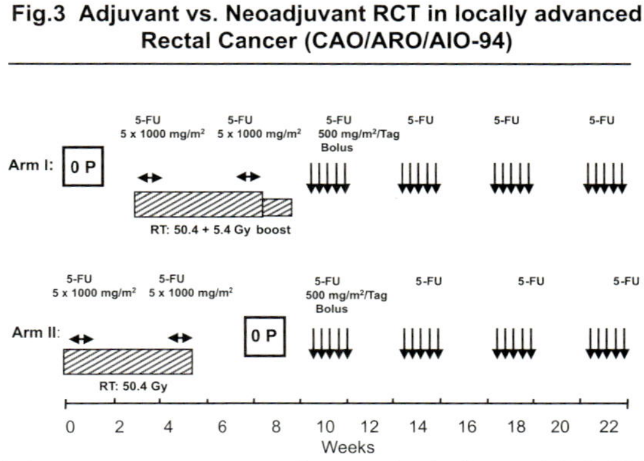

Figure 3. Design of the two-arm German Rectal Cancer Study (Protocol CAO ARO AIO 94) comparing preoperative with postoperative radiochemotherapy in locally advanced rectal cancer (UICC stage II III). (Sauer et al. 2003)

sphincter-sparing surgical procedures in low-lying tumors. Endpoints included local and distant control, 5-year overall and relapse-free survival, rate of curative (R0) resections and sphincter-saving procedures, toxicity of radiochemotherapy and surgical complications due to treatment mode.

Preliminary results were recently reported (Sauer et al. 2003): Compared with standard postoperative radiochemotherapy, preoperative combined modality therapy had a significant decrease in local failure (6% vs. 12%; $p=0.006$), acute toxicity (28% vs. 40%; $p=0.005$), chronic toxicity (10% vs. 23%; $p=0.04$), and in those 194 patients judged by the surgeon to require an APR, a significant increase in sphincter preservation (39% vs. 20%; $p=0.004$). With a median follow-up of 40 months, there was no difference in 5-year survival (74%).

The concurrent use of chemotherapy as part of the preoperative regimen is another important point, as it is not clear by now whether data from postoperative radiochemotherapy in resectable rectal cancer can be translated to the preoperative setting. The European Organization for Research and Treatment of Cancer (EORTC study 22921) has conducted a four-arm trial that treats all patients with preoperative radiation in conventional fractionation and tests whether preoperative concurrent radiochemotherapy, postoperative chemotherapy, or both are superior to preoperative radiation alone. Results of this trial are pending.

Conclusions and Future Perspectives

Is there a standard (neo-)adjuvant treatment of rectal cancer? The pros and cons have extensively been discussed in recent controversies. According to Consensus Conference recommendations in the USA and Germany, postoperative radiochemotherapy has been—until now—the treatment of choice in stage II and III resectable rectal cancer. Conversely, short-term preoperative radiotherapy has been widely adopted, especially in the northern countries of Europe.

New data have been collected and progress has been made both in surgery and perioperative radio-(chemo)therapy. Better knowledge of distal microscopic lymphatic spread within the mesorectum has led to the use of total mesorectal excision for mid and low rectal cancer. With this optimized surgery, local control rates have been markedly increased and local failure rates above 15%–20% are now no longer acceptable (Enker 1997). Technical advances in radiotherapy, including tumor- and radiobiologically optimized fractionation, 3D treatment planning and intensity-modulated radiation therapy will further allow application of more sophisticated treatment volume to reduce irradiation of normal tissue and increase the therapeutic index. Moreover, innovative ways of administration of chemotherapeutic agents such as continuous and chronomodulated infusion of 5-FU, as well as the emerging role of additional agents, e.g., capecitabine, oxaliplatin or irinotecan, need to be incorporated in multimodality regimens.

Evidently, the current monolithic approaches, established by studies more than a decade ago, to either apply the same schedule of postoperative radiochemotherapy to all patients with stage II III rectal cancer or to give preoperative intensive short-course radiation according to the Swedish concept for all patients with resectable rectal cancer irrespective of tumor stage and treatment goal (e.g., sphincter preservation) need to be questioned. The inclusion of different multimodal treatments in the surgical oncological concept, adapted to the tumor location and stage and to individual patient's risk factors is mandatory (Gunderson et al. 2002). Clearly, future developments will aim at identifying and selecting patients for the ideal treatment alternatives. Thus, clinicopathological (Nagtegaal and van Kriegen 2002) and molecular features as well as accurate preoperative imaging and staging methods (endorectal ultrasonography, magnetic resonance imaging) will take an important and integrative part in multimodality treatment of rectal cancer.

References

Beets-Tan RGH, Beets GL, Vliegen RFA et al (2001) Accuracy of magnetic resonance imaging in prediction of tumor-free resection margins in rectal cancer surgery. Lancet 357:497–504

Camma C, Giunta M, Fiorica F et al (2000) Preoperative radiotherapy for resectable rectal cancer. A meta-analysis. JAMA 248:1008–1015

Chan A, Wong A, Langevin J et al (1993) Preoperative concurrent 5-fluorouracil infusion, mitomycin C and pelvic radiation therapy in tethered and fixed rectal carcinoma. Int J Radiat Oncol Biol Phys 25:791–799

Enker WE (1997) Total mesorectal excision—the new golden standard of surgery for rectal cancer Ann Med 29:127–133

François Y, Nemoz CJ, Baulieux J et al (1999) Influence of the interval between preoperative radiation therapy and surgery on downstaging and the rate of sphincter-sparing surgery for rectal cancer: the Lyon R90-01 randomized trial. J Clin Oncol 17:2396–2402

Frykholm GJ, Glimelius B, Pahlman L (1993) Preoperative or postoperative irradiation in adenocarcinoma of the rectum: final treatment results of a randomized trial and an evaluation of late secondary effects. Dis Colon Rectum 36:564–572

Frykholm GJ, Pahlman L, Glimelius B (2001) Combined chemo-and radiotherapy vs. radiotherapy alone in the treatment of primary, nonresectable adenocarcinoma of the rectum. Int J Radiat Oncol Biol Phys 50:427–434

Grann A, Minsky BD, Cohen AM et al (1997) Preliminary results of preoperative 5-fluorouracil (5-FU),low dose leucovorin, and concurrent radiation therapy for resectable T3 rectal cancer. Dis Colon Rectum 40:515–522

Gunderson LL, Sargent DJ, Tepper JE et al (2002) Impact of T and N substages on survival and disease relapse in adjuvant rectal cancer: a pooled analysis. Int J Radiat Oncol Biol Phys 54:386-396

Hyams DM, Mamounas EP, Petrelli N et al (1997) A clinical trial to evaluate the worth of preoperative multimodality therapy in patients with operable carcinoma of the rectum: a progress report of NSABP R-03. Dis Colon Rectum 40:131–139

Junginger T, Hossfeld DK, Sauer R, Hermanek P (1999): Adjuvante Therapie bei Kolon- und Rektumkarzinom. Dt Ärztebl 96:698–700

Kapiteijn E, Marijnen CAM, Nagtegaal ID et al (2001) Preoperative radiotherapy combined with total mesorectal excision for resectable rectal cancer. N Engl J Med 345:638–648

Maghfoor I, Wilkes J, Kuvshinoff B et al (1997) Neoadjuvant chemoradiotherapy with sphincter-sparing surgery for low lying rectal cancer (abstract). Proc Am Soc Clin Oncol 1997;16:274

Mannerts GH, Martijn H, Crommelin MA et al (2000) Feasibility and first results of multimodality treatment, combining EBRT, extensive surgery, and IORT in locally advanced primary rectal cancer. Int J Radiat Oncol Biol Phys 47:425–433

Marijnen CAM, Nagtegaal ID, Klein Kranenbarg E et al (2001) No downstaging after short-term preoperative radiotherapy in rectal cancer patients. J Clin Oncol 19:1976–1984

Marijnen CAM, Nagtegaal ID, Kapiteijn E et al (2003) Radiotherapy does not compensate for positive resection margins in rectal cancer patients: report of a multicenter randomized trial. Int J Radiat Oncol Biol Phys 55:1311–1320

Marsh RD, Chu NM, Vauthey JN et al (1996) Preoperative treatment of patients with locally advanced unresectable rectal adenocarcinoma utilizing continuous chronobiologically shaped 5-fluorouracil infusion and radiation therapy. Cancer 78:217–225

Minsky BD (2002). Cancer of the colon, rectum and anus. ASTRO-refresher course 2002, Course Nr. 211

Minsky BD, Cohen AM, Kemeny N et al (1992) Enhancement of radiation induced downstaging of rectal cancer by fluorouracil and high-dose leucovorin chemotherapy. J Clin Oncol 10:79–84

Nagtegaal ID, van Kriegen JHJM (2002). The role of pathologists in the quality control of diagnosis and treatment of rectal cancer—an overview. Eur J Cancer 38:964–972

NIH Consensus Conference (1990) Adjuvant therapy for patients with colon and rectal cancer. JAMA 264:1444–1450

Rau B, Wust P, Gellermann J et al (1998) Preoperative radio-chemo-thermo-therapy in locally advanced rectal cancer. Strahlenther Onkol 174:556–565

Rödel C, Sauer R (2001) Perioperative radiotherapy and concurrent radiochemotherapy in rectal cancer. Semin Surg Oncol 20:3–12

Rödel C, Grabenbauer GG, Schick CH et al (2000) Preoperative radiation with concurrent 5-fluorouracil for locally advanced T4-primary rectal cancer. Strahlenther Onkol 176:161–167

Rödel C, Grabenbauer GG, Papadopoulos T et al (2003) Phase I II trial of capecitabine, oxaliplatin, and radiation for rectal cancer. J Clin Oncol 21:3098–3104

Roh MS, Petrelli N, Colangelo L et al (2001) Phase III randomized trial of preoperative versus postoperative multimodality therapy in patients with carcinoma of the rectum (NSABP R-03) (abstract). Proc Am Soc Clin Oncol 20:123a

Rouanet P, Fabre JM, Dubois JB (1995) Conservative surgery for low rectal carcinoma after high-dose radiation. Ann Surg 221:67–73

Sauer R for the German Rectal Cancer Study Group (2003) Adjuvant versus neoadjuvant combined modality treatment for locally advanced rectal cancer: first results of the German rectal cancer study (abstract 2). Int J Radiat Oncol Biol Phys 57:124

Swedish Rectal Cancer Trial (1997) Improved survival with preoperative radiotherapy in resectable rectal cancer. New Engl J Med 336:980–987

Valentini V, Coco C, Cellini N et al (1998) Preoperative chemoradiation for extraperitoneal T3 rectal cancer: acute toxicity, tumor response, and sphincter preservation. Int J Radiat Oncol Biol Phys 40:1067–1072

Van de Velde CJH (2002). Preoperative radiotherapy and TME-surgery for rectal cancer: detailed analysis in relation to quality control in a randomized trial (abstract). Proc Am Soc Clin Oncol 21:127a

Videtic GM, Fisher BJ, Perera FE et al (1998) Preoperative radiation with concurrent 5-fluorouracil continuous infusion for locally advanced unresectable rectal cancer. Int J Radiat Oncol Biol Phys 42:319–324

Wagman R, Minsky BD, Cohen AM et al (1998) Sphincter preservation with preoperative radiation therapy and coloanal anastomosis: long tern follow-up. Int J Radiat Oncol Biol Phys 42:51–57

Adjuvant Radiochemotherapy for Rectal Cancer

Martina Treiber, R. Krempien, H. P. Knaebel, J. Debus

M. Treiber (✉)
Department of Radiotherapy, University of Heidelberg, INF 400,
69120 Heidelberg, Germany
e-mail: martina_treiber@med.uni-heidelberg.de

Introduction

One of the basic questions for radiation oncologists is what we hope to achieve from treatments that are adjuvant to surgery. Can we achieve a better local control? Is there a decrease in metastatic disease? Can we see an effect on overall survival? Although some questions remain to be answered, some general recommendations for the treatment of rectal cancer can be given. Since the NIH recommendations in 1990, the majority of patients with rectal cancer are treated by a multimodality approach. Today surgery with total mesorectal excision (TME) is the standard therapy for cancers of the middle and low rectum in stages T1/2 N0. Radiochemotherapy (adjuvant or neoadjuvant) and short-term preoperative radiotherapy are both feasible approaches for the treatment of stage II and stage III rectal carcinomas. The superiority of any of these concepts is awaited clarifying by randomized trials. Patients with locally advanced rectal cancers (T4) should undergo long-term neoadjuvant radiochemotherapy with consecutive oncological resection.

Preoperative Versus Postoperative Radiotherapy or Radiochemotherapy

When both surgery and radiation are indicated in an adjuvant setting, different opinions exist regarding the preferred sequence of each modality. Potential advantages of preoperative irradiation and in long-term courses in combination with chemotherapy include the damaging effect on cells that may be spread locally or distantly at the time of resection and the downstaging of lesions in an attempt to improve the rate of sphincter preservation. The major advantage of postoperative radiotherapy or radiochemotherapy is that the staging is clear and there will be no over- or undertreatment. In this case, patients are treated with a high risk for local recurrence on the basis of pathological findings.

Recent Results in Cancer Research, Vol. 165

Preoperative Radiotherapy and Radiochemotherapy

Low-dose preoperative irradiation (less than 20 Gy in daily fractions from 1.8 to 2 Gy) showed no significant impact on either local or distant tumor control or survival. As best shown by the Medical Research Council trial (MRC) [15], which compared surgery alone with a preoperative irradiation with a total dose of 5 Gy in one fraction and 20 Gy in ten fractions. Although moderate-dose preoperative irradiation has shown improved local control in a randomized phase III European trial [5], improved survival was shown only in a subset analysis [10]. In both series, the dose delivered was 34.5 Gy (15 fractions, single dose 2.3 Gy, treatment time 19 days), which is equivalent to approximately 44 Gy in standard fractionation.

The Swedish phase III randomized trial showed that a significant improvement in local control could translate into improved survival as well [18]. The study randomized patients to surgery alone as a control arm (n=557), or to short-course high-dose preoperative irradiation with 25 Gy in five fractions (equivalent 45–50 Gy in 2-Gy single doses) followed by resection within 1 week (n=553). After a follow-up of 5 years, the rate of local relapse was 27% with surgery alone versus 11% with preoperative irradiation ($p<0.001$). The 5-year overall survival was 48% versus 58% ($p=0.004$), respectively. There was no impact on developing distant metastases with rates at 24% versus 23%.

Another Swedish randomized phase III trial [3] compared neoadjuvant, high-dose preoperative irradiation (25 Gy, five fractions, 1 week) to adjuvant postoperative irradiation (60 Gy, 30 fractions, 8 weeks, a split course with a break of 2 weeks). In the group of preoperative irradiated patients, the local relapse was less than in the postoperative group (13% vs. 22%, $p=0.02$). There was no significant difference in survival or distant metastasis rates.

A clear dose–response relationship in the relative reduction in local failure rates was observed in trials using 4×5 Gy [2] or 5×5 Gy [6]. In the Imperial Cancer Research Fund Trial [6] using 3×5 Gy, the effect on the recurrence rate was found to be of less magnitude than the other four trials. A recent meta-analysis showed a highly significant effect on the risk of local recurrence for patients with surgery alone compared to the radiotherapy-plus-surgery group [1]. From the Dutch multicenter study (randomized trial with 1,861 patients) it can be concluded that short-term preoperative radiotherapy further reduced the risk of local recurrence, although total mesorectal excision alone with quality control of the surgical technique can significantly decrease the risk of local recurrence [14].

The rationale for combining chemotherapy and radiotherapy is that chemotherapy agents such as 5-FU may have a radiosensitizing effect, and thus enhance the potential for locoregional control. In addition, by giving radiotherapy and chemotherapy simultaneously, rectum cancer is treated systemically for occult metastasis, and overall treatment time may also be decreased. Preoperative chemotherapy in combination with 5 Gy hyperfractionation for a short time such as in the Swedish literature does not have the same radiosensitizing effect as chemotherapy in combination with a radiation dose of 40–45 Gy in 5 weeks [3, 21]. Several studies have reported that the use of radiochemotherapy in a preoperative setting may increase the operability of T4-carcinomas and recurrent carcinomas and the prospects of preserving sphincter function in very low rectal cancer [4, 13, 17].

Postoperative Radiotherapy or Radiochemotherapy

Positive results are reported in randomized phase III adjuvant trials for resected high-risk rectal cancer [7, 8, 16, 20]. A decrease in local relapse and improvement in terms of both disease-free and overall survival with combined modality postoperative radiochemotherapy was shown. In the GTSG 7175 trial, patients were randomized to surgery alone and adjuvant therapy arms (postoperative irradiation, postoperative chemotherapy and postoperative combined radiochemotherapy) [7, 8]. Statistically significant advantages in disease-free and overall survival with the radiochemotherapy arm were achieved in a comparison with the surgery alone arm. Local relapse, an initial pattern of relapse, was significantly decreased with irradiation versus no irradiation. The best local control was achieved with combined radiochemotherapy (local relapse rate of 11% vs. 20% with irradiation alone). No impact on local control was seen with adjuvant chemotherapy alone, although rates of distant metastasis were lower in the arms that contained chemotherapy. In the two arms without chemotherapy, no single arm had a significant impact on the rate of distant metastasis.

In the GTSG 7180 and the O'Connell trial (NCCTG 864751) [9, 16], it was shown that a combination of 5-FU, methyl CCNU and radiotherapy did not produce a benefit. The NCCTG trial also tested the best method of giving 5-FU concomitant with irradiation. Interrupted bolus 5-FU (500 mg/m^2, 3 days, week 1 and 5 of EBRT) was compared with protracted low-dose infusion 5-FU (225 mg/m^2, 24 h, 7 days a week) in a randomized study (664 patients) [16]. In an interim analysis of disease control and time to relapse there was a significant advantage for patients who received protracted 5-FU chemotherapy during radiotherapy. Local relapse rates were 8% versus 12%, distant metastasis rates were 31% versus 40% and 4-year disease-free survival rates were 63% versus 53%. There was also a significant improvement in 4-year overall survival: 70% versus 60%.

The US Intergroup rectal adjuvant study tested various 5-FU bolus regimes in combination with radiotherapy. In the published final report [20], there was no difference in either overall survival or disease-free survival by drug regime. After 5 years, the disease-free survival for the total group was 54% and the overall survival was 64%; there was no difference by drug regime.

Pooled Analysis

Gunderson [12] created a pooled analysis from three randomized North American studies of adjuvant therapy in patients with rectal cancer. The study included 2,551 patients, all patients received postoperative radiotherapy, 96% were randomized to receive concurrent and maintenance chemotherapy. Five years of follow-up were available in 94% of patients and a 7-year follow-up in 84%. Overall survival and disease-free survival were dependent on both T and TN stage. Although in cases in an N2 situation, the T stage influenced 5-year overall survival (T1–2 69%; T3 48%, T4 38%). Gunderson identified three risk groups: (1) intermediate (T3N0 and T1–2N1); (2) moderately high (T4N0, T1–2N2 and T3N1) and high (T3N2, T4N1–2). For group one, 5-year overall survival was 74% and 81% and disease-free survival was 66% and 74%. In group two, the 5-year overall survival ranged from 61% to 69% and for group 3 overall survival ranged from 33% to 48%. Cumulative incidence rates of local relapse and distant metastases revealed similar differences to those seen in the survival analysis. The conclusion of the first pooled analysis was that patients with a single high-risk factor of extended tumor (T3–4) or nodal involvement (T1–2N1) have improved overall survival, disease-free survival and disease control when compared with those with both high-risk factors. Based on this analysis, there may be different treatment strategies indicated for the group of patients with intermediate risk (T3N0 and T1–2N1).

Side Effects

An optimal therapeutic ratio between local control and complications is achieved only with close interaction between the surgeon and the radiation oncologist and the use of sophisticated radiation techniques. In series that used conformal radiotherapy based on three-dimensional planning of irradiation, the incidence of small bowel obstruction requiring operative intervention was the same in patients receiving adjuvant postoperative irradiation (also in combination with chemotherapy) and those with surgery alone (6% vs. 5%) [19]. The incidence of acute enteritis was higher in the patients with combined radiochemotherapy versus radiotherapy alone. This did not translate into increased chronic intolerance. The incidence of severe small bowel stenosis was less than 6% with either adjuvant radiotherapy or radiochemotherapy. In O'Connell's study [16], acute gastrointestinal intolerance was higher with protracted venous infusion 5-FU than with bolus 5-FU during irradiation. Severe diarrhea occurred in 24% (protracted 5-FU) versus 14% (bolus 5-FU) of patients. Severe hematological problems were lower in the group of patients with protracted infusion (2% vs. 11%).

Another problem could be the unsatisfactory rectal function. The reasons could be decreased function of the nerve innovation of the sphincter (by operation or irradiation) or the increased frequency of bowel movements with resulting occasional stool incontinence and the need for antidiarrheal agents. It is not surprising that postoperative radiotherapy or radiochemotherapy may reduce compliance of the reconstructed stool reservoir and result in some dysfunction. The incidence of severe treatment-related dysfunction is low and the risk must be placed in proper perspective by considering the severe morbidity and dysfunction by pelvic relapse. Prospective quality of life studies with a particular emphasis on these endpoints need to be done.

Single-Modality Rectal Adjuvants

Neither radiotherapy nor chemotherapy as single adjuvant modalities achieve all suggested criteria of efficacy except for the Swedish preoperative irradiation trial [18]. Adjuvant irradiation reduces local recurrence in postoperative and preoperative trials, but this has no impact on overall survival in most series because of developing distant metastases. The only published trial in which single-modality adjuvant treatment improved both local control and survival was the large Swedish study with over 1,100 patients testing surgery alone versus preoperative radiotherapy [18]. No significant improvement in local control has been seen with single-modality adjuvant chemotherapy in any randomized study.

Combined-Modality Rectal Adjuvants

Only combined modality postoperative adjuvant treatments showed efficacy in all scientific endpoints [7, 8]. Bolus 5-FU was administered during irradiation and patients received additional chemotherapy after irradiation or in other trials before and after radiotherapy. In the US study, groups showed that MeCCNU does not provide additional benefit over bolus 5-FU [9, 16].

Systemic metastases, as an initial pattern of relapse, occurred in 26%–29% of patients despite combined radiochemotherapy [7]. It seems that metastases could be decreased with protracted infusion of 5-FU in combination with irradiation [16], but the magnitude of the problem is still significant. There is a need to evaluate the delivery of the most effective systemic therapy during as well as before and after irradiation to avoid delays of nearly 3 months between sequences of the most effective systemic therapy.

Conclusion

The standard of care for resectable rectal cancer patients who can tolerate a surgical procedure is surgical resection. However, since both local and systemic relapses are common after resection of rectal cancer, adjuvant treatment is indicated for many TN stages (Table 1). Over the last few years, there has been a shift to the regimes with preoperative radiotherapy or radiochemotherapy, especially in Europe. Before that time, patients with mobile, resectable mid and upper rectal cancers usually had surgical resection performed as the initial component of treatment, and consultations were obtained with radiotherapists and medical oncologists if high-risk features were found. Only patients with fixed T4N0–2 lesions were treated with preoperative radiochemotherapy. In this extended tumor stage, a boost with intraoperative radiotherapy with an electron irradiation (IOERT) was also used [11], especially if there was the likelihood of positive resection margins. Patients with a tumor very close to the sphincter also receive preoperative radiochemotherapy in an attempt to improve the percentage of patients in whom sphincter preservation could be accomplished.

Table 1. Treatment overview

Stage M0	Surgery	Radiotherapy/radiochemotherapy	
		Possible treatment	Our recommendation
T1–2 N0	Resection (TME) Low anterior resection if possible Abdominoperineal resection and regional lymph nodes Local excision of select lesions	–	–
T3 N0	Resection (TME) after/before RT/RCHT	Postop RCHT (45 Gy + 5.4 Gy boost)	Preop short-term RT (5×5 Gy, 1 week)
T4 N0	Resection after RCHT		Preop RCHT (45 Gy + 5-FU) Preop RCHT (41.1 Gy + 5-FU) + IORT (10 Gy)
T1–2 N1	Resection after/before RT/RCHT	Preop RCHT Postop RCHT	Preop short-term RT
T1–2 N2	Resection after/before RT/RCHT	Preop RCHT	Postop RCHT
T3 N1	Resection after/before RT/RCHT	Postop RCHT IORT (10 Gy)+ postop RCHT (45 Gy)	Preop short-term RT Preop RCHT Preop RCHT + IORT
T3 N2	Resection after/before RCHT	Postop RCHT IORT + postop RCHT	Preop RCHT Preop RCHT + IORT
T4 N1	Resection after RCHT	Postop RCHT IORT + postop RCHT	Preop RCHT Preop RCHT + IORT
T4 N2	Resection after RCHT	Postop RCHT IORT + postop RCHT	Preop RCHT Preop RCHT + IORT

TME, total mesorectal excision; RT, radiotherapy; RCHT, radiochemotherapy; IORT, intraoperative radiotherapy.

References

1. Colorectal Cancer Collaborative Group (2001) Adjuvant radiotherapy for rectal cancer: a systematic overview of 8,507 patients from 22 randomised trials. Lancet 358:1291–1304
2. Fisher B, Wolmark N, Rockette H, Redmond C, Deutsch M, Wickerham DL, Fisher ER, Caplan R, Jones J, Lerner H (1988) Postoperative adjuvant chemotherapy or radiation therapy for rectal cancer: results from NSABP protocol R-01. J Natl Cancer Inst 80:21–29
3. Frykholm GJ, Glimelius B, Pahlmann L (1993) Preoperative or postoperative irradiation in adenocarcinoma of the rectum: final treatment results of a randomized trial and evaluation of late secondary effects. Dis Colon Rectum 36:564–572
4. Gerard JP, Baulieux J, François Y, Grandjean JP, Romestaing P, Mornex F, Munoz P, Ayzac L (1998) The role of radiotherapy in the conservative treatment of rectal carcinoma—the Lyon experience. Acta Oncol 37:253–258

5. Gerard A, Buyse, Nordlinger B et al (1988) Preoperative radiotherapy as adjuvant treatment in rectal cancer: final results of randomized study (EORTC). Ann Surg 208:606–614
6. Goldberg PA, Nicholls RJ, Porter NH, Love S, Grimsey JE (1994) Long-term results of a randomised trial of short-course low-dose adjuvant pre-operative radiotherapy for rectal cancer: reduction in local treatment failure. Eur J Cancer 30A:1602–1606
7. Gastrointestinal Tumor Study Group (1985) Prolongation of the disease-free interval in surgical treated rectal carcinoma. N Engl J Med 312:1465–1472
8. Gastrointestinal Tumor Study Group (1986) Survival after postoperative combination treatment for rectal cancer. N Engl J Med 314:1294–1295
9. Gastrointestinal Tumor Study Group (1992) Radiation therapy and fluorouracil with or without semustine for the treatment of patients with surgical adjuvant adenocarcinoma of the rectum. J Clin Oncol 10:549–557
10. Gunderson LL (1999) Indications for and results of combined modality treatment of colorectal cancer. Acta Oncol 38:7–21
11. Gunderson LL, Nelson H, Martenson J et al (1997) Locally advanced primary colorectal cancer: intraoperative electron and external beam irradiation ± 5FU. Int J Radiat Biol Phys 37:601–614
12. Gunderson LL, Sargent DJ, Tepper JE et al (2002) Impact of T and N substage on survival and disease relapse in adjuvant rectal cancer: a pooled analysis. Int J Radiat Oncol Biol Phys 54:386–396
13. Hyams DM, Mamounas EP, Petrelli N, Rockette H, Jones J, Wieand HS, Deutsch M, Wickerham L, Fisher B, Wolmark N (1997) A clinical trial to evaluate the worth of preoperative multimodality therapy in patients with operable carcinoma of the rectum: a progress report of National Surgical Breast and Bowel Project Protocol R-03. Dis Colon Rectum 40:131–139
14. Kapiteijn E, Marijnen CA, Nagtegaal ID, Putter H, Steup WH, Wiggers T, Rutten HJ, Pahlman L, Glimelius B, van Krieken JH, Leer JW, van de Velde CJ (2001) Preoperative radiotherapy combined with total mesorectal excision for resectable rectal cancer. N Engl J Med 345:638–646
15. MRC Working Party (1984) The evaluation of low dose preoperative x-ray therapy in the management of operable rectal cancer: results of a randomly controlled trial. Br J Surg 71:21–25
16. OConnell MJ, Martenson JA, Wieland HS et al (1994) Improving adjuvant therapy for rectal cancer by combining protracted infusion fluorouracil with radiation therapy after curative surgery. N Engl J Med 331:502–507
17. Rouanet P, Fabre JM, Dubois JB, Dravet F, Saint AB, Pradel J, Ychou M, Solassol C, Pujol H (1995) Conservative surgery for low rectal carcinoma after high-dose radiation. Functional and oncologic results. Ann Surg 221:67–73
18. Swedish Rectal Cancer Trial (1997) Improved survival with preoperative radiotherapy in resectable rectal cancer. N Engl J Med 336:980–987
19. Tepper JE, O'Connell MJ, Petroni G et al (1997) Adjuvant postoperative 5-FU-modulated chemotherapy combined with pelvic radiation therapy for in rectal cancer. J Clin Oncol 15:2030–2039
20. Tepper JE, OConnell MJ, Niedziecki D et al (2002) Adjuvant therapy in rectal cancer: analysis of stage, sex and local control—Final report of Intergroup 0114. J Clin Oncol 20:1744–1750
21. Wannenmacher M, Herfarth C (2000) Belegtes zur präoperativen Therapie des Rektumcarcinoms. Chirurg 71:1440–1446

Intraoperative Radiotherapy for Rectal Carcinoma

Martina Treiber, S. Oertel, J. Weitz, R. Krempien, M. Bischof, M. Wannenmacher, M. Büchler, J. Debus

M. Treiber (✉)
Department of Radiotherapy, University of Heidelberg, INF 400,
69120 Heidelberg, Germany
e-mail: martina_treiber@med.uni-heidelberg.de

Introduction

Local recurrence following curative resection of rectal carcinoma is still a major problem. Recurrence rates of more than 30% have been reported in the past, but total mesorectal excision has reduced the incidence to considerably less than 10%. Still, the severe morbidity associated with local recurrence demands additional efforts to guarantee local control. Moreover, it may be hoped that a reduction of local recurrence translates into improved overall survival.

Postoperative adjuvant radiotherapy allows treatment after precise pathological staging, thus preventing over-therapy. The target area, however, includes radiosensitive tissues such as urinary bladder, ureters and intestines as well as a hypoxic postsurgical tumor bed with potentially reduced radiosensitivity. Neoadjuvant therapy can render resectability in locally advanced tumors and often facilitates sphincter preservation in low rectal cancer [19, 22]. It also reduces the spread of viable tumor cells and seems to decrease side effects concerning the small bowel. Finally radiosensitivity is expected to be better, because tumor cell oxygenation is not compromised preoperatively.

Many randomized trials have confirmed that adjuvant as well as neoadjuvant radiotherapy can reduce the incidence of local recurrence in UICC stage II and III rectal carcinoma by half [13] and neoadjuvant accelerated 5×5-Gy radiotherapy was associated with improved survival [20, 11].

Concept of Intraoperative Radiotherapy

To decrease acute and late toxicity of radiotherapy and to improve local control, institutes in the US, Europe, Russia and Japan have combined fractionated three-dimensional planned external beam radiotherapy (EBRT) with intraoperative radiotherapy (IORT) as a local boost technique. External beam radiotherapy is limited to 40–45 Gy in the pelvic area (only a small boost volume without irradiating small bowl can be treated up to a total dose of 50 Gy), because of the

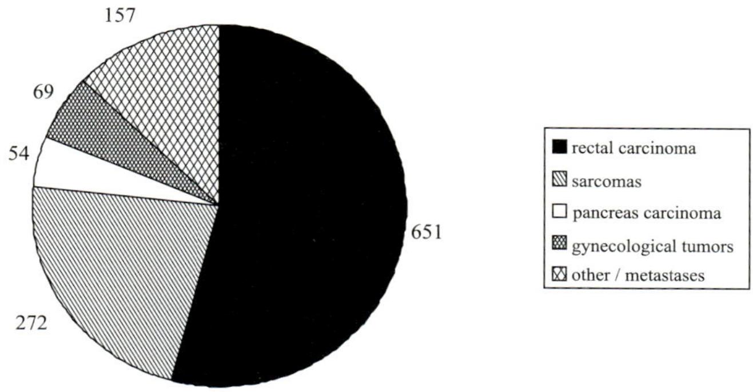

Figure 1. Overview of all patients treated with IORT in our department since 1991 (June 1991–June 2003), *n*=1,203

normal tissue tolerance. Tolerance of gastrointestinal tissues to fractionated EBRT is limited and depends on treated organ volume and irradiation dose. Tolerance dose for the small bowel is 40–45 Gy and for the colon 45–50 Gy [5]. Higher doses can be applied by IORT in order to reach the recommended 60 Gy. A single high dose irradiation such as IORT (dose range, 10–15 Gy) results in a higher biological effectiveness (2.5 times greater) compared to fractionated radiotherapy (1.8–2 Gy daily in five fractions per week). Higher doses can be given for microscopically or macroscopically incompletely resected tumors by IORT [15]. Besides potentially better local control rates, IORT patients save 2 weeks time compared to patients who are treated with an additional percutaneous conventional boost therapy with low daily single dose fractionation.

The target volume IORT for rectal carcinoma is determined by observations in patients who had re-operation after resection of primary rectal carcinoma. Recurrent carcinoma was most frequently found at the anastomosis and in the presacral area [6]. As a result, the presacral area and the lymphatic drainage up to the sacral promontory should be included in the IORT target volume.

Patients with rectal cancer who are candidates for IORT constitute a heterogeneous group. IORT can be integrated at different points in the treatment schedule. For locally advanced or recurrent carcinoma IORT is preferably used as an adjuvant treatment. It can also be applied in preirradiated patients. Figure 1 gives an overview of all patients (*n*=1,203) treated with IORT in our department since 1991.

Techniques and Dosage

In Heidelberg we use a dedicated operating unit equipped with a linear accelerator (electron beam) for intraoperative radiotherapy (Fig. 2). IORT is administered using special sterile chrome-plated brass applicators of different shapes, 5–12 cm in diameter, which are held fixed to the operation table. IORT is then delivered using a laser-guided air-docking system with electron energies of 8–18 MeV corresponding to a depth of 24–54 mm. The IORT dose is prescribed to the 90%

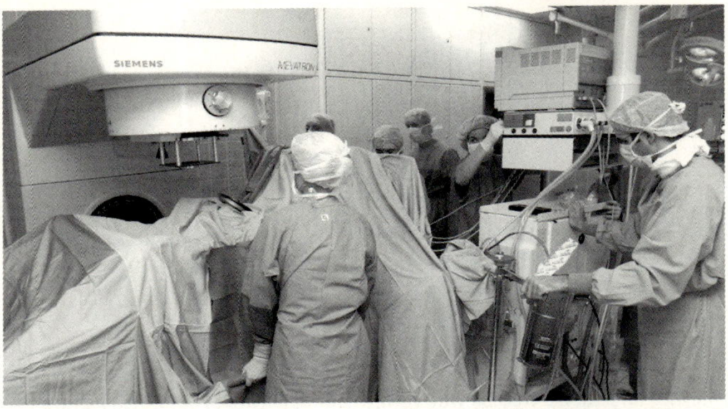

Figure 2. Dedicated IORT unit (linear accelerator Siemens Mevatron ME), University of Heidelberg

isodose and is delivered by a dose rate of 900 cGy per minute (Fig. 3). Surgical clips to identify the IORT volume facilitate 3D computed tomography planning of postoperative EBRT. EBRT is delivered at 1–4 weeks pre- or postoperatively in single fractions of 1.8 Gy (in combination with chemotherapy 5-FU/leucovorin) or with the new preoperative concept recommending 25 Gy in 1 week (5×5 Gy) by a linear accelerator with at least 6–23 MeV photons.

For patients who have not been preirradiated with 10 Gy, in case of residual or recurrent disease, up to 15 Gy are applied. The complete IORT procedure (positioning of the applicator, transportation to the accelerator, air-docking and irradiation) requires about 20 min, with a well-organized team of surgeons, radiation therapists and anesthesiologists.

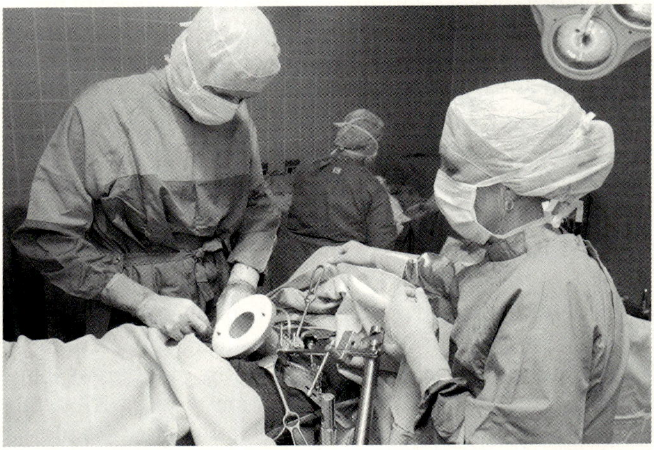

Figure 3. Rectal carcinoma: typical IORT situation

Morbidity and Toxicity

The most important dose-limiting factors to be considered in IORT are peripheral neuropathy and ureter stenosis. The frequency of complications depends on radiation doses and on the indication for IORT. Higher IORT-related complication rates (soft tissue or sacral damage and 10% pelvic neuropathy) were reported for patients with recurrent disease compared to those with primary disease (2% sacral injury) [23]. In the RTOG 8508 trial, 2-year actuarial risk of significant complications with primary or recurrent rectal carcinoma was 16%. There was no significant difference in complications in the IORT group compared with a non-randomized group who had surgery without IORT [12, 16]. In our experience with recurrent rectal cancer, morbidity was not significantly increased when IORT was added to EBRCT (external beam radiotherapy and additional chemotherapy) [21]. The risk of chronic gastrointestinal damage could be reduced from 7% to 0% in patients who were treated by combined radiotherapy (EBRCT plus IORT) [4, 21] due to dose reduction in the intestines. Still, only a randomized study will provide a reliable estimate of IORT-related complication rates, particularly in patients with recurrent disease.

Survival

Primary Advanced and Unresectable Rectal Cancer

A comparison of patients with completely resected tumors showed a reduction of local failure rates from 18% without IORT (n=66) to 11% when IORT was used (n=45). Patients with incomplete resection had a reduction of local failure from 83% without IORT to 35% with IORT. The 5-year overall survival rate for primary advanced rectal cancer patients within the IORT group was 63% for patients with negative margins and 32% for patients with positive margins [14]. Similar observations were made by other investigators [8, 9].

In our series of stage II and III primary rectal carcinoma, the 5-year overall survival was 64% and 41%, respectively. Local failure rates were inversely related to radiation doses: 32%, 40–48 Gy; 25%, 49–56 Gy; 5.2%, 66.4 Gy (41.4 + IORT 10 Gy; biological effective dose IORT 25 Gy). The 2-year and 3-year overall survival rates were significantly improved after IORT plus EBRCT in both primary and recurrent disease [3]. This results were confirmed by the IORT group in Rome, Italy [2].

Recurrent Rectal Cancer

Patients with local recurrence of rectal cancer represent a rather heterogeneous group with regard to tumor burden and prior treatment. Patients who already have had pelvic irradiation and chemotherapy receive IORT only (often at a reduced dose) during resection of recurrent tumor, while others, who were not preirradiated, can be treated with a full course of preoperative external beam radiochemotherapy followed by surgical resection plus IORT boost. Patients from the Mayo Clinic receiving 50–54 Gy before surgery plus 7.5–20 Gy IORT had local failure rates of 6% for complete resection, 18% for microscopically incomplete resection and 25% for gross residual disease [7]. Five-year overall survival was 27% for microscopic and 25% for macroscopic disease. Studies from the Massachusetts General Hospital in Boston, Massachusetts, USA, showed 5-year disease-free survival of 21% for completely resected patients, but only 7% for those whose tumors were incompletely resected [23].

The poor outcome for incompletely resected tumors was confirmed by a group from Eindhoven, the Netherlands [17]. They found that patients with gross residual disease had a significantly lower rate of 3-year local control (21% vs. 79%), disease-free survival (11% vs. 54%) and overall survival (35% vs. 74%) compared to those with negative or microscopically involved margins.

Our data showed a 5-year local control rate of 78% in patients with complete resection and 58% in patients with microscopic residues. In the group of incompletely resected tumors (R2), a marked increase in local failures was observed and the local control rate was reduced to 29%. The 5-year overall survival rate was low (39%) because of the high distant metastasis rate [21]. The IORT group in Münster, Germany, presented comparable results [10]. These days preoperative radiochemotherapy followed by radical surgical resection plus IORT is the preferred sequence of treatment in our institution.

Randomized Trials

A prospective multicenter trial in France includes UICC stage II and III rectal cancers. Following preoperative radiotherapy of 40 Gy, patients were randomized to either no further radiotherapy or intraoperative radiotherapy of 18 Gy (>10 MeV). Until 1996, 57 of 288 planned patients were entered. Postoperative morbidity was not significantly different between groups, but long-term results await completion of the trial [1]. Another randomized trial was performed in Russia, where 42 patients were randomized after preoperative radiotherapy to receive additional 20 Gy intraoperative boost irradiation (8–15 MeV) or not. At a median follow-up of 7 months (range, 1–15 months), two patients in the control group, but no patient in the treatment group had locoregional recurrence [18]. Again, long-term results have not yet been reported.

Outlook

Intraoperative radiotherapy represents an important component of multimodal therapy in rectal carcinoma. IORT makes it possible to give high irradiation doses to the tumor bed, resulting in better local control rates without an increase in side effects. Unfortunately, the potential therapeutic benefit of intraoperative electron beam radiotherapy has never been tested in large prospective, randomized and controlled trials. There were two main reasons for this: too few institutions were equipped with a dedicated unit for intraoperative radiotherapy and patients explicitly referred to receive IORT could hardly be randomized. Technical advances have made available a new generation of mobile accelerators such as the Novac 7 (Elektra) and others, which do not require special shielding of the operating room. This allows a more flexible use in different operating rooms. In our department, we have used a flexible mobile operation table (Maquet) to facilitate patient positioning to apply IORT over the last year. All these developments will allow a wider use of IORT in the future.

References

1. Bussieres E, Dubois JB et al (1997) IORT: a randomized trial in primary rectal cancer by the French Group of IORT. Front Radiat Ther Oncol 31:217–220
2. Doglietto GB, Ratto C et al (2001) Intraoperative radiotherapy (IORT) in the treatment of rectal cancer. Ann Ital Chir 72:567–571
3. Eble MJ, Kallinowski F et al (1994) Intraoperative radiotherapy of locally advanced and recurrent rectal cancer. Chirurgie 65:585–592
4. Eble MJ, Treiber M et al (1997) IORT for recurrent rectal carcinoma. Front Radiat Ther Oncol 31:229–233
5. Emami B, Lyman J et al (1991) Tolerance of normal tissue to therapeutic irradiation. Rad Oncol Biol Phys 21:109–122
6. Gunderson LL, Sosin H (1974) Areas of failure found at operation (second or symptomatic look) following "curative" surgery for adenocarcinoma of the rectum: clinicopathological correlation and implication for adjuvant therapy. Cancer 34:1278–1292
7. Gunderson LL, Nelson H et al (1996) Intraoperative electron and external beam irradiation with or without 5-Fluorouracil and maximum surgical resection for previously unirradiated, locally recurrent colorectal cancer. Dis Colon Rectum 39:1379–1395
8. Gunderson LL, Nelson H et al (1997) Locally advanced primary colorectal cancer: intraoperative electron and external beam irradiation plus 5FU. Int J Radiat Oncol Biol Phys 37:601–614
9. Harrison LB, Minsky BD et al (1998) High dose rate intraoperative radiation therapy (HDR-IORT) as part of the management strategy for locally advanced primary and recurrent rectal cancer. Int J Radiat Oncol Biol Phys 42:325–330
10. Hesselmann S, Micke O et al (2003) Intraoperative radiation therapy (IORT) in primary locally advanced and recurrent carcinoma of the rectum at a "non-dedicated" facility. Anticancer Res 23:1875–1881
11. Kapiteijn E, Marijnen CA et al (Dutch Colorectal Cancer Group) (2001) Preoperative radiotherapy combined with total mesorectal excision for resectable rectal cancer. N Engl J Med 345:638–646
12. Kim HK, Jessup JM et al (1997) Locally advanced rectal carcinoma: pelvic control and morbidity following preoperative radiation therapy, resection and intraoperative radiation therapy. Int J Radiat Oncol Biol Phys 38:777–783
13. Lehnert T, Herfarth C (1998) Multimodal therapy of rectal cancer. Chirurg 69:384–392
14. Nakfoor BM, Spiro IJ et al (1998) The impact of 5-fluorouracil and intraoperative electron beam radiation therapy on the outcome of patients with locally advanced primary rectal and rectosigmoid cancer. Ann Surg 228:194–200
15. Neve de W, Martijn H et al (1991) Incompletely resected rectum, rectosigmoid or sigmoid carcinoma: results of postoperative radiotherapy and prognostic factors. Int J Radiat Oncol Biol Phys 21:1297–1302
16. Noyes RD, Weiss SM et al (1993) Surgical complications of intraoperative radiation therapy: the Radiation Therapy Oncology Group experience. J Surg Oncol 50:209–215
17. Rutten HJT, Mannaerts GHH et al (2000) Intraoperative radiotherapy for locally recurrent rectal cancer in The Netherlands. Eur J Surg Oncol 26 [Suppl A]:S16–S20
18. Skoropad V, Berdov B et al (1995) Randomized trial of intraoperative radiotherapy for colorectal cancer. Eur J Cancer 31A:S157

19. Stockholm Colorectal Cancer Study Group (1996) Randomized study on preoperative radiotherapy in rectal carcinoma. Ann Surg Oncol 3:423–430
20. Swedish Rectal Cancer Trial (1997) Improved survival with preoperative radiotherapy in resectable rectal cancer. N Engl J Med 336:980–987
21. Treiber M, Lehnert Th et al (2004) Intraoperative radiotherapy – special focus: recurrent rectal carcinoma. Front Radiat Ther Oncol 38:1–5
22. Wagman R, Minsky BD et al (1998) Sphincter preservation with preoperative radiation therapy and coloanal anastomosis: long-term follow-up. Int J Radiat Oncol Biol Phys 42:51–57
23. Wallace HJ 3rd, Willett CG et al (1995) Intraoperative radiation therapy for locally advanced recurrent rectal or rectosigmoid cancer. J Surg Oncol 60:122–127

Indications and Effect on Survival of Standard Chemotherapy in Advanced Colorectal Cancer

Birgit Kallinowski

B. Kallinowski (✉)
Praxis for Gastroenterology and Oncology, Scheffelstr. 63, 68723 Schwetzingen, Germany
e-mail: birgit.kallinowski@web.de

Abstract

Since the introduction of combined systemic chemotherapy with 5-folinic-acid (FA) and/or oxaliplatin or irinotecan, the median survival in patients with advanced colorectal cancer has increased to more than 20 months. Novel agents in so-called targeted therapies such as monoclonal antibodies will further increase these excellent survival data in the near future.

Introduction

The role of systemic chemotherapy in patients with metastatic colorectal cancer (CRC) has been clearly established. However, only 10% of patients with metastatic CRC will survive more than 5 years. New combination therapies coming up in the last 5 years improved the median overall survival to nearly 20 months for the majority of patients. The main reason for this major breakthrough has been the integration of oxaliplatin and irinotecan in 5-FU-based chemotherapies. Furthermore, the substitution of intravenous 5-FU by oral 5-FU prodrugs such as tegafur and capecitabine in the mono- or combination therapy optimised the chemotherapeutic regimes as well. The following article is intended to give a short review of the present standard chemotherapeutic strategies in metastatic CRC and will give an outlook for future biologicals and targeted therapies.

Standard Principles in Palliative Chemotherapy for Colorectal Cancer

Data by Scheithauer et al. from the early 1990s demonstrated that chemotherapy prolongs survival time in patients with advanced CRC from 5 to 11 months compared to patients receiving best supportive care alone [1]. In addition the use of palliative chemotherapy often ameliorates tumour-associated symptoms and improves quality of life in these patients [2, 3]. This is also valid for older patients.

Recent Results in Cancer Research, Vol. 165

Another dogma for palliative chemotherapy which needs to be respected is that chemotherapy should be started as long as the asymptomatic patient is in good clinical condition, because a later start of chemotherapy in symptomatic patients worsens the prognosis [3]. The addition of folinic acid (FA) to 5-fluorouracil (5-FU) as a modulator has been superior to monotherapy with 5-FU. Response rates and time to progression, i.e. the progression-free survival (PFS) time, have been improved by the modulation of 5-FU by FA. However, the overall survival time for patients remained unchanged despite the modulation by FA [4]. The response rate is also dependent on the rate of 5-FU infusion. Maximal response rates and progression-free survival time with the same toxicity can only be achieved by ultrashort 5-FU infusion times of 2–4 min, the so-called bolus 5-FU. Longer infusion times of 10–20 min decrease the response rates from 27% to 13% and the PFS from 5.5 to 4.2 months [5]. Another progress in palliative chemotherapy was made when it was discovered that the infusional regime of 5-FU was more effective than the use of the bolus 5-FU. Due to the short half-life of bolus 5-FU, 5-FU is integrated mainly in RNA, while infusional 5-FU with its constantly low FU level mainly interferes with DNA synthesis. Weekly protocols with intermittent 24- or 48-h 5-FU infusions combined with FA significantly increased RR and PFS compared to the 5-FU bolus protocol, with a tendency for better overall survival (11.2 months versus 9.9 months with the bolus protocol). In addition, the infusional 5-FU protocols induce less gastrointestinal and hematological toxicity.

Oral 5-FU Prodrugs

Oral 5-FU prodrugs such as capecitabine and UFT imitate the continuous 5-FU infusion without the need for an intravenous port system. UFT consists of a combination of uracil and tegafur in a 4:1 ratio. UFT needs to be taken three times per day fasting with the addition of folinic acid, whereas capecitabine needs to be taken only twice a day without FA. Both prodrugs are less toxic compared to intravenous 5-FU referring to neutropoenia, diarrhoea and mucositis. However, capecitabine more often induces a hand-foot syndrome than its oral counterpart UFT. In randomised prospective trials comparing capecitabine and UFT and the Mayo protocol, the PFS and the overall survival with a median of 12 months were not different (Table 1) [6–8]. However, capecitabine has been demonstrated to be at least as effective as 5-FU bolus protocols with a response rate of 25.8% versus 11.6%. These response rates have usually been only achieved by infusional 5-FU regimes.

Combination Therapy with 5-FU/FA and Irinotecan and/or Oxaliplatin

The dramatic breakthrough with response rates in excess of 50% and median survival times of more than 20 months in patients with metastatic CRC were achieved in the last 3 years by the combination of infusional 5-FU/FA with the camptothecin

Table 1. Oral fluoropyrimidines versus bolus 5-FU/FA: phase III trials

Authors	Treatment	Patients (n)	Response rate (%)	Survival (months)	PFS (months)
Hoff et al. 2001	Capecitabine	302	25.8*	12.5	4.3
	Bolus 5-FU/FA	303	11.6	13.3	4.7
Cutsem et al. 2001	Capecitabine	301	18.9	13.2	5.2
	Bolus 5-FU/FA	301	15.0	12.1	4.7
Douillard et al. 2002	UFT/FA	409	12.0	12.4	3.5
	Bolus-5-FU/FA	407	15.0	13.4	3.8
Carmichael et al. 2002	UFT/FA	190	11.0	12.2	3.4
	Bolus 5-FU/FA	190	9.0	10.3	3.5

*$p<0.05$.
PFS, progression-free survival.

Table 2. 5-FU combination therapies: phase III trials

Author and publication source	Patients (n)	Response rate (%)	
		5-FU/LV	Combination
De Gramont et al. JCO 2000	420	22	57 (Oxaliplatin)*
Giacchetti et al. JCO 2000	200	16	53 (Oxaliplatin)*
Grothey et al. ASCO 2002	252	23	49 (Oxaliplatin)*
Douillard et al. Lancet 2000	387	31	49 (Irinotecan)*
Saltz et al. NEJM 2000	666	27	49 (Irinotecan)*
Köhne et al. ASCO 2003	440	30	50 (Irinotecan)*

*$p<0.001$.

analogue irinotecan (CPT-11) and the platin analogue oxaliplatin (Table 2) [9–12]. The typical clinical side effects of the topoisomerase-inhibitor CPT-11 include a cholinergic syndrome, which can be successfully treated by atropine, whereas the limiting side effect with prolonged treatment with oxaliplatin consists of peripheral neuropathy. The question of whether a patient with metastatic CRC should be initially started on a combination chemotherapy or not is still controversially discussed. However, any oncologist should take into consideration that the use of a primary combined chemotherapy in advanced CRC induces a significantly better short-term (60 days mortality 11]) and long-term survival compared to a 5-FU-based monotherapy. Given these data, we prefer that patients presenting with a high tumour load and a poor performance status should be initially started on a combination therapy whenever possible.

Optimal Sequence of First- and Second-Line Chemotherapy in Metastatic Colorectal Cancer

Another question concerning which combination therapy should be used as first- or second-line therapy has been already investigated by Tournigand and colleagues [14] in a phase III trial in 2001 (Table 3). There was no difference detected for either sequence. Initial response rates of 56% for FOLFIRI followed by FOLFOX nor for FOLFOX and of 54% for the sequence FOLFOX–FOLFIRI and an equal overall survival time of 20–21 months were found in both groups. However, preliminary data presented on the ASCO meeting in 2003 by Goldberg and colleagues favoured FOLFOX as first-line chemotherapy because the overall survival (OS) with 19.5 months was better compared to FOLFIRI (OS, 14.8 months) and/or IROX (OS, 17.4 months). In summary, according to recent data a combination therapy of infusional 5-FU either with oxaliplatin or irinotecan should be the first-line therapy for any patient with metastatic CRC whenever possible.

Table 3. Sequence of combination therapies in metastatic colorectal cancer

	FOLFIRI *n*=109	FOLFOX *n*=81	FOLFOX *n*=111	FOLFIRI *n*=69
RR	56%	15%	54%	4%
RR +SD	79%	63%	81%	35%
PFS	14.4 months		11.5 months	
OS	20.2 months		21.5 months	
2-year survival	41%		45%	

RR, response rate; SD, stable disease; PFS, progression-free survival; OS, overall survival.

New Agents

In conclusion, with the new available chemotherapeutic regimes median overall survival times of more than 20 months can now be achieved. Despite these promising results, novel targeted therapies such as EGF receptor inhibitors, VEGF inhibitors, Cox-2 inhibitors, Farnesyltransferase inhibitors and small molecules such as antisense olignonucleotides are presently under investigation in huge phase III multicentre trials hoping to increase not only response rates up to 70%, but also the overall survival time in patients with advanced colorectal cancer.

References

1. Scheithauer B, Rosen H, Kornek GV et al (1993) Randomized comparison of combination chemotherapy plus supportive care with supportive care alone in patients with metastatic colorectal cancer . BMJ 306:752–755

2. Glimelius B, Hoffmann K, Graf W et al (1995) Cost-effectiveness of palliative chemotherapy in advanced gastrointestinal cancer. Ann Oncol 6:205–207
3. Nordic Gastrointestinal Tumor Adjuvant Therapy Group (1992) Expectancy or primary chemotherapy in patients with advanced asymptomatic colorectal cancer: a randomized trial. J Clin Oncol 10:904–911
4. Advanced Colorectal Cancer Meta-Analysis Project (1992) Modulation of fluorouracil by leucovorin in patients with advanced colorectal cancer: evidence in terms of response rate. J Clin Oncl 10:896–903
5. Glimelius B, Jakobsen A, Graf W et al (19987) Bolus injection (2–4 min) versus short-term (10–20 min) infusion of 5-fluorouracil in patients with advanced colorectal cancer: a prospective randomised trial. Nordic Gastrointestinal Tumour Adjuvant Therapy Group. Eur J Cancer 34:674–678
6. Carmichael J, Popiela T, Radstone D et al (1999) Randomized comparative study of ORZEL (oral uracil/Tegafur (UFTTM) plus leucovorin (LV) versus parenteral 5-fluorouracil (5-FU) plus LV in patients with metastatic colorectal cancer. Proc Am Soc Clin Oncol 18:264A
7. Hoff P, Ansar R, Batist G et al (2001) Comparison of oral capecitabine versus intravenous fluorouracil plus leucovorin as first-line therapy in 605 patients with metastic colorectal cancer: results of a randomized phase III study. J Clin Oncol 19:2282–2292
8. Van Cutsem E, Twelfes C, Cassidy J et al (2001) Oral capecitabine compared with intravenous fluorouracil plus leucovorin in patients with metastatic colorectal cancer: results of a large phase III study. J Clin Oncol 19:4097–4106
9. De Gramont A, Figer A, Seymour M et al (2000) Leucovorin and fluorouracil with or without oxaliplatin as first-line treatment in advanced colorectal cancer. J Clin Oncol 18:2938–2947
10. Giacchetti S, Perpoint B, Zidani R et al (2000) Phase III multicenter randomized trial of oxaliplatin added to chronomodulated fluorouracil-leucovorin as first-line treatment of metastatic colorectal cancer. J Clin Oncol 18:136–147
11. Grothey A, Deschler B, Kroening H et al (2002) Phase III study of bolus 5-fluorouracil (5FU/folinic acid (FA Mayo) vs weekly high-dose 24 h 5-FU infusion/FA + oxaliplatin (OXA) in advanced colorectal cancer. Proc Am Soc Clin Oncol21:219A
12. Douillard J, Cunningham D, Roth A et al (2000) Irinotecan combined with fluorouracil compared with fluorouracil alone as first-line treatment for metastatic colorectal cancer: a multicentre randomised trial. Lancet 355:1041–1047
13. Saltz L, Cox J, Blanke C et al (2000) Irinotecan plus fluorouracil and leucovorin for metastatic colorectal cancer. Irinotecan Study Group. N Engl J Med 343:905–914
14. Tournigand C, Louvet C, Quinaux E et al (2001) FOLFIRI followed by FOLFOX versus FOLFOX followed by FOLFIRI in metastatic colorectal cancer: final results from a phase IIII study. Proc Am Soc Clin Oncol 0:214A

New Chemotherapeutic Strategies in Colorectal Cancer

Markus Moehler, Andreas Teufel, Peter R. Galle

M. Moehler (✉)
Department of Internal Medicine, Johannes-Gutenberg University Mainz,
Langenbeckstr. 1, 55131 Mainz, Germany
e-mail: moehler@mail.uni-mainz.de

Abstract

Since colorectal cancer is the second most prevalent cancer worldwide, its treatment remains a major challenge for researchers, gastroenterologists and oncologists. Despite curative resections, half of all patients diagnosed with colorectal cancer die because of their underlying disease. Integral chemotherapeutic components of standard regimens are 5-fluorouracil (5-FU), its modulation by folinic acid and irinotecan or oxaliplatin. All these drugs sequentially given have results in terms of median overall survival of more than 20 months in the palliative treatment of advanced colorectal cancer. Oral fluoropyrimidines, currently under clinical investigation, are likely to substitute continuous 5-FU. Inhibitors of growth factor receptors or their signaling may further prolong disease-free and overall survival rates. Preliminary evidence exists that improved adjuvant and neoadjuvant chemotherapy strategies may further improve the prognosis, mainly because more patients are able to go for primary or secondary surgery with curative intent.

Introduction

Colorectal cancer is the second most prevalent cancer and the third leading cause of cancer deaths worldwide [1]. Despite curative resections, many patients develop later recurrence or metachronic metastases. Many other patients already present with metastatic or surgically not resectable disease at the time of diagnosis. More than half of all colorectal cancer patients die as a result of its metastatic disease [2]. Therefore, there is an urgent need to improve the treatment options for colorectal cancer. This chapter first reviews the established concepts of adjuvant and palliative protocols. Second, it integrates the chemotherapeutic agents irinotecan and oxaliplatin into these treatment combinations. Third, we focus on the upcoming innovative strategies of oral fluoropyrimidines and biological targeting to further increase the patients' quality of life and the neoadjuvant protocols for a better likelihood of curative procedures (Fig. 1).

Recent Results in Cancer Research, Vol. 165

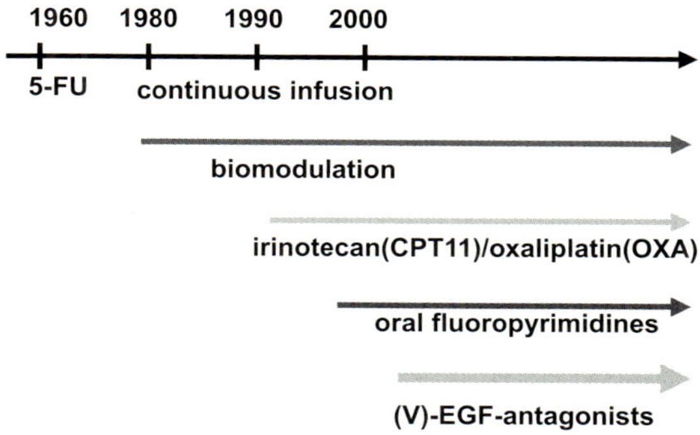

Figure 1. Treatment strategies of colorectal cancer during the last 40 years

Established Concepts of Adjuvant and Palliative Treatment Protocols

For over 40 years, the antimetabolite 5-fluoruracil (5-FU) and its modulation by folinic acid (FA) has been the standard of care [3]. Palliative chemotherapy has been shown to be more effective than best supportive care in prolonging survival and improving quality of life. In a north central cancer treatment group (NCCTG) trial, 429 patients were randomized to one of six regimens: 5-FU alone, 5-FU plus high-dose or low-dose FA, 5-FU plus high-dose or low-dose methotrexate or 5-FU plus cisplatin [4]. Herein, FA/5FU protocols were the superior regimens, with no significant advantage over high-dose or low-dose FA regarding the response rates and the 1-year survival rate. In other studies, two major FA-modulated 5-FU regimens have been employed as standards at the end of the last century in western countries [5, 6]:

1. The Mayo Clinic protocol
   5-FU 425 mg/qm daily and FA 20 mg/qm daily administered for 5 consecutive days, repeated every 4 weeks for two cycles and then every 5 weeks thereafter (6 months).
2. The Roswell Park regimen
   5-FU 500 mg/qm and FA 500 mg/qm, administered once weekly, for 6 consecutive weeks and repeated every 8 weeks.

Continuous 5FU Is Superior to Bolus 5-FU

As 5-FU has a short plasma half-life and as its efficacy and toxicity can be influenced by continuous infusions, prolonged or high-dose 5-FU protocols have been thoroughly evaluated. In Europe, different 5-FU infusion protocols have been established, with still widely used concepts on the part of the Spanish, the French or the German study groups. A recent pooled metaanalysis of 1,219 patients comparing continuous infusions with bolus administration of 5-FU reported a significantly higher response rate and modest improvement in survival (median, 12.1 months vs. 11.3 months; p=0.04) [7]. In infusional regimens, the toxicity profile is to some extent altered with less hematological toxicity but more frequent hand-foot syndrome. In the US however, the European enthusiasm was tempered mainly because of concerns about catheter-associated complications and the possible patient inconvenience. However, according to the data of Goldberg and Tournigand, American treatment strategies may also likely change to the more common use of 5-FU continuous infusions in oxaliplatin or irinotecan combinations [8, 9].

Adjuvant Chemotherapy Is of Benefit for UICC III (Dukes' C) Patients

Many randomized trials have clearly demonstrated the benefits of adjuvant therapy in node-positive UICC III (Dukes' C) colon cancer [10]. Standard of care is either the Mayo Clinic Protocol or the Roswell park regimen for 6 months in Western countries. However, the role of adjuvant chemotherapy following curative resection of node-negative colon cancer with large tumors (T3/T4; UICC II, Dukes' B) is still in dispute [11]. The debate was stimulated by two conflicting meta-analyses, in which one of the NSABPs demonstrated similar treatment benefits for UICC II and III, although fewer recurrences were noted because of the improved prognosis at UICC II. The authors concluded that adjuvant chemotherapy should be considered since a significant proportional reduction in mortality was found [12]. However, the implication is still difficult because of the heterogeneity of the treatment arms. In contrast, a separate meta-analysis showed no survival advantage for adjuvant therapy in UICC II patients, only a modest 2% absolute rest reduction in 5 years survival, concluding that adjuvant therapy should not be routinely offered to patients with UICC II disease [13]. Hopefully, prospective data will help to settle this ongoing controversy. Upcoming results of European trials are awaited with interest. Until then, patients with node-negative disease should be evaluated for discussion about the available data so that they may participate in the treatment decision.

State-of-the-Art in Colorectal Cancer

For Adjuvant Treatment in UICC III Colon Cancer, FA/5-FU Is Not Enough

Several ongoing, randomized studies in colon cancer are attempting to define the role of new agents in adjuvant treatment. Recently reported data from the adjuvant Mosaic study may therefore gain further clinical plausibility. In this trial, oxaliplatin in the FOLFOX regimen induced an additional 23% relative risk reduction in a 3-year relapse-free survival compared with infusional FA/5-FU alone [14, 15]. However, the overall survival could not yet been shown to be significantly different (Fig. 2). Optimism also seems to be justified relative to the outcome of the pan-European trial on adjuvant colon cancer (PETACC3/V-307) comparing irinotecan with FA/5-FU (FOLFIRI) to infusional FA/5-FU alone. Other studies

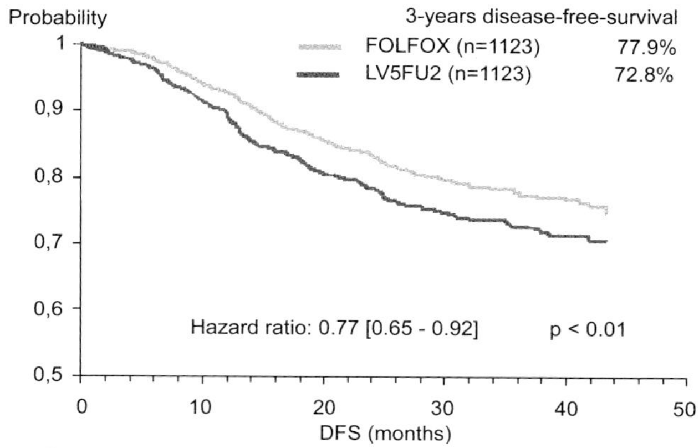

Figure 2. Disease-free survival by FOLFOX in adjuvant colon cancer

are the US/NCI Intergroup comparing weekly bolus FA/5-FU with or without irinotecan, while a French trial is comparing LV5FU2 alone and the same regimen plus irinotecan [16].

For Palliative Therapy, Irinotecan/Oxaliplatin with *Continuous* FA/5FU Is the Standard of Care

FA/5-FU remained the most widely used chemotherapeutic agent for treatment of metastatic disease. However, in recent years there were at least six large phase III trials which changed definitely the common treatment praxis. Four main studies of irinotecan or oxaliplatin combined with FA/5-FU versus FA/5-FU alone showed the significant superiority of the combination regimens in regard to progression-free survival (Table 1) [17–20]. Additionally, the overall survival was better for the irinotecan/FA/5-FU combinations [17, 18]. Very recently, Goldberg presented

Table 1. Main studies of irinotecan/oxaliplatin combined with FA/5-FU versus FA/5-FU alone

Regime	RR	PFS	OS	Author
Douillard/AIO	23%	4.4	14.1	Douillard
+ Irinotecan	35%	6.7	17.4	Lancet 2000
FL (Saltz)	21%	4.3	12.6	Saltz
+ Irinotecan	39%	7.0	14.8	NEJM 2000
LV5FU2	22%	6.6	14.7	De Gramont
+ Oxaliplatin	57%	9.0	16.2	JCO 2000
FUCM/LV	16%	6.1	19.9	Giacetti
+ Oxaliplatin	53%	8.7	19.4	JCO 2000

Table 2. Infusion regimens and overall survival according to Tournigand [9]

	Arm A		Arm B	
	FOLFIRI	FOLFOX	FOLFOX	FOLFIRI
n	109	89	111	69
RR	56%	15%*	54%	4%
PFS	8.5	4.2**	8.0	2.5 months
Total PFS	14.2 months		10.9 months	
OS	21.5 months		20.6 months	

*p=0.05; **p=0.003.
PFS, progression-free survival; OS, overall survival.

data that oxaliplatin/*continuous* FA/5-FU was superior to irinotecan/*bolus* FA/5-FU (IFL) [8]. Merging these data, it is of utmost importance to treat all metastatic colorectal cancer patients with combinations of irinotecan or oxaliplatin combined with *continuous* FA/5-FU (FOLFIRI or FOLFOX). In second-line therapy, patients should receive oxaliplatin after irinotecan or vice versa [9].

Giving all three drugs as sequences resulted in a median survival of more than 20 months. This has been reached in the randomized phase III trial by Tournigand and colleagues (Table 2) [9]. They compared the sequence FOLFIRI followed by FOLFOX with the reverse sequence in advanced colorectal cancer. Thus this trial is extremely important, as patients with both sequences had comparable survival rates with 21.5 months for FOLFIRI and FOLFOX versus 20.6 months allocated to FOLFOX and then FOLFIRI. Response rates in first-line chemotherapy were about 56% and 54%, respectively. As other studies have revealed, patients refractory to first-line treatment should definitely receive a second-line therapy, which is oxaliplatin after irinotecan and irinotecan after oxaliplatin [9].

In addition to the agents discussed, several other drugs have shown activity in CRC. These include raltitrexed, trimetrexate, ethyniluracil, MTA and S1 [21]. However, it is also likely (at least in the near future) that applications of these drugs will be based on combination regimens with irinotecan or oxaliplatin.

Future Challenges in Colorectal Cancer

At present, there are three immediate challenges for the treatment of colorectal cancer:

- Do oral fluoropyrimidines substitute 5-FU infusions without losing efficacy in the combinations with irinotecan/oxaliplatin?
- How much will the combined use of chemotherapy with molecular targeted agents against growth factor receptors improve treatment options?
- Do local procedures (i.e., local resection, RFTA, PEI) additionally induce a better long-term survival or even cure after downsizing with improved neoadjuvant chemotherapy?

Oral Fluoropyrimidines May Substitute Infusional 5-FU Regimens

Since the gastrointestinal mucosa contains dihydropyrimidine dehydrogenase (DPD) [22], one of the enzymes that catabolize 5-FU, it was questionable whether 5-FU can be given orally. It seemed that individuals who have greater concentrations of DPD in their intestinal mucosa inactivate more of 5-FU, which leads to lower plasma drug concentrations.

Strategies have been developed to improve the oral absorption of 5-FU including on the one hand the coadministration of drugs that inhibit the action of DPD [22] or on the other hand the oral administration of prodrugs of 5-FU that are absorbed intact and are activated metabolically after intestinal absorption. Three of these compounds have been compared individually with loading bolus FA/5-FU in prospectively randomized phase II and III trials as first-line therapy for colorectal cancer [14, 23].

Capecitabine represents a member of the prodrug group which is absorbed intact through the mucosa. In the liver, it is subsequently metabolized to doxifluridine. The enzyme thymidine phosphorylase, which is selectively expressed in tumor tissue, leads to the final conversion of doxifluridine into 5-FU, exploiting a higher 5-FU activity at the tumor site [24]. In clinical trials, capecitabine monotherapy has been demonstrated to have a favorable safety profile that is typical of infused 5-FU [24]. Given its toxicity profile (i.e. hand and foot syndrome), capecitabine acts biologically similarly to continuous 5-FU infusion [24, 26]. The majority of adverse events were mild to moderate, with a low incidence of alopecia and myelosuppression. With a dosage of 1,250 mg/qm twice daily, for 2 weeks of treatment followed by 1 week of rest, capecitabine has been approved by the FDA and most European nations as monotherapy of metastatic colorectal cancer [24]. Currently, combination protocols with oxaliplatin or irinotecan are under investigation in phase II and III trails to determine whether they can substitute their 5-FU combinations, like FOLFOX or FOLFIRI [14, 25–27].

Inhibition of Growth Factor Receptors and Their Signaling Will Be Integrated into the Chemotherapeutic Concepts

The regulation and expression of growth factors and/or their receptors have been extensively studied in the development and prognosis of colorectal cancer [28, 29]. The epidermal growth factor receptor (EGFr) is a commonly expressed transmembrane glycoprotein which signals pathways affecting mainly cellular proliferation. Similar to EGFR, the vascular endothelial growth factor (VEGF) receptor is localized in the cell membrane and consists of two transmembrane proteins [30]. After binding the ligands, receptor dimerization activates intracellular tyrosine kinases, triggering further signaling reactions regulating cell growth and survival. Tumor cells overexpressing EGFR or VEGFR may in addition produce endogenous receptor ligands, leading to an autocrine-stimulated proliferation. Thus, the blockade of growth factors and its signaling pathways are of mutual interest as targets for anticancer therapy.

Table 3. Response rates and overall survival by cetuximab plus irinotecan (CPT) in irinotecan-refractory colorectal cancer patients

	Cetux/Iri	Cetux
CR/PR	22.9%	10.8%
Tumor control	55.5%	32.4%
Survival		
Progression-free	4.1 months	1.5 months
Overall	8.6 months	6.9 months

In the laboratory, monoclonal antibodies to EGFR inhibited proliferation of cells that simultaneously produce both EGFR and its activating ligand. The Cetuximab (C225, Erbitux) is an immunoglobulin G1 chimeric antibody antagonizing the EGF receptor [31]. Based on its first scientific background, a phase II study evaluated the activity and safety of cetuximab plus irinotecan in irinotecan-refractory colorectal cancer patients, with a major response rate of 22.5%. Subsequently, Cunningham confirmed in the same patient population during a later randomized phase II trial that both cetuximab alone and cetuximab plus irinotecan had response rates of 10.8% for cetuximab alone and 22.9% for cetuximab plus irinotecan (Table 3) [32, 33]. Additionally, preliminary phase II data for the combination of cetuximab with oxalipaltin or irinotecan plus infusional FA/5-FU in first-line treatment in EGFR-positive metastatic colorectal cancer patients showed response rates and tumor control rates of up to 70% and 90%, respectively [34, 35]. In this study, secondary resections of liver metastases were possible in three patients and had been planned in another two [34]. Comparably, cetuximab combined with irinotecan/biweekly FA/5-FU achieved a tumor control in 89% in EGFR-positive colorectal cancer patients [35].

The most common toxicity of cetuximab was an acne-like rash, which occurrs in approximately 75% for patients. A recent meta-analysis investigated the relationship between the presence and severity of the rash and survival [33]. Here, skin rash could be identified as an important clinical gate marker of efficacy. Therefore, further prospective trials are initiated to evaluate skin rash and other biological markers for the dosing and response of such EGF antagonists.

Even as many VEGF or VEGFR antagonists (e.g., Iressa, PTK787, SU5416, SU6668) are currently under investigation [36], the VEGF antibody bevacizumab (rhuMab against VEGF-A), presented the most promising results in a randomized phase II study with three arms: bolus FA/5-FU (Roswell-Park schedule) without rhuMab VEGF, with 5 or 10 mg/kg rhuMab VEGF-A biweekly in metastatic colorectal cancer [37]. With FA/5-FU plus 5 mg/kg bevacizumab, the response rate was 40%, progression-free survival was 9.0 months, and median survival was 21.5 months, both higher than with FA/5-FU alone or with FA/5-FU combined with the high dose of 10 mg/kg rhuMab VEGF [37].

Recently, impressive results of the first phase III trial in 813 chemonaive metastatic colorectal cancer patients randomized to irinotecan/*bolus* FA/5-FU (IFL) versus IFL plus bevacizumab were reported (Table 4) [38]. The response

Table 4. Irinotecan/*bolus*FA/5-FU (IFL) versus IFL plus bevacizumab (BV) in chemonaive metastatic colorectal cancer patients

	IFL/placebo (*n*=412)	IFL/BV (*n*=403)
Overall survival	15.6 months	20.3 months
Progression-free survival	6.2 months	10.6 months
Response rate	35%	45%
Hypertension	2.3%	11%

rate (35% vs. 45%), progression-free survival (6.2 vs. 10.6 months) and overall survival (15.6 vs. 20.3 months) were all in favor of the combination. There were no additional significant toxicities, except of grade III hypertension with bevacizumab (10.9% vs. 2.3%), but no significant increase in bleeding or thrombotic events. Thus, the concept of anti-angiogenic treatment has been proven for the first time in a phase III study [38].

Neoadjuvant Chemotherapy May Additionally Improve Individual and Overall Survival

Increasing numbers of liver metastases may now be considered surgically resectable [28]. Various factors explain this trend [39]: progress in surgical techniques, better knowledge of the functional anatomy of the liver, detection of metastases at an earlier stage, introduction of new therapeutic approaches (e.g., cryosurgery, radiofrequency ablation) and use of improved chemotherapy before resection [40–43]. This neoadjuvant chemotherapy approach with FA/5-FU plus oxaliplatin or irinotecan [44] reduced the size of metastases, so that additional 50%–60% of metastases that previously seemed unresectable could be resected [39, 44, 45]. After complete surgery of (liver) metastasis, approximately 30% of patients can be expected to survive 5 years or longer [46]. Thus, the advantage of better downsizing may also have an effect on the outcome of the patient population itself. Randomized prospective trials testing this neoadjuvant chemotherapy approach further with FA/5-FU plus irinotecan or oxaliplatin are currently ongoing [47].

A recent study showed that neoadjuvant chemotherapy with oxaliplatin-based therapy may induce sinusoidal obstructions in the liver, associated with sinusoidal fibrosis and veno-occlusive lesions, occasionally with nodular or regenerative hyperplasia [48]. To our knowledge, these changes after oxaliplatin have not been systematically investigated in other chemotherapeutic protocols. As no targeted liver biopsy studies have yet been performed in patients who received oxaliplatin-based chemotherapy, it is difficult to justify the role of these new-found abnormalities. To date, oxaliplatin has proven to be safe and its side effects have been easy to manage with appropriate awareness from the patient and care providers. However, as at least three-quarters of patients had specific liver lesions after oxaliplatin, the clinical consequences of these sinusoidal lesions need to be reevaluated with respect to the potential impairment of liver regeneration after extended resections [48].

References

1. Parkin DM (2001) Global cancer statistics in the year 2000. Lancet Oncol 2:533–543
2. Landis SH, Murray T, Bolden S, Wingo PA (1999) Cancer statistics, 1999. CA Cancer J Clin 49:8–31
3. Anonymous (1992) Modulation of fluorouracil by leucovorin in patients with advanced colorectal cancer: evidence in terms of response rate. Advanced Colorectal Cancer Meta-Analysis Project. J Clin Oncol 10:896–903
4. Poon MA et al (1989) Biochemical modulation of fluorouracil: evidence of significant improvement of survival and quality of life in patients with advanced colorectal carcinoma. J Clin Oncol 7:1407–1418
5. Poon MA et al (1991) Biochemical modulation of fluorouracil with leucovorin: confirmatory evidence of improved therapeutic efficacy in advanced colorectal cancer. J Clin Oncol 9:1967–1972
6. Patel K et al (2004) Weekly 5-fluorouracil and leucovorin: achieving lower toxicity with higher dose-intensity in adjuvant chemotherapy after colorectal cancer resection. Ann Oncol 15:568–573
7. Anonymous (1998) Efficacy of intravenous continuous infusion of fluorouracil compared with bolus administration in advanced colorectal cancer. Meta-analysis Group In Cancer. J Clin Oncol 16:301–308
8. Goldberg RM et al (2004) A randomized controlled trial of fluorouracil plus leucovorin, irinotecan, and oxaliplatin combinations in patients with previously untreated metastatic colorectal cancer. J Clin Oncol 22:23–30
9. Tournigand C et al (2004) FOLFIRI followed by FOLFOX6 or the reverse sequence in advanced colorectal cancer: a randomized GERCOR study. J Clin Oncol 22:229–237
10. Moertel CG (1994) Chemotherapy for colorectal cancer. N Engl J Med 330:1136–1142
11. Maughan TS (2001) Adjuvant chemotherapy for colorectal cancer. Br J Cancer 85:1422–1424
12. Mamounas E et al (1999) Comparative efficacy of adjuvant chemotherapy in patients with Dukes' B versus Dukes' C colon cancer: results from four National Surgical Adjuvant Breast and Bowel Project adjuvant studies (C-01, C-02, C-03, and C-04). J Clin Oncol 17:1349–1355
13. Anonymous (1999) Efficacy of adjuvant fluorouracil and folinic acid in B2 colon cancer. International Multicentre Pooled Analysis of B2 Colon Cancer Trials (IMPACT B2) Investigators. J Clin Oncol 17:1356–63
14. Maung K (2003) Integrating oxaliplatin and capecitabine in adjuvant therapy of high-risk colorectal cancer. Clin Colorectal Cancer 3:150–153
15. Andre T, Boni C, Mounedji-Boudiaf L, Navarro M, Tabernero J, Hickish T, Topham C, Zaninelli M, Clingan P, Bridgewater J, Tabah-Fisch I, de Gramont A; Multicenter International Study of Oxaliplatin/5-Fluorouracil/Leucovorin in the Adjuvant Treatment of Colon Cancer (MOSAIC) Investigators (2004) Oxaliplatin, fluorouracil, and leucovorin as adjuvant treatment for colon cancer. N Engl J Med 350:2343–2351
16. Wils J, O'Dwyer P, Labianca R (2001) Adjuvant treatment of colorectal cancer at the turn of the century: European and US perspectives. Ann Oncol 12:13–22
17. Saltz LB et al (2000) Irinotecan plus fluorouracil and leucovorin for metastatic colorectal cancer. Irinotecan Study Group. N Engl J Med 343:905–914
18. Douillard JY et al (2000) Irinotecan combined with fluorouracil compared with fluorouracil alone as first-line treatment for metastatic colorectal cancer: a multicentre randomised trial. Lancet 355:1041–1047
19. Giacchetti S et al (2000) Phase III multicenter randomized trial of oxaliplatin added to chronomodulated fluorouracil-leucovorin as first-line treatment of metastatic colorectal cancer. J Clin Oncol 18:136–47
20. De Gramont A et al (2000) Leucovorin and fluorouracil with or without oxaliplatin as first-line treatment in advanced colorectal cancer. J Clin Oncol 18:2938–2947
21. Sobrero A et al (2000) New directions in the treatment of colorectal cancer: a look to the future. Eur J Cancer 36:559–566
22. Heslin MJ et al (2003) Dihydropyrimidine dehydrogenase (DPD) rapidly regenerates after inactivation by eniluracil (GW776C85) in primary and metastatic colorectal cancer. Cancer Chemother Pharmacol 52:399–404
23. Wilke H (2002) Future treatment options with capecitabine in solid tumours. Eur J Cancer 38 [Suppl 2]:21–25

24. Van Cutsem E et al (2001) Oral capecitabine compared with intravenous fluorouracil plus leucovorin in patients with metastatic colorectal cancer: results of a large phase III study. J Clin Oncol 19:4097–4106
25. Grothey A, Schmoll HJ (2001) New chemotherapy approaches in colorectal cancer. Curr Opin Oncol 13:275–286
26. Rothenberg ML (2002) Current status of capecitabine in the treatment of colorectal cancer. Oncology (Huntingt) 16:16–22
27. Kerr D (2002) Capecitabine/irinotecan in colorectal cancer: European early-phase data and planned trials. Oncology (Huntingt) 16:12–15
28. Folprecht G, Kohne CH (2004) The role of new agents in the treatment of colorectal cancer. Oncology 66:1–17
29. Baselga J, Albanell J (2002) Epithelial growth factor receptor interacting agents. Hematol Oncol Clin North Am 16:1041–1063
30. Tebbutt NC, Cattell E, Midgley R, Cunningham D, Kerr D (2002) Systemic treatment of colorectal cancer. Eur J Cancer 38:1000–1015
31. Herbst RS, Kim ES, Harari PM (2001) IMC-C225, an anti-epidermal growth factor receptor monoclonal antibody, for treatment of head and neck cancer. Expert Opin Biol Ther 1:719–732
32. Saltz LB et al (2004) Phase II trial of cetuximab in patients with refractory colorectal cancer that expresses the epidermal growth factor receptor. J Clin Oncol 22:1201–1208
33. Cunningham D, Humblet Y, Siena S, Khayat D, Bleiberg H, Santoro A, Bets D, Mueser M, Harstrick A, Verslype C, Chau I, Van Cutsem EN (2004) Cetuximab monotherapy and cetuximab plus irinotecan in irinotecan-refractory metastatic colorectal cancer. Engl J Med 351:337–345
34. Taberno JM et al (2004) An international phase II study of cetuximab in combination with oxaliplatin/5-fluorouracil (5-FU)/folinic acid (FA) (FOLFOX-4) in the first-line treatment of patients with metastatic colorectal cancer (CRC) expressing Epidermal Growth Factor Receptor (EGFR). Preliminary results (abstract). Proceedings of ASCO 22:3512
35. Rougier P et al (2004) Cetuximab+FOLFIRI as first-line treatment for metastatic colorectal CA (abstract). Proceedings of ASCO, 22:3513
36. Douglass EC (2003) Development of ZD1839 in colorectal cancer. Semin Oncol 30:17–22
37. Kabbinavar F et al (2003) Phase II, randomized trial comparing bevacizumab plus fluorouracil (FU)/leucovorin (LV) with FU/LV alone in patients with metastatic colorectal cancer. J Clin Oncol 21:60–65
38. Hurwitz HLF et al (2004) Bevacizumab plus irinotecan, fluorouracil, and leucovorin for metastatic colorectal cancer.. N Engl J Med 350:2335–2342
39. Bismuth H et al (1996) Resection of nonresectable liver metastases from colorectal cancer after neoadjuvant chemotherapy. Ann Surg 224:509–520; discussion 520–522
40. Giovannini M Percutaneous alcohol ablation for liver metastasis. Semin Oncol 29:192–5 (2002)
41. Livraghi T et al (2003) Treatment of focal liver tumors with percutaneous radio-frequency ablation: complications encountered in a multicenter study. Radiology 226:441–451
42. Kessler A et al (2002) Minimally invasive techniques in the treatment of liver tumors. Isr Med Assoc J 4:1106–1110
43. Scaife CL et al (2003) Feasibility of adjuvant hepatic arterial infusion of chemotherapy after radiofrequency ablation with or without resection in patients with hepatic metastases from colorectal cancer. Ann Surg Oncol 10:348–354
44. Pozzo C, Basso M, Cassano A, Quirino M, Schinzari G, Trigila N, Vellone M, Giuliante F, Nuzzo G, Barone C (2004) Neoadjuvant treatment of unresectable liver desease with irinotecan and 5-fluorouracil plus folinic acid in colorectal cancer patients. Ann Oncol 15:933–939
45. Giacchetti S et al (1999) Long-term survival of patients with unresectable colorectal cancer liver metastases following infusional chemotherapy with 5-fluorouracil, leucovorin, oxaliplatin and surgery. Ann Oncol 10:663–669
46. Penna C, Nordlinger B (2003) Surgery and local treatments of liver metastases from colorectal cancer: how to improve results. Scand J Surg 92:90–96
47. Lorenz M et al (1999) Relevance of neoadjuvant and adjuvant treatment for patients with resectable liver metastases of colorectal carcinoma. Langenbecks Arch Surg 384:328–338
48. Rubbia-Brandt L et al (2004) Severe hepatic sinusoidal obstruction associated with oxaliplatin-based chemotherapy in patients with metastatic colorectal cancer. Ann Oncol 15:460–466

Active Specific Immunotherapy in Colon Cancer

A. J. M. van den Eertwegh

A.J.M. van den Eertwegh (✉)
Department of Medical Oncology, Vrije Universiteit Medical Center,
De Boelelaan 1117, 1081 HV Amsterdam, The Netherlands
e-mail: vandeneertwegh@Vumc.nl

Abstract

Colorectal cancer is one of the leading causes of cancer-related mortality. After a series of clinical trials, the adjuvant 5-FU-based chemotherapy has established a definitive role in the management of stage III colon cancer. While the precise role for chemotherapy in stage II disease remains under investigation, less toxic treatment modalities such as active specific immunotherapy (ASI) have emerged as potentially attractive alternatives. In a randomized trial it was demonstrated that ASI, using autologous tumor cells and BCG, had a significant clinical benefit in the adjuvant treatment of stage II colon cancer. In addition, it was found that the delayed-type cutaneous hypersensitivity reactions (DTH) against autologous cells correlated significantly with survival, confirming its suitability for immunomonitoring. Nowadays, 5-FU-based chemotherapy is a standard treatment for stage III colon cancer and because there is preclinical evidence for synergism between chemotherapy and ASI, we performed a phase II study to investigate whether the combined treatment with 5-FU and ASI is tolerable and feasible. We demonstrated that 5-FU treatment hardly affected the DTH response against autologous tumor cells and that the combination treatment was well tolerated. A randomized phase III trial is now warranted to show that the combination of ASI and chemotherapy is superior to chemotherapy alone.

Colon Cancer

Colorectal cancer is a leading cause of cancer death in Western societies [5]. Most patients present with surgically resectable disease, but unfortunately in a significant number of these patients metastases will occur in the years following surgery. Only a low percentage of patients with recurrent disease may be cured by radical resection of metastases and the majority will ultimately die of their disease [5]. In general, surgical cure of colorectal cancer is only possible if the malignancy has not spread beyond the regional lymph nodes. Stage II colon cancer patients, whose

Recent Results in Cancer Research, Vol. 165

tumors invade through the muscularis propria or serosa, have a 5-year survival rate of approximately 75%, while the survival rate of stage III patients with lymph node metastases is between 25% and 60%, depending on the number of positive nodes [5]. Different types of adjuvant treatments have been developed as auxiliary weapons to surgery aiming at eradicating the so-called micro-metastases [19]. So far, chemotherapy has been the only modality that has evolved to a standard treatment for stage III colon cancer. Preclinical studies suggest that immunotherapy is most effective in patients with low residual disease [3], and although the clinical results are very promising, particularly for ASI, this new modality is not yet a standard adjuvant treatment for colon cancer [8].

Adjuvant Chemotherapy

The early adjuvant trials were retrospective and under-powered and failed to show any therapeutic benefit with respect to recurrence rate or survival [4]. In 1990 the intergroup trial showed that adjuvant treatment with 5-FU/levamisole resulted in 33% reduction in the odds of death and a 41% decrease in recurrences as compared with surgery alone or surgery plus levamisole [16]. These results were confirmed by three large randomized phase III trials investigating 5-FU and leucovorin as adjuvant treatment [17, 20, 25]. Nowadays, 5-FU/leucovorin is considered as standard adjuvant therapy for stage III colon cancer patients.

For the adjuvant treatment of stage II colon cancer, the precise role of chemotherapy is still not defined. The intergroup 0035 trial failed to demonstrate a survival benefit from 5-FU/leucovorin chemotherapy in stage II patients, although a reduction in recurrences comparable with that documented for stage III patients was observed [18]. Even in an international multicenter pooled analysis of stage II colon cancer trials with a total accrual of 1,016 patients, no significant benefit in overall survival could be demonstrated [7]. Several possible reasons for this discrepancy in clinical benefit have been suggested. Because of the relatively low frequency of death in stage II patients, most adjuvant trials contain an insufficient number of patients to be able to address the study's primary questions with adequate statistical power. Patients participating in these trials are relatively old and have co-morbidity and consequently a relatively large percentage of non-cancer-related deaths. This dilutes the observed survival difference and makes the detection of a significant survival benefit very difficult.

To circumvent this problem, future studies should focus on stage II colon cancer patients with high-risk prognostic factors (e.g., microsatellite instability and p53 mutation, tumor-positive sentinel node), to make it easier to identify a subset of patients that may benefit from adjuvant chemotherapy.

Adjuvant Immunotherapy

Immunotherapeutical approaches for colorectal cancer have substantially evolved over the past years from treatments with nonspecific immune stimulants to more tumor-specific therapies. Nonspecific immune stimulating therapies such as Bacillus Calmette-Guérin (BCG) [21] and levamisole [16, 17] were tested in randomized trials and were found to have no clinical benefit in the treatment of high-risk colon cancer patients. Therefore, research is now moving towards more tumor-specific immunotherapies such as colon cancer-specific antibodies [9] or active vaccination strategies. In this article we will review the promising results of ASI, using autologous tumor cells and BCG, in the adjuvant treatment of colon cancer.

Adjuvant Active Specific Immunotherapy

ASI differs from nonspecific immune-based therapies in that the goal is not general but rather specific activation of the immune system to eliminate tumor cells without affecting surrounding normal tissue [22]. It is generally assumed that specific vaccination should result in activation of the two main arms of the immune system, namely the humoral (antibody-producing B cells) and the cellular immune response (T cells). B cells recognize the tumor antigens in their native protein state at the cell surface, whereas T lymphocytes recognize proteins as peptide fragments, presented in the context of major histocompatibility complex (MHC) antigens on the surface of the tumor cells. There are two types of T cells, CD4 and CD8, which recognize antigens through a specific T-cell receptor. These antigens are presented by a group of specialized cells called antigen-presenting cells (APCs). A variety of cells are capable of processing and presenting antigens, including B cells, monocytes, macrophages, and dendritic cells (DCs). DCs are the most efficient APCs, expressing costimulatory molecules and high levels of MHC class I and class II molecules required for the activation of CD8- and CD4-positive T cells, respectively. CD4-positive T cells, also called helper T cells, secrete cytokines that regulate B cells, cytotoxic cells and other immune cells, but can also have a cytotoxic activity. CD8-positive cytotoxic T cells (CTL) are at this moment considered to be the most potent cells to eradicate specifically tumor cells. The purpose of most vaccination strategies is to activate this specific subset of T cells. DCs are essential for the specific activation of T cells and these cells are found in the lymphoid organs, blood and skin. The most convenient way to load these APCs with tumor antigens is via an intradermal injection. An adjuvant such as BCG is co-administered to activate the skin DCs and these APCs will subsequently migrate to the draining lymph nodes, where they will encounter and activate the tumor-specific T cells.

A logical strategy of immunization is the use of whole tumor-cell preparations. One of the main advantages of this approach is that all potential tumor antigens of the patients' carcinoma are presented to the immune system. Hanna et al. established a guinea pig hepatocarcinoma model for the study of ASI as adjuvant treatment [10]. They demonstrated the value of a vaccine prepared from viable metabolically active tumor cells mixed with BCG organisms. A correct ratio of BCG organisms to tumor cells and an optimal vaccination schedule enabled them to control hematogenous and lymphatic metastases from surgically excised primary tumors.

On the basis of these preclinical studies, Hoover et al. conducted a trial using irradiated autologous tumor cells and BCG in patients with stage II and stage III colorectal cancer [14]. After surgical resection of their primary tumors, patients were randomized to vaccination or observation and stratified by both disease type and stage. Three to 4 weeks after surgery, patients were vaccinated with two weekly vaccinations with tumor cells and BCG. One week later, a third vaccine was administered, not containing BCG. An intention-to-treat analysis showed no significant clinical benefit, but a subgroup analysis of overall and disease-free survival in colon cancer patients showed a significant trend for ASI being superior to surgery alone. Side effects were minimal and the most prominent were ulcerations at the site of the first two vaccinations caused by BCG. Immunized patients showed DTH reactions to autologous tumor cells that were stronger than background responses to autologous mucosal cells, suggesting the presence of tumor-specific immunity. The absence of a survival benefit in the rectal cancer group was thought to be caused by the radiotherapy that was given close to the vaccination-draining lymph nodes. However, it is important to realize that because of the low number of vaccinated rectal cancer patients, this low-powered study does not allow a reliable analysis of the efficacy of ASI in rectal cancer. Nowadays, rectal cancer patients are being irradiated before removal of the carcinoma, which precludes ASI in its current form.

These promising results were reason to conduct a large phase III study with stage II and stage III colon cancer patients under the auspices of the Eastern Cooperative Oncology Group (ECOG) [13]. This study differed from the Hoover study in that each site performed its own vaccine manufacturing because of large numbers of subjects and wide geographic distribution of the sites involved. From a practical point of view, this meant that some centers were making only a few vaccines in a year. The fact that these centers were not making vaccines on a daily basis could have had a negative effect on the quality of vaccines. In an intent-to-treat analysis of all randomized patients, there were no significant differences between the two treatment arms in time to recurrence or overall survival. In the ECOG study, 12% of all vaccines failed to meet quality control specifications (cell number/viability), and 15% of the vaccinated patients failed to have adequate DTH reactions. It was hypothesized that the poor quality of a part of the vaccinations could have caused the disappointing results of this study. Therefore, a survival analysis was performed on patients who were treated with vaccines that met standardized criteria and developed antitumor immunity (DTH response to third vaccine >5 mm) and compared to control patients. In this subgroup analysis, a significant improvement in overall survival was demonstrated in patients treated with ASI, suggesting that optimal immunization strategies are essential for a successful adjuvant treatment of colon cancer patients. This was supported by the observation that the size of DTH response to autologous tumor cells correlated with survival, which was also observed by our group in metastatic melanoma [1]. The development of a DTH response could also reflect the immune status of patients. However, in a separate study it was demonstrated that stage II + III colon cancer patients had normal skin reactions against recall antigens, indicating that these patients with no or a low tumor burden had a normal immune status, which makes the latter possibility not so likely [13].

A third phase III study was conducted by the Vrijt University Medical Center Amsterdam in the Netherlands involving 254 patients with stage II and stage III colon cancer [24]. This pivotal study differed from the previous clinical trials in that treated patients received a booster with irradiated tumor cells alone, administered 6 months after surgical resection. In contrast to the previous study, a centralized manufacturing laboratory supported the 12 participating hospitals, which prepared 98% quality-approved vaccines, and 97% of the vaccinated patients had DTH responses greater than 5 mm. In an intent-to-treat analysis, ASI significantly reduced the rate of disease recurrence by 44% in patients with stage II and stage III colon cancer, but the overall survival was not significantly better. The major impact was seen in stage II disease in which there was 61% risk reduction for recurrences and a trend toward improved overall survival. These data may indicate that the centralized method of vaccine manufacturing, or a facility that makes vaccines on a daily basis, is very important for vaccine quality and successful immunization. It is also possible that the extra vaccination after 6 months may have contributed to the positive results in the latter trial. The relatively low number of stage II patients in this trial did not make it possible to detect a small survival difference. Furthermore, the absence of a significant survival benefit could also be explained by the same arguments as were discussed for the adjuvant chemotherapy trials. The relatively high non-colon-cancer-related mortality in this aged patient group together with the relatively good overall survival rate of stage II colon cancer patients requires a very large randomized study to detect a survival benefit for any adjuvant treatment.

Therefore, a meta-analysis was performed that included the above-mentioned three randomized trials [12]. In the intent-to-treat meta-analysis of all 723 patients who received either a three- or a four-vaccine regimen, recurrence-free survival was significantly improved by ASI. In the meta-analysis of patients who met quality control specifications and protocol eligibility, recurrence-free survival was significantly improved and disease-specific survival approached significance when compared with controls. In general, patients with a distant recurrence will eventually die from colon cancer. However, even though recurrences were significantly reduced by ASI, no significant survival benefit could be demonstrated in the intent-to-treat meta-analysis, which might be explained by the same statistical difficulties for chemotherapy trials in stage II colon cancer, as discussed above. In conclusion, these studies showed that ASI has minimal side effects and that the most pronounced clinical benefit can be seen in stage II colon cancer.

In stage III colon cancer patients, ASI did not result in a significant clinical benefit, which could be explained by the lack of statistical power of these studies. Furthermore, the residual tumor load in stage III patients is probably larger than in stage II patients, which could be relevant since it is known that ASI is more effective in a minimal residual disease setting [10].

In preclinical models, ASI and chemotherapy were shown to have a synergistic antitumor effect [12]. Apart from the capacity to directly destroy micro-metastases, ASI has been demonstrated to disrupt the characteristically compact structure of metastatic foci, enabling chemotherapy to reach deeper into the cancer tissue. Furthermore, chemotherapy reduces the tumor burden, thereby increasing the chances of ASI to eliminate the residual malignant cells. In preparation for a large phase III trial, we performed a feasibility study on the combination of ASI and chemotherapy in stage III colon cancer. We showed that the combination ASI and 5-FU/leucovorin did not result in more toxicity and that the ASI-induced antitumor immunity (DTH response) was hardly impaired by consecutive chemotherapy [2]. A randomized trial should prove that these two modalities have a synergistic antitumor effect.

Future Developments

One of the consequences of using colon tumor tissue for the production of autologous tumor cell vaccines is the inherent presence of small amounts of the normal colonic bacterial flora in the vaccines. The assumption that this does not present a clinically relevant threat to the health of the patients receiving the vaccines is supported by the observation that no serious infections have occurred after more than 2,000 colon tumor vaccinations in the VU University Medical Center in the past 14 years. However, recent guidelines of the American Food and Drug Administration prescribe that anything that is injected into a patient needs to be sterile. To obtain sterility we slightly changed the production process of the vaccines. An important side effect of the adjuvant BCG is ulceration that can last more than 3 months. After healing, a scar at the site of vaccination remains visible. The last decade new potent adjuvants were developed which were in preclinical studies at least as good as BCG. Nowadays most vaccination studies use granulocyte-macrophage colony stimulating factor (GM-CSF) as an immunostimulating agent. This cytokine is able to recruit Langerhans cells and promote the maturation of these cells into potent APCs through up-regulation of MHC class II, co-stimulatory molecules and cytokine production [6]. It increases antibody responses and cellular immunity after immunization. Another interesting adjuvant is Cytosine-phosphate Guanine (CpG) 7909, a single-stranded phosphorothioate oligodeoxynucleotide (ODN), which is a potent stimulator of both the innate and adaptive immune response [15]. CpG 7909 is a very potent adjuvant that promotes Th1 humoral and cellular immune responses with very little toxicity, particularly no ulcerations. Besides its enhancing effect on antibody production, CpG 7909 promotes the effector arm of the humoral response as well. The combination of GM-CSF and CPG7909 was found to give superior antitumor-immunity as compared to GM-CSF alone [23]. In the near future, we will investigate in a phase II trial whether the combination of CPG 7909 and GM-CSF at least equals the results of our previous studies using BCG alone. For this purpose the DTH response against autologous tumor cells will be used as measure for antitumor immunity. If results of the phase II study show that modified ASI is at least as effective as found in previous studies, we will proceed with a randomized trial in stage II colon cancer comparing modified ASI with no treatment.

Conclusions

It took several decades before the toxic adjuvant treatment with 5-FU/leucovorin was established as a standard treatment for stage III colon cancer. Specific immunotherapies have a low toxicity profile and randomized clinical trials suggest a promising role for ASI in the adjuvant treatment of colon cancer. ASI with autologous tumor cells have been investigated in three randomized trials and a meta-analysis confirmed that ASI has the greatest clinical in stage II colon cancer. Because of new guidelines of the American Food and Drug Administration requiring sterile vaccines and the emerging of new potent adjuvants, it is expected that a new formulation of vaccines will be developed and studied in a large randomized trial to demonstrate its efficacy in colon cancer. In stage III colon cancer, it was demonstrated that a combined modality treatment with ASI and chemotherapy is well tolerated and that chemotherapy hardly affects the antitumor immunity induced by the tumor cell vaccination. A randomized phase III trial is warranted to show that the combination of ASI and chemotherapy is superior to chemotherapy alone.

References

1. Baars A, Claessen AM, van den Eertwegh AJ, Gall HE, Stam AG, Meijer S, Giaccone G, Meijer CJ, Scheper RJ, Wagstaff J, Vermorken JB, Pinedo HM (2000) Skin tests predict survival after autologous tumor cell vaccination in metastatic melanoma: experience in 81 patients. Ann Oncol 11:965–970
2. Baars A, Claessen AM, Wagstaff J, Giaccone G, Scheper RJ, Meijer S et al (2002) A phase II study of active specific immunotherapy and 5-FU/leucovorin as adjuvant therapy for stage III colon carcinoma. Br J Cancer 86:1230–1234
3. Berd D (1998) Cancer vaccines: reborn or just recycled? Semin Oncol 25:605–610
4. Buyse M, Zeleniuch-Jacquotte A, Chalmers TC (1988) Adjuvant therapy of colorectal cancer. Why we still don't know. JAMA 259:3571–3578
5. DeVita VT, Hellman S, Rosenberg, SA (2001) Cancer. Principles & practice of oncology, 6th edn. Lippincott Williams & Wilkins, Baltimore
6. Disis ML, Bernhard H, Shiota FM, Hand SL, Gralow JR et al (1996) Granulocyte-macrophage colony-stimulating factor: an effective adjuvant for protein and peptide-based vaccines. Blood 88:202–210
7. No authors listed (1999) Efficacy of adjuvant fluorouracil and folinic acid in B2 colon cancer. International Multicentre Pooled Analysis of B2 Colon Cancer Trials (IMPACT B2) Investigators. J Clin Oncol 17:1356–1363
8. Foon KA (2001) Immunotherapy for colorectal cancer. Curr Oncol Rep 3:116–126
9. Green MC, Murray JL, Hortobagyi GN (2000) Monoclonal antibody therapy for solid tumors. Cancer Treat Rev 26:269–286
10. Hanna MG Jr, Brandhorst JS, Peters LC (1979) Active specific immunotherapy of residual micrometastasis: an evaluation of sources, doses and ratios of BCG with tumor cells. Cancer Immunother 7:165–173
11. Hanna MG Jr, Key ME (1982) Immunotherapy of metastases enhances subsequent chemotherapy. Science 217:367–369

12. Hanna MG, Hoover HC, Vermorken JB, Harris JE, and Pinedo HM (2001) Adjuvant active specific immunotherapy of stage II and stage III colon cancer with an autologous tumor cell vaccine: first randomized phase III trials show promise. Vaccine 19:2576–2582
13. Harris JE, Ryan L, Hoover HC Jr, Stuart RK, Oken MM, Benson AB III, Mansour E, Haller DG, Manola J, Hanna MG Jr (2000) Adjuvant active specific immunotherapy for stage II and III colon cancer with an autologous tumor cell vaccine: Eastern Cooperative Oncology Group Study E5283. J Clin Oncol 18:148–157
14. Hoover HC Jr, Brandhorst JS, Peters LC, Surdyke MG, Takeshita Y, Madariaga J, Muenz LR, Hanna MG Jr (1993) Adjuvant active specific immunotherapy for human colorectal cancer: 6.5-year median follow-up of a phase III prospectively randomized trial. J Clin Oncol 11:90–399
15. Krieg AM (2002) CpG motifs in bacterial DNA and their immune effects. Ann Rev Immunol 20:709–760
16. Moertel CG, Fleming TR, Macdonald JS, Haller DG, Laurie JA, Goodman PJ, Ungerleider JS, Emerson WA, Tormey DC, Glick JH et al. (1990) Levamisole and fluorouracil for adjuvant therapy of resected colon carcinoma. N Engl J Med 322:352–358
17. Moertel CG, Fleming TR, Macdonald JS, Haller DG, Laurie JA, Tangen CM, Ungerleider JS, Emerson WA, Tormey DC, Glick JH et al (1995) Fluorouracil plus levamisole as effective adjuvant therapy after resection of stage III colon carcinoma: a final report. Ann Intern Med 122:321–326
18. Moertel CG, Fleming TR, Macdonald JS, Haller DG, Laurie JA, Tangen CM, Ungerleider JS, Emerson WA, Tormey DC, Glick JH et al (1995) Intergroup study of fluorouracil plus levamisole as adjuvant therapy for stage II/Dukes' B2 colon cancer. J Clin Oncol 13:2936–2943
19. Moore HC, Haller DG (1999) Adjuvant therapy of colon cancer. Semin Oncol 26:545–555
20. O'Connell MJ, Mailliard JA, Kahn MJ, Macdonald JS, Haller DG, Mayer RJ, Wieand HS (1997) Controlled trial of fluorouracil and low-dose leucovorin given for 6 months as postoperative adjuvant therapy for colon cancer. J Clin Oncol 15:246–250
21. Panettiere FJ, Goodman PJ, Costanzi JJ, Cruz AB Jr, Vaitkevicius VK, McCracken JD, Brownlee RW, Laufman L, Stephens RL, Bonnet J et al (1988) Adjuvant therapy in large bowel adenocarcinoma: long-term results of a Southwest Oncology Group Study. J Clin Oncol 6:947–954
22. Pardoll DM (1998) Cancer vaccines. Nat Med 4:525–531
23. Sandler AD, Chihara H, Kobayashi G, Zhu X, Miller MA, Scott DL, Krieg AM (2003) CpG oligonucleotides enhance the tumor antigen-specific immune response of a granulocyte macrophage colony-stimulating factor-based vaccine strategy in neuroblastoma. Cancer Res 63:394–399
24. Vermorken JB, Claessen AM, van Tinteren H, Gall HE, Ezinga R, Meijer S, Scheper RJ, Meijer CJ, Bloemena E, Ransom JH, Hanna MG Jr, Pinedo HM (1999) Active specific immunotherapy for stage II and stage III human colon cancer: a randomised trial. Lancet 353:345–350
25. Wolmark N, Rockette H, Fisher B, Wickerham DL, Redmond C, Fisher ER, Jones J, Mamounas EP, Ore L, Petrelli NJ et al (1993) The benefit of leucovorin-modulated fluorouracil as postoperative adjuvant therapy for primary colon cancer: results from National Surgical Adjuvant Breast and Bowel Project protocol C-03. J Clin Oncol 11:1879–1887

Radiofrequency Ablation in Metastatic Disease

Andreas Lubienski

A. Lubienski (✉)
Department of Diagnostic Radiology, University Hospital Heidelberg,
Im Neuenheimer Feld 110, 69120 Heidelberg, Germany
e-mail: lubienski@med.uni-heidelberg.de

Abstract

The liver is the most common site of metastas from colorectal cancer. Hepatic metastases are the major cause of morbidity and mortality in those patients. Surgical resection provides the greatest potential for cure in patients with secondary liver tumors but can be offered to only a small number of patients (5%–20%). In selected patients image-guided radiofrequency ablation (RFA) takes over the role as curative treatment option, especially in patients who are technically not eligible for surgery. Technical aspects, criteria for patient selection, aspects concerning follow-up imaging and results of percutaneous radiofrequency ablation in liver metastases from colorectal cancer are discussed.

Introduction

Colorectal cancer is one of the most frequent solid tumors, especially in Western countries, being responsible for approximately 10% of cancer-related deaths [1]. With regard to liver metastases, synchronous development accounts for approximately 15%–25% [2]. In about 60% of all patients with colorectal cancer liver metastases occur [2]. Surgical resection provides the greatest potential for cure in patients with secondary liver tumors but can be offered to only a small number of patients (5%–20%) [3]. Survival rates range from 25% to 40% at 5 years [3] with an operative mortality to about 2% in patients that undergo extended hepatic resection [4]. In colorectal liver metastases, survival ranges from 4.5 to 15 months, which can be prolonged by liver resection with curative intent to about 37 months [5, 6]. In about 60%–75% of all resected patients (R0 resection), recurrent liver metastases develop [7]. Under these circumstances, any technique capable of destroying hepatic metastases that surgery cannot excise is highly desirable. Systemic chemotherapy for liver metastases results in less than 25% of patients at best achieving a response; especially significant improvements in patient survival are marginal [8]. Local ablative techniques are deemed to destroy viable liver tumor, which leads

Recent Results in Cancer Research, Vol. 165

to longer survival and potential cure due to local tumor control. Several interstitial treatment modalities such as radiofrequency ablation (RFA), laser-induced thermotherapy (LITT), microwave ablation (PMCT), high-intensity focused ultrasound (HIFU), cryoablation and percutaneous ethanol injection (PEI) have been introduced as therapy options for nonresectable colorectal liver metastases. This review will focus on the role of RFA in the treatment of hepatic metastasis from colorectal cancer.

Patient Selection

So far no clear, commonly accepted indications are given for radiofrequency ablation in liver tumors. Therefore as a first step a group of experts was constituted during the 1983 Annual Meeting of the German Radiological Society as a Working Group on Radiofrequency Ablation (IGRA) within the Interventional Working Group (AGIR) of the German Radiological Society (DRG). The main purpose was

Table 1. Recommendations for RFA in colorectal liver metastases according to IGRA

Preinterventional diagnostic work-up according to IGRA
Staging according to the guidelines established by the German Cancer Society including coloscopy
High-field MRI (1.5 T) with liver-specific contrast media or biphasic contrast CT (maximum 2 weeks before RFA)
Histologic (bioptic) diagnosis whenever the differential diagnosis of the focal liver lesion is unclear; alternative PET scan
Serum tumor markers (CEA)
Indications for RFA according to IGRA
Multicentricity: maximum 3.5 cm in diameter (no limitation concerning number of nodules if treatment intention is complete ablation [R0])
Unicentricity: maximum 5.0 cm in diameter (repositioning required)
Systemic tumorous progression: no indication for RFA only
Extrahepatic tumor manifestation with no dynamic changes or treatment opportunity (bone, lung) is no absolute contraindication
Quick >50%, platelets >60,000/mcl
Informed consent
Further recommendations
Neoadjuvant chemotherapy has not proven effective so far; combined treatment including RFA and neoadjuvant or adjuvant chemotherapy should be performed under study conditions

to build up a nationwide registry of patients treated with radiofrequency ablation for liver tumors and work out standards for clinical use. The recommendations of this group concerning preinterventional patient work-up, indications and treatment recommendations for radiofrequency ablation in colorectal liver metastases are listed in Table 1 [9]. Prior to therapy there should always be multidisciplinary consent concerning the use of radiofrequency ablation as a treatment option. Only patients with nonresectable liver tumors should be treated. A combined approach—first partial resection, second radiofrequency ablation of the residual tumor foci—is also possible. If the patient definitely rejects surgery, radiofrequency is accepted as the alternative treatment option. If necessary RFA should be part of a multimodal treatment concept. An additional systemic or local therapy is not an exclusion criteria for RFA. Moreover RFA is not a substitute for systemic treatment such as chemotherapy.

Technique

The use of radiofrequency current in living tissue producing heat was first described by d'Arsonval in 1891 [10]. Rossi and McGahan pioneered the application of RFA to primary and metastatic liver tumors [11, 12].

The basic principle of radiofrequency thermal ablation is to convert RF waves into heat. At low-power settings, the alternating current (375–480 kHz) delivered by the RF generator causes agitation of the ions in the adjacent tissue via an uninsulated electrode tip which is placed in the region of interest. Ionic vibration generates frictional heat as the ions attempt to follow the change in direction of the rapidly alternating current that extends into adjacent tissues by conduction. At high-power settings, fast ion destruction through desiccation and charring of the superficial tissue is observed. Heat production in this situation is minimal [13]. In order to destroy tumorous tissue, temperatures between 65 and 100°C have to be maintained for a certain period of time. Thermal damage to cells begins at 42°C, with exposure times required for cell death ranging from 3 to 50 h dependent on the tissue type. With increasing tissue temperatures, an exponential decrease in exposure time is needed for cellular destruction. Irreversible protein denaturation occurs at 60°C and cell death becomes inevitable. Thermal coagulation begins at 70°C and tissue desiccation at 100°C [14].

The first RFA probes were single, monopolar needles resulting in ellipsoid thermolesions because the highest temperature at the electrode surface is at the proximal and distal end of the probe. The lesion diameter was restricted to a maximum of 1.6 cm [11]. To date, several RF systems with different electrode designs are available, all of them monopolar (Table 2). The single, expanded—with multiple retractable lateral-exit jackhooks on the tip—or clustered electrode is placed under image guidance (Fig. 1) within the tumor and grounding electrodes are required to close the electrical circuit. Maximum reproducible lesion size without repositioning in a single session is limited to approximately 4–5 cm [15]. As the electrical energy passes through the body between the probe and the neutral electrodes, a certain amount of applied energy is not used for thermoablation

Table 2. Monopolar RF systems

Manufacturer/generator	Power	Control mode	Ablation mode	Electrode
Radionics CC-1 Cosman	200 W 480kHZ	Impedance	Pulsed Saline cooled	Single Cluster®
Radiotherapeutics RF 3000	200 W 460 kHz	Impedance	Stepwise	LeVeen®
RITA Model 1500	150 W 460 kHz	Impedance Temperature	Stepwise	Starburst®
Berchtold Elektrotom 106	60 W 375 kHz	Impedance	Saline infusion	HITT®

but increases the body temperature by up to 1.5°C and furthermore may lead to skin burns at the site of the grounding pads [16]. In addition, surgical clips or pacemaker electrodes may be a source of heating if they are involved to the electrical circuit and, thus, are a relative contraindication to monopolar RF ablation. Recent data suggested that bipolar RF systems do not have these limitations. Both electrodes are located within the tumor and the current does not exceed the target volume. The radiofrequency current exclusively flows between the electrodes placed in the tissue being treated. The necrosis area produced by bipolar electrodes is still elliptical rather than spheroid. So far predominantly experimental studies contributed to the evaluation of bipolar arrays [17]. A recent clinical study showed the effectiveness of a bipolar RF device in different tumor entities [18].

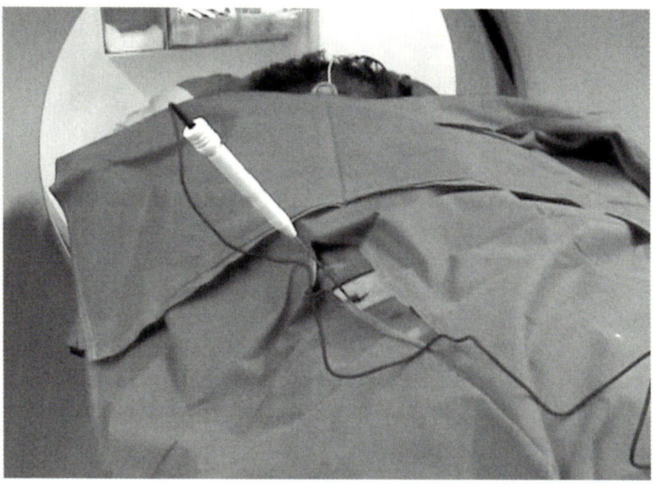

Figure 1. RF needle placement under CT guidance

Follow-Up Imaging

Follow-up imaging is usually performed with dynamic contrast-enhanced computed tomography (CT) and magnetic resonance imaging (MRI) since animal studies suggested superiority in monitoring RF lesions compared to ultrasound [19] (Fig. 2). Because of the characteristics of metastatic liver lesions of colorectal cancer—relatively hypovascular compared to the normal liver tissue—interpretation of follow-up scans are sometimes difficult since contrast enhancement of viable tumor foci may not be great. In addition, a peripheral hyperemic halo surrounding an area of hypoattenuation is seen on contrast-enhanced follow-up CT or MRI scans after radiofrequency ablation. The halo may be caused by an inflammatory reaction and hemorrhagic granulation tissue along the edge of the area of necrosis [20]. Especially in tumors that initially enhanced with contrast, this rim enhancement after treatment might be confused with residual enhancing tumor. Usually the hyperemic halo disappears by 1–3 months [21]. Then a more accurate assessment of treatment outcome can be performed. Complete coagulation necrosis corresponds to a hypoattenuated area and fails to enhance after contrast injection. On MRI, the treated tumor is characterized by low signal intensity on T2-weighted images, whereas viable tumor is shown to be hyperintense

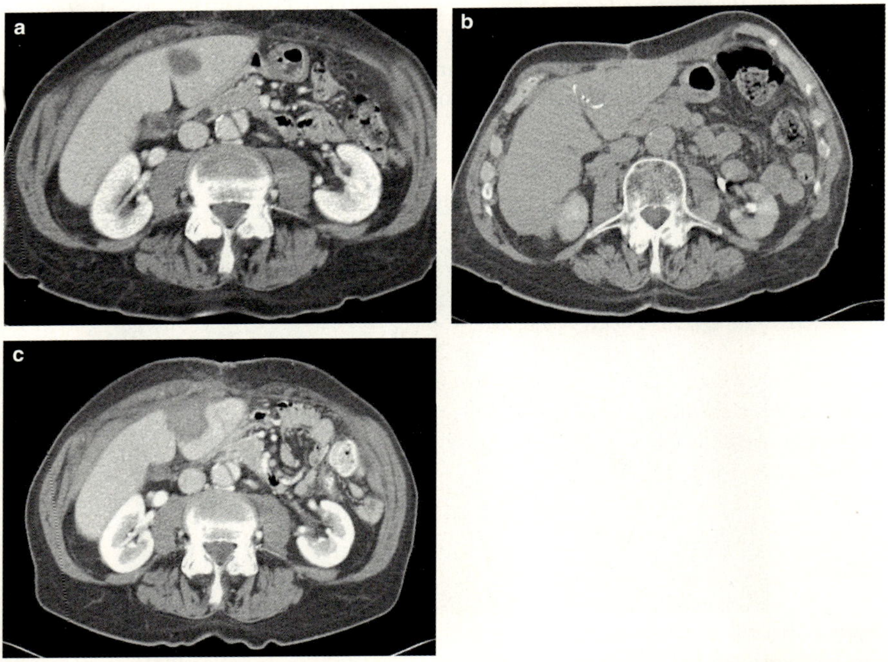

Figure 2. a Preinterventional diagnostic CT showing metastatic disease in liver segment four. **b** RF electrode with expanded hooks is placed within the metastatic nodule. **c** Follow-up CT-imaging after 3 months with no evidence of residual tumor foci and sufficient safety margin

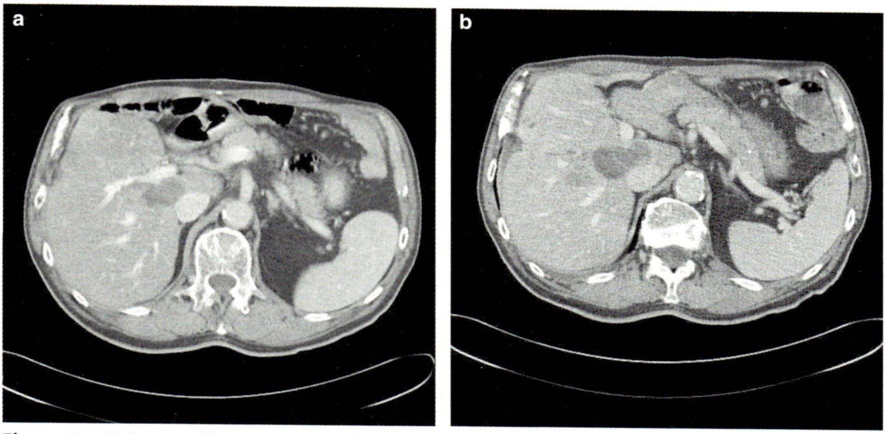

Figure 3. **a** Follow-up CT imaging 3 months after RFA with no evidence of residual tumor in liver segment one. **b** Follow-up CT-imaging 6 months after RFA showing a recurrent tumor nodule at the periphery of the RF lesion indicative of an incomplete primary RFA with insufficient safety margin

Table 3. Postinterventional diagnostic work-up according to IGRA

Clinical status every 6 months, lung X-ray, probably abdominal ultrasound
High-field MRI (1.5 T) with liver specific contrast media or biphasic contrast CT (1–30 days after RFA) concerning residual tumor foci
High-field MRI (1.5T) with liver-specific contrast media or biphasic contrast CT (every 3 months the 1st year after RFA)
No local or heterotopic recurrence after 12 months, follow-up imaging at 6-month intervals possible
Serum tumor markers (CEA) every 3–6 months

on T2-weighted images [22]. Image findings correspond well to histopathologic analysis [20]. Biopsies of ablated areas to prove complete necrosis are generally unreliable and therefore not recommended [23]. Follow-up scans are usually performed at 3-months intervals and are often combined with serum tumor markers such as CEA (Table 3) [9]. Any increase in lesion size or irregularity or residual enhancement should be carefully interpreted in terms of residual tumor foci or recurrent metastases (Fig. 3). It is mandatory to look for evidence of both intra- and extrahepatic spread.

Results

Despite a high number of published studies, the analysis of clinical results of percutaneous radiofrequency ablation in colorectal liver metastases is hampered by several problems. Many reports presented data that involve different tumor entities including primary and metastatic liver tumors with different tumor sizes.

Treatment was performed with different types of RF generators and needle designs and additional therapies such as resection, regional or systemic chemotherapy, and other local ablative techniques have been used in combination with RF ablation. Finally the studies have different endpoints and follow-up durations, as well as criteria for evaluating results. A systematic review on the outcomes of RFA for unresectable hepatic metastases reveals a dearth of long-term follow-up data. Seidenfeld et al. [24] found only seven articles that provided data on disease-free or recurrence-free survival, rates of hepatic relapse, and median or percent survival at 1–5 years after treatment. Five studies reported 86%–94% survival at 1 year, but only one study reported survival at 2 years or longer [25]. In a recent study by Solbiati et al. [23], the results from 109 patients with 172 metastatic lesions who underwent RFA under ultrasound guidance were analyzed. The median follow-up was 3 years a local tumor control was achieved in 70% of the lesions. Local recurrence—including residual tumor foci—occurred in 30% that were again treated by RFA so that the entire rate of local tumor control reached 78%. New metastases developed in 50.4% of the patients at a median time to recurrence of 12 months after RFA. The overall 2- and 3-year survival rates were 67% and 33%, respectively, and the median survival 30 months. This compares favorably with data reported by Gillams [26] with a median survival of 34 months and a 3-year survival of 36%. Survival of 36% at 3 years in inoperable patients is similar to patients undergoing resection for operable metastatic disease showing a 3-year survival of 42%–44% [27, 5]. In another larger series, 88 hepatic metastases in 47 patients were treated with percutaneous RFA. At a mean follow-up of 13.7 months, 79% of the patients were alive, 42% had no evidence of new or recurrent malignant hepatic disease, but only 27% were completely tumor-free [28].

A recent paper by Mulier et al. [29] reviewed the world literature until the end of 2001 concerning complications after radiofrequency ablation. A total of 3,670 patients were analyzed, including 2,898 patients having had a percutaneous approach for radiofrequency ablation. Mortality was found to be 0.5%, with sepsis, liver failure and cardiac complications the most important ones. De Baere et al. [30] reported 1.4% with portal vein thrombosis responsible for the highest number of fatal outcomes. The entire complication rate of 10.6% is comparable to 7.2% presented by Mulier et al. [29] In detail, Mulier et al. [29] had intraperitoneal bleeding in 0.8%, subcapsular hematoma in 0.6%, biliary tract damage in 0.6%, pulmonary complications in 0.6%, pad skin burns in 0.6%, visceral damage in 0.5%, liver failure in 0.4%, hepatic vascular damage in 0.4% and cardiac complications in 0.3%. Interestingly, de Baere et al. [30] showed that abscess occurred significantly more frequently in patients bearing a bilioenteric anastomosis, which is confirmed by the data of Livraghi et al. [31]. Seeding was shown to have a rate of 0.3% reported by Mulier et al. [29] in contrast to 12.5% from Llovet et al. [32], whereas de Baere et al. [30] also reported seeding to be rare with 0.5%. Minor complications are usually not listed in the published data; consequently, the true complication rate may be even higher. Some late complications such as bile duct strictures and electrode track seeding may have been missed because of the short follow-up in many studies.

Conclusions

Percutaneous radiofrequency ablation (RFA) is an emerging treatment tool in patients suffering from nonresectable liver tumors with survival rates for inoperable patients reaching the rates of resected patients. Reasons for the use of RFA more frequently than other minimal invasive tumor therapies include the advantageous relation between probe diameter and efficacy, reliable size of coagulation necrosis and cost-effectiveness of RF systems [9]. In contrast, operative approaches to liver metastases allow more accurate assessment for the presence of extrahepatic spread, better evaluation of intrahepatic disease especially in conjunction with intraoperative ultrasound, and isolation of the liver from adjacent organs that may be injured. Therefore percutaneous RFA should still be used in patients not eligible for surgery. The worldwide reported complication and mortality rates (7.2% and 0.5%) for percutaneous radiofrequency ablation [29] indicate that the complication risk should not be underestimated but they also confirm that RF ablation is a relatively low-risk procedure for the treatment of focal liver tumors. With adequate knowledge, many complications are preventable. It is conceivable when RFA is used for larger tumor volumes that complication rates may rise.

References

1. Geoghegan JG, Scheele J (1999) Treatment of colorectal liver metastases. British J of Surg 86:158–169
2. Landis SH, Murray T, Bolden S, Wingo PA (1999) Cancer statistics, 1999. CA Cancer J Clin 49:8–31
3. Choti MA, Bulkley GB (1999) Management of hepatic metastases. Liver Transplant Surg 5:65–80
4. Redaelli CA, Dufour JF, Wagner M, Schilling M, Hüsler J, Krähenbühl L, Büchler MW, Reichen J (2002) Preoperative galactose elimination capacity predicts complications and survival after hepatic resection. Ann Surg 235:77–85
5. Jaeck D, Bachellier PGM, Boudjema K, Vaillant JC, Balladur P, Nordlinger B (1997) Long-term survival following resection of colorectal hepatic metastases. Association Francaise de Chirurgie. Br J Surg 84:977–980
6. Lehnert T, Golling M (2001) Indikationen und Ergebnisse der Lebermetastasenresektion. Radiologe 42:40–48
7. Ott R, Wein A, Hohenberger W (2001) Lebermetastasen – primäre oder multimodale Therapie? Chirurgerie 71:887–897
8. Kemeny N, Huang Y, Cohen AM, Shi W, Conti JA, Brennan MF, Bertino JR, Turnbull AD, Sullivan D, Stockman J, Blumgart LH, Fong Y (1999) Hepatic arterial infusion of chemotherapy after resection of hepatic metastases from colorectal cancer. N Engl J Med 341:2039–2048
9. Tacke J (2003) Percutaneous radiofrequency ablation – clinical indications and results. Fortschr Röntgenstr 175:156–168
10. Siperstein AE, Gitomirski A (2000) History and technological aspects of radiofrequency thermoablation. Cancer J 6 [Suppl 4]:S239–S303
11. Rossi S, Fornari F, Paties CT, Buscarini L (1990) Thermal lesions induced by 480 kHz localized current field in guinea pig and pig liver. Tumori 76:54–57
12. McGahan JP, Brock JM, Tesluk H, Gu WZ, Schneider P, Browning PD (1992) Hepatic ablation with use of radiofrequency electrocautery in the animal model. J Vasc Interv Radiol 3:291–297
13. Organ LW (1976–1977) Electrophysiologic principles of radiofrequency lesion making. Appl Neurophysiol 39:69–76

14. Goldberg SN, Gazelle GS, Halpern EF, Rittman WJ, Mueller PR, Rosenthal DI (1996) Radiofrequency tissue ablation: importance of local temperature along the electrode tip exposure in determining lesion shape and size. Acad Radiol 3:212–218
15. Pereira PL, Trübenbach J, Schmidt D (2003) Radiofrequency ablation: basic principles, techniques and challenges. Fortschr Röntgenstr 175:20–27
16. Livraghi T, Solbiati L, Meloni MF et al (2003) Treatment of focal liver tumors with percutaneous radio-frequency ablation: complications encountered in a multicenter study. Radiology 226:441–451
17. Desinger K, Stein T, Tschepe J et al (1996) Investigations on radiofrequency current application in bipolar technique for interstitial thermotherapy (RF-ITT). Minimal Invasive Medizin 7:92–97
18. Tacke J, Mahnken A, Roggan A, Günther RW (2004) Multipolar radiofrequency ablation: first clinical results. Fortschr Röntgenstr 176:324–329
19. Cha CH, Lee FT Jr, Gurney JM et al (2000) CT versus sonography for monitoring radiofrequency ablation in a porcine liver. Am J Roentgenol 175:705–711
20. Goldberg SN, Gazelle GS, Compton CC, Mueller PR, Tanabe KK (2000) Treatment of intrahepatic malignancy with radiofrequency ablation: radiologic-pathologic correlation. Cancer 88:2452–2463
21. Choi H, Loyer EM, DuBrow RA, Kaur H, David CL, Huang S, Curley S, Charnsangavej C (2001) Radio-frequency ablation of liver tumors: assessment of therapeutic response and complications. Radiographics 21:S41–S54
22. Sironi S, Livraghi T, Meloni F, DeCobelli F, Ferero CG, Del Maschio A (1999) Small hepatocellular carcinoma treated with percutaneous RF ablation: MR imaging follow-up. Am J Roentgenol 173:1225–1229
23. Solbiati L, Ierace T, Tonolini M, Osti V, Cova L (2001) Radiofrequency thermal ablation of hepatic metastases. Eur J Ultrasound 13:149–158
24. Seidenfeld J, Korn A, Aronson N (2002) Radiofrequency ablation of unresectable liver metastases. J Am Coll Surg 195:378–386
25. Solbiati L, Ierace T, Goldberg SN, Sironi S, Livraghi T, Fiocca R, Servadio G, Rizzatto G, Mueller PR, Del Maschio A, Gazelle GS (1997) Percutaneous US-guided radio-frequency tissue ablation of liver metastases: treatment and follow-up in 16 patients. Radiology. 202:195–203
26. Gillams A (2001) Thermal ablation of liver metastases. Abdominal Imaging 26:361–368
27. Jenkins LT, Millikan KW, Bines SD, Staren ED, Doolas A (1997) Hepatic resection for metastatic colorectal cancer. Am Surg 63:605–610
28. Bowles BJ, Machi J, Limm WM, Severino R, Oishi AJ, Furumoto NL, Wong LL, Oishi RH (2001) Safety and efficacy of radiofrequency thermal ablation in advanced liver tumors. Arch Surg 136:864–869
29. Mulier S, Mulier P, Ni Y, Miao Y, Dupas B, Marchal G, De Wever I, Michel L (2002) Complications of radiofrequency coagulation of liver tumours. Br J Surg 89:1206–1222
30. De Baere T, Risse O, Kuoch V, Dromain C, Sengel C, Smayra T, El Din MG, Letoublon C, Elias D (2003) Adverse events during radiofrequency treatment of 582 hepatic tumors. AJR 181:695–700
31. Livraghi T, Solbiati L, Meloni MF, Gazelle GS, Halpern EF, Goldberg SN (2003) Treatment of focal liver tumors with percutaneous radio-frequency ablation: complications encountered in a multicenter study. Radiology 226:441–451
32. Llovet JM, Vilana R, Bru C, Bianchi L, Salmeron JM, Boix L, Ganau S, Sala M, Pages M, Ayuso C, Sole M, Rodes J, Bruix J Barcelona Clinic Liver Cancer (BCLC) Group (2001) Increased risk of tumor seeding after percutaneous radiofrequency ablation for single hepatocellular carcinoma. Hepatology 33:1124–1129